T0172400

SHORT-TERM PLAY THERAPY
FOR CHILDREN

Also from Heidi Gerard Kaduson and Charles E. Schaefer

Contemporary Play Therapy:
Theory, Research, and Practice
Edited by Charles E. Schaefer and Heidi Gerard Kaduson

Separation Anxiety in Children and Adolescents:
An Individualized Approach to Assessment and Treatment
Andrew R. Eisen and Charles E. Schaefer

Short-Term Play Therapy for Children

THIRD EDITION

Edited by
HEIDI GERARD KADUSON
CHARLES E. SCHAEFER

THE GUILFORD PRESS
New York   London

© 2015 The Guilford Press
A Division of Guilford Publications, Inc.
370 Seventh Avenue, Suite 1200, New York, NY 10001
www.guilford.com

All rights reserved

No part of this book may be reproduced, translated, stored in
a retrieval system, or transmitted, in any form or by any means,
electronic, mechanical, photocopying, microfilming, recording,
or otherwise, without written permission from the publisher.

Printed in the United States of America

This book is printed on acid-free paper.

Last digit is print number: 9 8 7 6 5 4 3 2

The authors have checked with sources believed to be reliable in their efforts to
provide information that is complete and generally in accord with the standards
of practice that are accepted at the time of publication. However, in view of the
possibility of human error or changes in behavioral, mental health, or medical
sciences, neither the authors, nor the editors and publisher, nor any other party
who has been involved in the preparation or publication of this work warrants
that the information contained herein is in every respect accurate or complete, and
they are not responsible for any errors or omissions or the results obtained from
the use of such information. Readers are encouraged to confirm the information
contained in this book with other sources.

Library of Congress Cataloging-in-Publication Data

Short-term play therapy for children / edited by Heidi Gerard Kaduson, Charles
E. Schaefer. -- Third edition.
    pages cm.
Includes bibliographical references and index.
ISBN 978-1-4625-2027-5 (hardback); ISBN 978-1-4625-2784-7 (paperback)
1. Play therapy. 2. Children--Counseling of. 3. Family psychotherapy.
4. Child psychotherapy. I. Kaduson, Heidi. II. Schaefer, Charles E.
RJ505.P6S53 2015
618.92'891653--dc23
                                                              2015010854

*To the efficacious and affordable delivery
of play therapy services*

About the Editors

Heidi Gerard Kaduson, PhD, RPT-S, specializes in evaluation and intervention services for children with a variety of behavioral, emotional, and learning problems. She is past president of the Association for Play Therapy and Director of The Play Therapy Training Institute, Inc., in Monroe Township, New Jersey. She has lectured internationally on play therapy, attention-deficit/hyperactivity disorder, and learning disabilities. Dr. Kaduson's coedited books with Charles E. Schaefer include *101 Favorite Play Therapy Techniques, 101 More Favorite Play Therapy Techniques,* and *Contemporary Play Therapy.* She maintains a private practice in child psychotherapy in Monroe Township, New Jersey.

Charles E. Schaefer, PhD, RPT-S, is Professor Emeritus of Psychology at Fairleigh Dickinson University. He is cofounder and director emeritus of the Association for Play Therapy, which recognized him with its Lifetime Achievement Award. In addition to his coedited volumes with Heidi Gerard Kaduson, Dr. Schaefer's more than 60 books include *The Therapeutic Powers of Play, Foundations of Play Therapy, Play Therapy with Adolescents,* and *Separation Anxiety in Children and Adolescents.* He maintains a private practice in child psychotherapy in Hackensack, New Jersey.

Contributors

Meena Dasari, PhD, Department of Psychology, New York University School of Medicine, New York, New York

Tracie Faa-Thompson, MA, Turn About Pegasus, Northumberland, United Kingdom

Amy Frew, PhD, LMFT, clinical counseling and supervision, Brentwood, Tennessee

Paris Goodyear-Brown, MSSW, RPT-S, Paris and Me, LLC: Counseling for Kids, Antioch, Tennessee

Sarah Hamil, LCSW, RPT-S, ATR-BC, School of Social Work, Union University, Jackson, Tennessee

Esther B. Hess, PhD, RPT-S, Center for the Developing Mind, Los Angeles, California

Kimberly M. Jayne, EdD, Counselor Education, University of New Mexico, Albuquerque, New Mexico

Heidi Gerard Kaduson, PhD, RPT-S, The Play Therapy Training Institute, Inc., Monroe Township, New Jersey; private practice, Monroe Township, New Jersey

Susan M. Knell, PhD, Spectrum Psychological Associates, Cleveland, Ohio

Garry L. Landreth, EdD, RPT-S, LPC, Department of Counseling and Center for Play Therapy, University of North Texas, Denton, Texas

Norma Leben, LCSW, RPT-S, Morning Glory Treatment Center for Children, Pflugerville, Texas

Evangeline Munns, CPsych, RPT-S, CACPT-S, private practice, King City, Ontario, Canada

Violet Oaklander, PhD, The Violet Oaklander Institute, Los Angeles, California

Terry Pifalo, MPS-CAT, ATR, Dee Norton Lowcountry Children's Center, Charleston, South Carolina

Scott Riviere, MSW, KIDZ, Inc., Lake Charles, Louisiana

Elizabeth R. Taylor, PhD, RPT-S, College of Education, Texas Christian University, Fort Worth, Texas

Susan G. Timmer, PhD, CAARE Diagnostic and Treatment Center, UC Davis Children's Hospital, Sacramento, California

Anthony J. Urquiza, PhD, RPT, CAARE Diagnostic and Treatment Center, UC Davis Children's Hospital, Sacramento, California

Risë VanFleet, PhD, Family Enhancement and Play Therapy Center, Boiling Springs, Pennsylvania

Pamela Wolfberg, PhD, Department of Special Education and Communication Disorders, San Francisco State University, San Francisco, California

Sharon Rea Zone, LCSW, CAARE Diagnostic and Treatment Center, UC Davis Children's Hospital, Sacramento, California

Preface

SHORT-TERM PSYCHOTHERAPY

Clearly we are living in a time in which cost control and the numerous stresses on families make it imperative that child mental health professionals provide most of their psychotherapy services in a short-term manner. "Short-term therapy" refers to interventions designed to produce therapeutic change within a brief amount of time (i.e., 1–20 sessions). Often short-term therapy is time-limited in that the number of sessions is specified by the therapist at the start of treatment. This deliberate time limit adds a sense of intensity and urgency and creates expectancies in both the therapist and the client as to when change will occur.

The following are among the major reasons why child clinicians need to offer short-term therapies for their clients:

1. *They are effective.* Brief interventions with children that have been empirically evaluated have been found to be superior to no interventions at all and as effective as longer term varieties, regardless of the therapists' theoretical orientations (Andrade, Lambert, & Bickman, 2000; Bloom, 2002).

2. *They are cost-effective.* Short-term therapies are compatible with the managed-care, cost-accountability climate that exists today. Cost control is a major and legitimate consideration for the delivery of mental health services today.

3. *They appeal to parents with limited time availability.* The crowded life schedules of working parents and their children make long-term psychotherapy burdensome and stressful for them in terms of both time and energy.

4. *They work with a wide range of childhood disorders.* Short-term therapies have proven effective for numerous internalizing (Jalali, Ahmadi,

& Aghael, 2011; Scheidlinger & Batkin-Kahn, 2005) and externalizing (Carpentier, Silovsky, & Chaffin, 2006; Cole, Treadwell, Dosani, & Frederickson, 2013) disorders of children and adolescents.

   5. *Their effects are maintained.* Treatment gains for short-term interventions tend to be maintained (Hampe, Noble, Miller, & Barrett, 1973; Schuhman, Foote, Eyberg, & Boggs, 1998; Gallagher-Thomson, Hanley-Peterson, & Thompson, 1990).

   6. *There are fewer "no-shows" and "dropouts."* It is easier for clients to commit to and follow through with brief treatments and those with a defined endpoint. This reduces premature terminations and session cancellations. Also, brief treatment shortens waiting lists, which tends to reduce dropout rates (Sloves & Peterlin, 1986).

   7. *They are suitable to different theoretical models.* There are now forms of short-term therapy for all the major theoretical orientations, including child-centered (Ryan, 2001; Osterweil, 1986), Adlerian (Wood, 2003), cognitive-behavioral (McGinn & Sanderson, 2001), psychodynamic (Muratori, 2002; Shefler, 2000), and solution-focused (Concoran & Stephenson, 2000; Taylor, 2009).

   8. *Time-limited group therapy is particularly cost-effective.* Time-limited (10–15 sessions) group treatment for children and adolescents has proven to be effective across a range of disorders (Lomonaco, Scheidlinger, & Aronson, 1998; Springer & Misurell, 2010; Schaefer, 1999). Among the advantages of such time-limited groups are that the clinician can treat more than one child at a time, which reduces the cost of therapy.

   9. *Time-limited parent training groups have a strong evidence base.* Short-term parent training that integrates relationship play therapy with behavior management training (Landreth & Bratton, 2006; McNeil & Hembree-Kigin, 2010) has become the treatment of choice for disruptive behaviors of young children.

   10. *Short-term interventions avoid overtreatment.* For mild-to-moderate behavior problems of children, short-term therapy has strong and growing empirical support. It is important for therapists, in consultation with parents, to know when to stop the therapy so as not to overtreat (Bloom, 2002).

SHORT-TERM PLAY THERAPY

All theoretical models of play therapy—both directive and nondirective—can now be applied in a short-term manner. In this updated third edition of *Short-Term Play Therapy for Children*, contributors describe in detail how to conduct brief play therapy within such diverse orientations as child-centered play therapy, release play therapy, cognitive-behavioral play therapy, Theraplay, solution-focused play therapy, integrative play therapy, parent training (filial therapy, child–parent relationship therapy, parent–child interaction therapy), Gestalt play therapy, animal-assisted play therapy, Floortime, and group play therapies. Short-term play interventions for a broad range and different intensities of childhood disorders are included, including internalizing problems (e.g., anxieties, phobias, trauma and grief reactions), externalizing problems (e.g., anger, deviant sexual behaviors, oppositional/defiant behaviors, attention-deficit/hyperactivity disorder), developmental disorders (e.g., autism spectrum disorder), and peer relationship difficulties.

The chapter contributors provide the reader with both clinical guidance and case examples for conducting the latest applications of short-term play interventions. Most of the chapters in this third edition are new, while a few have been revised and updated from the second edition. The book covers short-term play therapies for individuals, groups, and families. The prescriptive approach to treatment exemplified in this book enables therapists to tailor and individualize brief interventions to meet the needs of their clients with specific problems.

In summary, the current mental health zeitgeist necessitates that the delivery of psychotherapy be primarily short term. Accordingly, the contributors in this volume describe a number of effective ways to implement play therapy in a short-term manner. This book should be of interest to child and play therapists of all theoretical orientations and levels of experience who wish to deepen their knowledge of current, short-term play therapy approaches.

REFERENCES

Andrade, A., Lambert, W., & Bickman, L. (2000). Dose effect in child psychotherapy: Outcomes associated with negligible treatment. *Journal of the American Academy of Child and Adolescent Psychiatry, 3*(2), 161–168.

Bloom, B. (2002). Brief psychotherapy with children and adolescents: Recent treatment outcome studies. *Brief Treatment and Crisis Intervention, 2*(3), 482–488.

Carpentier, M., Silovsky, J., & Chaffin, M. (2006). Randomized trial of treatment for children with sexual behavior problems. *Journal of Consulting and Clinical Psychology, 74*(3), 482–488.

Cole, R., Treadwell, S., Dosani, S., & Frederickson, N. (2013). Evaluation of a short-term, cognitive-behavioral intervention for primary age children with anger-related difficulties. *School Psychology International, 34*(1), 82–100.

Concoran, J., & Stephenson, M. (2000). The effectiveness of solution-focused therapy with child behavior problems: A preliminary report. *Families in Society*, *81*, 468–474.

Gallagher-Thomson, D., Hanley-Peterson, P., & Thompson, L. (1990). Maintenance of gains versus relapse following brief psychotherapy for depression. *Journal of Consulting and Clinical Psychology*, *58*(3), 371–374.

Hampe, E., Noble, H., Miller, L. C., & Barrett, C. L. (1973). Phobic children one and two years post-treatment. *Journal of Abnormal Psychology*, *82*, 446–453.

Jalali, S., Ahmadi, M., & Aghael, A. (2011). The effect of cognitive-behavioral group play therapy on social phobia of 5–11 year old children. *Journal of Research in Behavioral Sciences*, *9*(2), 11–20.

Landreth, G., & Bratton, S. (2006). *Child parent relationship therapy (CPRT): A 10 session filial therapy model*. New York: Routledge.

Lomonaco, S., Scheidlinger, S., & Aronson, S. (1998). Time-limited group treatment of children. *American Journal of Psychotherapy*, *52*, 240–247.

McNeil, C., & Hembree-Kigin, T. (2010). *Parent–child interaction therapy* (2nd ed.). New York: Springer.

McGinn, L., & Sanderson, N. (2001). What allows cognitive-behavioral therapy to be brief: Overview, efficacy, and crucial factors facilitating brief treatment. *Clinical Psychology: Science and Practice*, *8*(1), 23–37.

Muratori, F. (2002). Efficacy of brief dynamic psychotherapy for children with emotional disorders. *Psychotherapy and Psychosomatics*, *71*, 28–38.

Osterweil, Z. (1986). Time-limited play therapy. *School Psychology International*, *7*, 224–230.

Ryan, V. (2001). Non-directive play therapy with children experiencing psychic trauma. *Clinical Child Psychology, Psychiatry*, *6*(3), 437–453.

Schaefer, C. E. (1999). *Short-term psychotherapy groups for children: Adapting group processes for specific problems*. Northvale, NJ: Aronson.

Scheidlinger, S., & Batkin-Kahn, G. (2005). In the aftermath of September 11th: Group interventions with traumatized children revisited. *International Journal of Group Psychotherapy*, *55*(3), 335–354.

Schuhman, E., Foote, R., Eyberg, S., & Boggs, S. (1998). Efficacy of parent–child interaction therapy: Interim report of a randomized trial with short-term maintenance. *Journal of Clinical Child Psychology*, *27*(1), 34–45.

Shefler, G. (2000). Time-limited psychotherapy with adolescents. *Journal of Psychotherapy Practice Research*, *9*(2), 88–94.

Sloves, R., & Peterlin, K. (1986). The process of time-limited psychotherapy with latency-aged children. *Journal of the American Academy of Child Psychiatry*, *25*(6), 847–854.

Springer, C., & Misurell, J. (2010). Game-based cognitive-behavioral therapy: An innovative group treatment program for children who have been sexually abused. *Journal of Child and Adolescent Trauma*, *3*(3), 163–180.

Taylor, E. (2009). Sandtray and solution-focused therapy. *International Journal of Play Therapy*, *18*(1), 56–68.

Wood, A. (2003). Alfred Adler's treatment as a form of brief therapy. *Journal of Contemporary Psychotherapy*, *33*(4), 287–301.

Contents

PART I. INDIVIDUAL PLAY THERAPY

Part I

~

INDIVIDUAL PLAY THERAPY

Chapter 1

ॐ

Release Play Therapy for Children with Posttraumatic Stress Disorder

Heidi Gerard Kaduson

*I*n order to have the proper perspective on how posttraumatic stress disorder (PTSD) affects children, one must first understand what a trauma is. A psychic trauma is an emotional shock or wound that has long-lasting effects. It results when an individual is exposed to an overwhelming event and is rendered temporarily helpless and unable to use ordinary coping and defensive operations of the ego in the face of intolerable danger, anxiety, or instinctual arousal (Eth & Pynoos, 1995). There has been much research on PTSD with war veterans, but the research is minimal with regard to PTSD and play therapy (Kaduson, 2011). There are many traumatic experiences, as there might have always been: however, with technology, children are now subject to more of them than ever before.

PTSD is a psychiatric disorder that can occur following the experiencing or witnessing of life-threatening events such as military combat, natural disasters, terrorist incidents, serious accidents, or violent personal assaults like rape. Adults who suffer from PTSD often relive the experience through nightmares and flashbacks, have difficulty sleeping, and feel detached or estranged; these symptoms can be severe enough and last long enough to significantly impair a person's daily life.

Contemporary research on the biology of PTSD has confirmed that there are profound and persistent alterations in physiological reactivity and stress hormone secretion in people with PTSD. The brain is an analyzing and amplifying device for maintaining a person's internal and external environment (MacLean, 1988), and if emotional arousal is intense and persists, as has often been experienced by trauma survivors, the person may develop conditioned emotional and biological responses with long-term effects. High levels of emotional arousal are likely responsible for the observation that traumatic experiences initially are imprinted as sensations or states of physiological arousal that often cannot be transcribed into personal narratives (van der Kolk & Fisler, 1995).

PTSD is not a new disorder. Written accounts of similar symptoms go back to ancient times. Careful research and documentation of PTSD began in earnest after the Vietnam War. The National Vietnam Veterans Readjustment Study estimated in 1988 that the prevalence of PTSD in the group studied was 15.2% at that time and that 30% had experienced the disorder at some point since returning from Vietnam (Zatzick et al., 1997).

PTSD has subsequently been observed in all veteran populations that have been studied, including World War II, the Korean conflict, and Persian Gulf populations, and in United Nations peacekeeping forces deployed to other war zones around the world. There are remarkably similar findings of PTSD in military veterans in other countries. For example, Australian Vietnam veterans experience many of the same symptoms that American Vietnam veterans experience (Creamer & Forbes, 2004).

PTSD is not only a problem for veterans, however. Although there are unique culture- and gender-based aspects of the disorder, it occurs in men and women, adults and children, Western and non-Western cultural groups, and all socioeconomic strata. A national study of American civilians conducted in 1995 estimated that the lifetime prevalence of PTSD was 5% in men and 10% in women (Kessler, Sonnega, Bromet, Hughes, & Nelson, 1995).

PTSD was formally recognized as a psychiatric diagnosis in the third edition of the *Diagnostic and Statistical Manual of Mental Disorders* (DSM-III; American Psychiatric Association, 1980). At that time, little was known about what PTSD looked like in children and adolescents. Today we know children and adolescents are susceptible to developing PTSD, and we know that PTSD has different age-specific features. Although a diagnosis of PTSD required the patient to have the symptoms for over a month's duration, a diagnosis of acute stress disorder, in DSM-IV (American Psychiatric Association, 1994), covers those children who have symptoms like PTSD, but for a duration of at least 2 days and less than 1 month. DSM-5 (American Psychiatric Association, 2013), refines the diagnostic criteria so that different types of traumatic events can be separated out as acute stress disorder. With this diagnosis,

Exposure to actual or threatened death, serious injury or sexual viola-
tion occur in one (or more) of the following ways:

1. Directly experiencing the traumatic events(s).
2. Witnessing in person, the event(s) as it occurred to others.
3. Learning that the event(s) occurred to a close family member or close
   friend.
4. Experiencing repeated or extreme exposure to aversive details of the
   traumatic event(s) (e.g., first responders collecting human remains,
   police officers repeatedly exposed to details of child abuse). (American Psychiatric Association, 2013, p. 280)

It cannot be diagnosed until 3 days after a traumatic event, although it may
progress to PTSD after 1 month. Also noted in DSM-5 is that the forms of
experiencing can vary across development. Unlike adults and adolescents,
young children may report nightmares without content that clearly reflect
aspects of the trauma (e.g., waking in fright in the aftermath of the trauma
but being unable to relate the content of the nightmare to the traumatic
event). Children with a mental age younger than 6 are more likely than
older children to express reexperiencing symptoms through play that refers
directly or symbolically to the trauma.

A diagnosis of PTSD means that an individual has experienced an
event that involved a threat to his or her own or another's life or physical
integrity and that this person responded with intense fear, helplessness,
or horror. A number of traumatic events have been shown to cause PTSD
in children and adolescents. Children and adolescents may be diagnosed
with PTSD if they have survived natural or human-made disasters such as
floods; violent crimes such as kidnapping, rape, murder, suicide of a parent,
sniper fire, and school shootings; motor vehicle accidents such as automobile and plane crashes; severe burns; exposure to community violence; war;
peer suicide; and sexual and physical abuse.

A few studies of the general population have examined rates of exposure for PTSD in children and adolescents. Results of these studies indicate
that 15–43% of girls and 14–43% of boys have experienced at least one
traumatic event in their lifetimes. Of those children and adolescents who
have experienced a trauma, 3–15% of girls and 1–6% of boys could be
diagnosed with PTSD (Giaconia et al., 1995; Cuffe et al., 1998).

Rates of PTSD are much higher in children and adolescents recruited
from at-risk populations. The rates of PTSD in these at-risk children and
adolescents vary from 3–100%. For example, studies have shown that as
many as 100% of children who witness a homicide of a parent or sexual
assault develop PTSD (Kilpatrick & Williams, 1997). Similarly, 90% of
sexually abused children (Hamblen, 2004), 77% of children exposed to
a school shooting (Ackerman, Newton, McPherson, Jones, & Dykman,

1998), and 35% of urban youth exposed to community violence develop PTSD (Margolis & Gordis, 2000).

Certainly not all children develop PTSD. There are, however, many factors that have been shown to increase the likelihood that children will develop PTSD:

- Quality of pretrauma attachment relationships and overall adjustment.
- Amount of social support (the more, the better).
- Type of disaster (human-made disaster leads to more PTSD than natural disaster).
- Human aggression (abuse, etc., leads to more severe symptoms of PTSD).
- Degree to which trauma is life-threatening (the less, the better).
- Parents' reactions (the less distressed, the better).
- Degree to which primary attachment figures are available and supportive.
- Communication (the more open, the better).
- Cumulative stressors (the fewer, the better).
- Degree of exposure (the more direct the exposure, the more likely PTSD).

In general, children and adolescents who report experiencing the most severe traumas also report the highest levels of PTSD symptoms. Family support and parental coping have also been shown to affect PTSD symptoms in children. Studies show that children and adolescents with greater family support and less parental distress have lower levels of PTSD symptoms. Finally, children and adolescents who are farther away from the traumatic event report less distress (Pynoos et al., 1987).

In terms of gender, several studies suggest that girls are more likely than boys to develop PTSD (Pfefferbaum et al., 1999, 2000). However, DSM-5 (American Psychiatric Association, 2013) also notes that the increased risk for the disorder in females may be attributable in part to a greater likelihood of exposure to the types of traumatic events with a high conditional risk for acute stress disorder, such as rape and other interpersonal violence. A few studies have examined the connection between ethnicity and PTSD. Although some studies find that minorities report higher levels of PTSD symptoms, researchers have shown that this is due to other factors such as differences in levels of exposure. It is not clear how a child's age at the time of exposure to a traumatic event impacts the occurrence or severity of PTSD. Some studies find a relationship; others do not. Differences that do occur may be due to differences in the way PTSD is expressed in children and adolescents of different ages or developmental levels (Vernberg & Varela, 2001; Shelby, 1997).

Researchers and clinicians are beginning to recognize that PTSD may not present itself in children the same way it does in adults. Criteria for PTSD now include age-specific features for some symptoms (DeWolfe, 2004; Pynoos & Nader, 1993):

Infancy through Preschool

1. Helplessness and passivity; lack of usual responsiveness
2. Generalized fear
3. Heightened arousal and confusion
4. Cognitive confusion
5. Difficulty in talking about event; lack of verbalization
6. Difficulty in identifying feelings
7. Sleep disturbances, nightmares
8. Separation fears and clinging to caregivers
9. Regressive symptoms (e.g., bed wetting, loss of acquired speech and motor skills)
10. Inability to understand death as permanent
11. Anxieties about death
12. Grief related to abandonment by caregiver
13. Somatic symptoms (e.g., stomachaches, headaches)
14. Startle response to loud/unusual noises
15. "Freezing" (sudden immobility of body)
16. Fussiness, uncharacteristic crying, and neediness
17. Avoidance of or alarm responses to specific trauma-related reminders involving sights and physical sensations

School-Age Children (Ages 6–11 Years)

1. Responsibility and guilt
2. Repetitious traumatic play and retelling
3. Reminders triggering disturbing feelings
4. Sleep disturbances, nightmares
5. Safety concerns, preoccupation with danger
6. Aggressive behavior, angry outbursts
7. Fear of feelings and trauma reactions
8. Close attention to parents' anxieties
9. School avoidance
10. Worry and concern for others
11. Changes in behavior, mood, and personality

12. Somatic symptoms (complaints about bodily aches and pains)
13. Obvious anxiety and fearfulness
14. Withdrawal and quieting
15. Specific, trauma-related fears; general fearfulness
16. Regression to behavior of a younger child
17. Separation anxiety with relation to primary caretakers
18. Loss of interest in activities
19. Confusion and inadequate understanding of traumatic events most evident in play rather than in discussion
20. Unclear understanding of death and the causes of "bad" events
21. Magical explanations to fill in gaps in understanding
22. Loss of ability to concentrate and attend at school, with lowering of performance
23. "Spacey" or distractible behavior

Preadolescents and Adolescents (Ages 12–18 Years)

1. Self-consciousness
2. Life-threatening reenactment
3. Rebellion at home or school
4. Abrupt shift in relationships
5. Depression, social withdrawal
6. Decline in school performance
7. Trauma-driven acting-out behavior: sexual acting-out or reckless, risk-taking behaviors
8. Effort to distance from feelings of shame, guilt, and humiliation
9. Flight into driven activity and involvement with others or retreat from others in order to manage inner turmoil
10. Accident-proneness
11. Wish for revenge and action-oriented responses to trauma
12. Increased self-focusing and withdrawal
13. Sleep and eating disturbances; nightmares

Very young children may exhibit few PTSD symptoms. This may be because eight of the PTSD symptoms require a verbal description of one's feelings and experiences. Instead, young children may report more generalized fears such as stranger or separation anxiety, avoidance of situations that may or may not be related to the trauma, sleep disturbances, and a preoccupation with words or symbols that may or may not be related to the trauma. These children may also display posttraumatic play in which they repeat themes of the trauma. In addition, children may lose an acquired developmental skill (such as toilet training) as a result of experiencing a traumatic event.

Clinical reports suggest that elementary school-age children may not experience visual flashbacks or amnesia for aspects of the trauma. However, they do experience "time skew" and "omen formation," which are not typically seen in adults. Time skew refers to a child's mis-sequencing trauma-related events when recalling the memory. Omen formation is a belief that there were warning signs that predicted the trauma. As a result, children often believe that if they are alert enough, they will recognize warning signs and avoid future traumas. School-age children also reportedly exhibit posttraumatic play or reenactment of the trauma in play, drawings, or verbalizations. Posttraumatic play is different from reenactment in that posttraumatic play is a literal representation of the trauma, involves compulsively repeating some aspect of the trauma, and does not tend to relieve anxiety but to actually increase it (Terr, 1991). An example of posttraumatic play is an increase in shooting games after exposure to a school shooting. Posttraumatic reenactment, on the other hand, is more flexible and involves behaviorally re-creating aspects of the trauma (e.g., carrying a weapon after exposure to violence).

While the development and course of PTSD is well documented, there is now abundant evidence for what DSM-IV called "delayed onset" but is now called "delayed expression", with the recognition that some symptoms typically appear immediately and that the delay is in meeting full criteria (DSM-5, p. 276).

PTSD in adolescents may begin to more closely resemble PTSD in adults.

However, there are a few features that have been shown to differ. As discussed earlier, children may engage in traumatic play following a trauma. Adolescents are more likely to engage in traumatic reenactment, in which they incorporate aspects of the trauma into their daily lives. In addition, adolescents are more likely than younger children or adults to exhibit impulsive and aggressive behaviors.

Besides PTSD, children and adolescents who have experienced traumatic events often exhibit other types of problems. Perhaps the best information available on the effects of traumas on children comes from a review of the literature on the effects of child sexual abuse. In this review, it was shown that sexually abused children often have problems with fear, anxiety, depression, anger and hostility, aggression, sexually inappropriate behavior, self-destructive behavior, feelings of isolation and stigma, poor self-esteem, difficulty in trusting others, and substance abuse. These problems are often seen in children and adolescents who have experienced other types of traumas as well. Children who have experienced traumas also often have relationship problems with peers and family members, problems with acting out, and problems with school performance.

Along with associated symptoms, there are a number of psychiatric disorders that are commonly found in children and adolescents who have been traumatized. A commonly co-occurring disorder is major depression. Other disorders include substance abuse; other anxiety disorders such as separation anxiety, panic disorder, and generalized anxiety disorder; and externalizing disorders such as attention-deficit/hyperactivity disorder, oppositional defiant disorder, and conduct disorder.

TREATMENT INTERVENTIONS FOR PTSD

Although some children show a natural remission of PTSD symptoms over a period of a few months, a significant number of children continue to exhibit symptoms for years if left untreated. Few studies focus on PTSD treatments to determine which are most effective for children and adolescents. A review of the studies of PTSD treatments for adults shows that cognitive-behavioral therapy (CBT) is an effective approach. CBT for children generally blends both cognitive and behavioral interventions, including having the child directly discuss the traumatic event (exposure), anxiety management techniques such as relaxation and assertiveness training, and correction of inaccurate or distorted trauma-related thoughts (Berliner & Saunders, 1996; Foa & Rothman, 1998). Although there is some controversy regarding exposing children to the events that scare them, exposure-based treatments seem to be most relevant when memories or reminders of the trauma distress a child. Children can be exposed gradually and taught relaxation so that they can learn to relax while recalling their experiences. Through this procedure, they learn that they do not have to be afraid of their memories. CBT also involves challenging children's false beliefs, such as "the world is totally unsafe." The majority of studies have found that it is safe and effective to use CBT for children with PTSD (Mannarino, Cohen, & Berman, 1994; Mannarino & Cohen, 1996; March & Mulle, 1998).

CBT is often accompanied by psychoeducation and parental involvement. Psychoeducation in this case is education about PTSD symptoms and their effects. It is as important for parents and caregivers to understand the effects of PTSD as it is for children. Research shows that the better parents cope with the trauma, and the more they support their children, the better their children will function. Therefore, it is important for parents to seek treatment for themselves in order to develop the necessary coping skills that will help their children.

Psychological first aid has been prescribed for children exposed to community violence and can be used in schools and traditional settings. Psychological first aid involves clarifying trauma-related facts, normalizing the children's PTSD reactions, encouraging the expression of feelings, teaching problem-solving skills, and referring the most symptomatic children for additional treatment (Pynoos & Nader, 1988).

Eye movement desensitization and reprocessing (EMDR) combines cognitive therapy with directed eye movements (Shapiro, 1998). Although EMDR has been shown to be effective in treating both children and adults with PTSD, studies indicate that it is the cognitive intervention rather than the eye movements that accounts for the change. Medications have also been prescribed for some children with PTSD. However, due to the lack of research in this area, it is too early to evaluate the effectiveness of medication therapy.

But what about the child who cannot "talk" about it? Such children are considered to be fine because they are not showing the symptoms in a verbal sense. Children will tend to play out traumas on their own if they can. It may be that no adult will ever see the play. However, if the support system is weak for these children (parent pathology), or if the trauma was too intense and too frequent, then they may not even attempt to play out the trauma on their own. Children do heal themselves through their play if they can. But if conditions prevent such play, then that is when release play therapy (RPT) shows the most promise and positive clinical results (Kaduson, 1997).

There has been great interest and activity over the years devoted to the study of the child's play as a basis for psychotherapy. Treating children's problems by exploiting their own methods of treating themselves has a sound basis, analogous to a study of the cure of disease by determining the organism's own methods of protection (Kaduson, 1997). Because many of the symptoms that children have are seen in their play, it is the natural course of intervention.

THERAPEUTIC POWERS OF PLAY

One of the most important aspects of play therapy is the actual therapeutic powers of play (Schaefer, 1993). Certainly, when we are talking about PTSD, there are clear indications that the following therapeutic powers are at work in helping children assimilate a trauma and gain mastery over the event through their own means of communication, namely, play.

Communication is one of the most important powers of play. Play is to the child what verbalization is to the adult—the most natural medium of self-expression. Because play is the language of the child, it allows the child to "speak" to us without words. There are two types of communication: unconscious and conscious. Children play out unconscious material without direct awareness at first. They reveal thoughts, feelings, and conflicts that they are totally unaware of. Children project their feelings onto miniature figures or puppets, thereby allowing their unconscious thoughts to rise to consciousness. Play provides a window into the otherwise invisible inner world of children. The play is "as if " it were real, so children are protected from flooding of the event when they are not ready for it. Conscious material is also communicated through play because children use their natural expression (play) to communicate events, traumas, and so forth, without using words. Play allows children to enact those thoughts and feelings of which they are aware but cannot express in words. This helps them to report their traumas in a nonthreatening way.

Abreaction is the reliving of past stressful events and the emotions associated with those events, even if a child could not express those emotions at the actual time of the trauma. Children use abreactive play to work through their traumas and assimilate the material a piece at a time. This concept was used by Sigmund Freud (1920/1955) to help explain how trauma victims resolve their experiences. Repressed memories are brought to consciousness and relived with the appropriate release of affect. Freud applied the concept to children, and he noted (1920/1955) that play offers young children a unique opportunity to accomplish this mental work. According to Freud, the posttraumatic anxiety can be resolved only if the therapist is able to get the child to relive the trauma with appropriate release of affect. This assimilation model fits well with the work of Piaget (1950), in that the traumatic experience is gradually assimilated into a schema (frame of reference) that is developed by the therapist–client interaction (Schaefer, 1993).

In abreaction, children have to do the opposite of what they want to do. They want to avoid processing the trauma. This can be done by (1) avoidance of knowledge of the event (amnesia), (2) avoidance of affect (numbing), (3) avoidance of behavior (phobic responses), and/or (4) avoidance of any communication about the event (Kaduson, Cangelosi, & Schaefer, 1997). Of course, the problem with such avoidance is that one cannot process the traumatic experience unless one relives it. The best way to expose young children to traumatic memories is through structured play.

Abreaction is enhanced through the act of repetition. Freud (1914/1958) maintained that children unconsciously re-create, in their play, situations related to the original traumatic event, and the frequency of the play is related to the intensity of the trauma. Therefore, every new repetition of play weakens the negative response associated with the trauma and seems to strengthen the child's sense of mastery of the event.

By means of the brief intervention of RPT, the play therapist can, in the playroom, present the child with miniature play objects representing the trauma scene and can encourage the child to play out the trauma. In this way the children can reexperience an event or a relationship in a different way, and with a more positive outcome than that of the original event. For children to benefit from play reenactment of past traumas, a number of therapeutic processes must be present (Ekstein, 1966):

1. Miniaturization of experiences by use of the small play objects.
2. Active control and domination of events that are possible in play.
3. Piecemeal assimilation of a traumatic event by repetitiously playing out that event.

As children play in later sessions with the play therapist, different distressing details of the trauma are likely to be emphasized until, piecemeal, the event is brought into complete awareness and the reality of it accepted and integrated into the psyche.

Mastery is another therapeutic power of play that impels children to play out their traumas. Because play is a self-motivated activity, it tends to satisfy children's innate need to explore and master the environment (Berlyne, 1960). When children have experienced a traumatic event, their sense of efficacy is diminished. Yet through the play in RPT, children become competent and feel satisfied by their sense of efficacy.

Also at work with mastery is systematic desensitization (Wolpe, 1958). Children's play can reduce anxiety through the process of exposing them to a fearful situation while they are relaxed in play. The pleasure of play can counteract and neutralize the fearfulness, so that the children can perform the desired behavior of working through the event. The repetition of play allows for the desensitization of the traumatic experience so that the child gains a sense of power and mastery at the same time.

Catharsis is the release of tension and affect. It also refers to the arousal and discharge of strong emotions (positive and negative) for therapeutic relief (Schaefer, 1993). In RPT, children can release the intense feelings of anger, grief, or anxiety that have been difficult or impossible to express before, either due to the intensity of the trauma or because of the lack of a support system that would allow such expression. This discharge results in a sense of relief.

Fantasy compensation also allows children to create their own realities. In the world of imagination, children do not have to be satisfied with current realities or their own limitations. In RPT, children can have the power through their fantasy to compensate for their real-life weaknesses, hurts, losses, or fears and satisfy unmet needs while playing out the traumatic situation repetitively and safely in the playroom.

Pretending gives children power over their world, even when they do not have much actual control in real-life situations (Schaefer, 1993). It is the one area in which children can make reality conform to their wishes. Therefore, when they revisit a traumatic event through play, they can modify the circumstances to fill their own needs, place a support system around themselves even if it didn't exist during the trauma, and make the ending turn out better than they experienced in the first place.

With the therapeutic powers in play, RPT can give children and adults a chance to assimilate a traumatic situation slowly and with enjoyment as they face the frightening event through their play.

ORIGINS OF RPT

David Levy (1932) originated RPT during a time when he was observing many children experiencing the same responses to night terrors or night-mares. It was already known that children handle their own emotional difficulties through their imaginative play. When they play, they get rid of tensions arising out of anxiety. Presumably, if children's behaviors were appropriate during the event that caused the anxiety, no tension residuals would have remained (Levy, 1932). When a child's method of dealing with the anxiety is unsuccessful, symptoms of the presence of the anxiety are still at hand.

During his research, Levy found that the reasons that the children did not naturally abreact certain situations had do with a number of factors: (1) the strength of the stimulus (because fears are of varying intensity and duration); (2) the summation of events (several traumas may occur simulta-neously or in close time relation); (3) the children's sensitivity to the stimu-lus (at different ages, different effects may occur with certain situations); (4) children may have been sensitized through a specific past experience that intensifies the response; and (5) whether any children who experienced a traumatic situation had any psychological problems prior to the event.

TYPICAL RESPONSES
TO A TRAUMATIC SITUATION

Based on the foregoing discussion, an example is used to illustrate how children naturally abreact. Although many children go through daily dif-ficulties, it is their play and the conditions of the situation that allow them to "work it through" in their play. The following example illustrates this procedure.

Julie, a 5-year-old girl, was playing with her friend (also a 5-year-old) in the ocean close to shore. They were both jumping in the waves and screaming with delight. Julie's mom wanted to take a picture of the two children, so she walked toward the water and called for Julie and her friend to get close together for the picture. Mom was directing Julie to move a bit farther out in the ocean so that she could frame the shot better. Without

Mom's knowledge, and in a split second, Julie fell into a sinkhole in the ocean and went underwater. People around her saw this and began grabbing for her in the water. The ocean's water was not clear, so it was difficult for them to see her. Mom's immediate response was to move the camera, thinking that Julie was fooling around. In a few seconds, it was clear to Julie's mom that something had happened. She started screaming for help, and the lifeguard came quickly. He took Julie out of the water, and she immediately vomited the salt water onto the beach. Mom held her while they both cried, and then they went back to their blanket. At this point, Julie's friend was just watching from her own blanket about 5 feet away.

Mom sat on the blanket, holding Julie; then, without notice, Julie pulled away and started digging furiously in the sand to make a hole big enough to put her doll in. After she covered the doll with sand, she pulled it out again, and repeated the same action again and again while her mother watched. After about five repetitions, Julie asked her mother to get her some water. Mom just took a bucket and ran to the water's edge to scoop up the water. She filled the bucket and returned to the blanket. Julie then dug another hole, put water in the hole, and then the doll. She covered the doll completely with water and repeated this action several times. She then wanted more water, so Mom went to the ocean again and filled the bucket. During this short time, Julie's friend asked her innocently if she wanted to go back into the ocean. Julie said, "Not yet." When Mom returned again with the water, Julie took her doll, put the doll in the bucket of water, and then pulled her out quickly and made her "vomit" onto the sand. Julie repeated this three times. Then she threw her doll in the air and grabbed her friend's hand, and they both returned to the water, playing as if nothing had ever happened.

Julie was able to naturally abreact because she had all of the conditions that made it easy for her to repetitively revisit her scary situation without feeling out of control. The trauma was of short duration and intensity (although she had swallowed some water, she was never unconscious), her support system was strong (people helping immediately, as well as her mother's being right there and holding her), and this had never happened to Julie before. She was able to play it out right away without someone stopping her, perhaps by saying, "Don't worry honey, it's OK now. You don't need to do that." Whenever these words are spoken, it stops a child from doing what is naturally helpful to work through a fearful situation.

OTHER CLINICAL ISSUES

Among the many clinical issues that must be addressed when working with children diagnosed with PTSD are countertransference and termination.

Countertransference issues are very common in treating children who have been traumatized, including, but not limited to, overidentification with the helplessness of the child and the unfairness of the circumstances, denial, excessive distancing and "vicarious traumatization." It is very important for the play therapist to remain empathic, sympathetic, and objective throughout the therapy, despite the difficulties in doing so. Supervision is helpful to ensure that personal feelings do not interfere with the therapy for the child.

In addition, RPT should be used where mastery play seems appropriate for child trauma cases. In that regard, the cases selected for this type of treatment must be "post" the traumatic incident. If the therapist suspects that there is ongoing abuse or traumatic situations may still prevail, RPT should not be used. In those cases, there are many different approaches, including, but not limited to, cognitive-behavioral play therapy (Knell, 1993; Kaduson, 2006), child-centered play therapy (VanFleet, 2010), and others. It would be inappropriate to use RPT if the child is severely depressed, resists play reenactment, shows no affect during the play, exhibits no diminution of fear reaction over the course of an exposure play session, or exhibits overvalued ideation (i.e., believes the fears are realistic) (Schaefer, 1994).

When using RPT, it is important to help keep the play focused on the traumatic situation so that the child can slowly assimilate the experience, and get to a point of mastery before termination begins. Abreactive or mastery play has been successful when two considerations are met (Caplan, 1981):

1. The play reduces to tolerable limits physiological and psychological manifestations of emotional arousal during and shortly after the stressful event.
2. The play mobilizes the child's coping resources so that the child can reduce the threat and find substitute sources of gratification for what was lost in the trauma.

To assess that the emotional processing is complete during or following play therapy, the play therapist can present relevant trauma stimuli in play or conversation to evoke an emotional reaction. If a strong negative response is elicited, it indicates that the emotional processing has not been successfully completed and further sessions are needed before termination. In many clinical cases, the child just might express that the play is finished, or he or she may seem totally disinterested in the thematic play that had been the focus of the RPT. Although rare, one-session treatment has been documented where it appears that the child just needed to be "heard."

RPT FOR CHILDREN WITH PTSD

In order to work with a child who is diagnosed with PTSD, it is very important for the therapist to get enough information from the intake with the parents, caretakers, or whoever was present so that the therapist can help the child play through the event, rather than avoid the thoughts and feelings associated with it. Although the intake information may not be totally accurate, if the therapist can replicate the situation closely enough, children can play through the event slowly so that they can assimilate the feelings at a pace that they can tolerate. This is always a short-term approach. If the conditions are right, a child might be able to play it out in one to 10 sessions. The therapist will be very directive even while following the lead of the child. As illustrated shortly, a child may play "around" the event or withdraw from the actual play when his or her anxiety becomes too great. It is the therapist's responsibility to help the child get closer to the event, and to keep in the event, by using humor or other creative means to join the child in the experience. This can give the child more ego strength and allow for a greater feeling of safety and an opportunity to revisit something that was very scary the first time around.

It is important in RPT to remain playful and lighthearted even if the situation was so frightening that the child may have dissociated or stopped playing at all. If that happens, the child is in a severe state of PTSD. Because during the event the child felt hopeless and helpless, his or her only protection was to dissociate. This does not mean that the child cannot play about it at some time, but it does mean that at the time of the trauma, the child was frozen and experienced so much fright that he or she removed the ability to feel at all. It might not be noticed by any of the adults in the child's life, but in many cases the behavior of the child changes to one of oppositional defiance. The onset is slow, but since parents seem to fight opposition, it doesn't become an issue until there is an escalated behavior pattern. This is a common presenting problem of oppositional defiant disorder (ODD), while the underlying cause is really unknown until treatment, as will be illustrated with Martin.

CASE ILLUSTRATION

Martin was a 5-year-old boy who was referred due to his oppositional behavior and diagnosed with ODD. His parents were seen first for the intake without Martin. They were interviewed regarding family history on both sides of the family, including grandparents, aunts, uncles, and cousins of Martin. Martin's parents had divorced 2 years earlier, but they had maintained a good relationship and shared custody. He was an only child, and his family history was unremarkable. There was some anxiety on both sides, but nothing severe that might impact Martin directly or indirectly. During the intake both parents were asked specific questions about Martin, his sleep patterns, sensory issues, eating habits, academics and school reports, friends, relationships with peers and adults, gross motor skills, fine motor skills, and typical day in his life. All seemed to be within the normal range, although he was above "grade level," and he had started reading on his own. He goes to school in the morning, and since both parents work, he is dropped off at his paternal grandmother's house where he stays until either parent finishes work and picks him up. When asked what kind of discipline the parents used individually, both said they had tried everything, and nothing worked. He used to be easy to manage and didn't have the "terrible twos," but recently his behavior had escalated from just not doing what he was told, to become very angry and throwing things at both homes (although not with his grandmother). School had not reported any difficulties in kindergarten. After all information was gathered through this interview, the parents were given possible examples of why children become defiant, including attention getting, learned history of parental response to action, or reuniting of parents in this particular case. With that being said, Martin's parents would take parent-training sessions, if needed, as part of his treatment.

The next session was the intake for Martin. This was done with a nondirective approach, indicating to Martin that this was a special playroom, and he could do almost anything he wanted in here, and if there was something he could not do, the therapist would let him know. He entered the playroom and remarked at how many things there were to play with. He immediately gravitated to the dinosaurs, and he made an entire family with them. He said that the daddy dinosaur was the biggest, then the mommy, and last was the little one. He named that dinosaur Junior. He created two separate forests where each of the adult dinosaurs lived, and Junior would fly through the air to visit each of his parents everyday. He gave voice to Junior, but the parents were just put into their respective forests to hang out at home. Junior was the dinosaur, who made all the rules for the parents, and they had to listen to him or he would time them out. He laughed when I reflected that the biggest dinosaur was afraid of the little one, and he said both of them were afraid of Junior because he was smarter than they were. He also decided that Junior could make rain happen, and even thunderstorms, so that the parents had to get wet or run for cover. Junior was protected by his flying ability, and both parents did not know how to fly. He said that they worked at staying still. He was giving more and more power to Junior the entire session, which reflected that this was an important part of his play. He was in charge and feeling empowered by the play. After the

5-minute warning that we had to stop soon, he did put some closure on this play by saying that the sun will come out later so that the parents can come out and play or go to work. I reflected that he could make all things happen just the way he wanted them to, and he agreed. He transitioned out of the playroom very easily, and as I walked him to his mother in the waiting room, he said, "Wow, that was fun. Hey, next time let's play about when I swallowed the quarter."

Following that comment, Martin's parents were contacted so that this event could be verified. They said that because both of them work, Martin stayed at Grandma's house after preschool. Grandma, however, was wheelchair-bound, and certainly Martin was helping her out as well. One day, however, Martin did indeed swallow a quarter, and while he was having difficulty breathing, it was not possible for his grandmother to do anything but call 911. Both parents were not reachable by cell phone, although voicemail messages were left. The emergency medical team (EMT) arrived, and they took Martin to the hospital, and unfortunately, he had to go alone because his grandmother could not accompany him. He seemed very calm according to the EMT. They reported to the parents that he was very brave and handled everything well. He was only 3½ years old. I asked for the complete details of the trauma, and I explained that since his oppositional behavior began right after this incident, it was possible that this was the key to the acute onset of what was thought to be ODD. When I had reviewed the normal limitations of preschoolers, and the fact that normal behavior would be to cry, scream, or be very scared, I told them I would like to do RPT with him on the next visit to let him work through this incident other than verbally.

Before Martin entered the playroom on the following visit, I had set up an entire Playmobil hospital and ambulance, along with "Grandma's house," and the types of instruments that Martin had seen when he was taken into the hospital. His parents didn't arrive until an hour later. Martin came into the playroom, thrilled to see all of the toys, and immediately said that this will be the little boy (picking up a boy Playmobil doll with his hair color). He said that we will now play about when this boy swallowed a quarter. He put the story into third person, which is what most preschoolers would do to assimilate traumatic experiences slowly. Martin jumped into the play with ease, and when I asked what the little boy's name was, he responded, "Little boy." Martin took the little boy and put him into the ambulance first, leaving out the entire grandmother's house where the incident actually occurred. This was a red flag that the fear possibly began after the event, rather than during. As he was putting the child on the gurney, I asked him, "Is Mommy or Daddy with him?" He questioned what I said as if he never heard the words before (Mommy? Daddy?), and then recanted and said, "Oh yeah, Mommy, Mommy and Daddy are with him." Still strapping the boy into the gurney, Martin made the sound of an ambulance siren. Then after strapping him in, he had the ambulance drive to the hospital, again making the sound of an ambulance siren.

He would start telling me about things as he played, whenever it became too frightening. So as the ambulance went to the hospital, Martin told me that the attendants in the ambulance were called "hospitalees." He interpreted this from hearing the EMT talking to each other to find out which hospital they should go to. They kept naming different hospitals, so he thought that was their names. As soon as he arrived at the emergency room, he was taken out of the ambulance, put in triage and then after x-rays they did the procedure right in the emergency room before moving Martin to his own bed in the pediatric ward. What Martin played, however, was that the little boy was put in a wheelchair, and then moved to find out "if his heart was beating." During this segment, once again the siren was the background even when he was being wheeled to different areas. He did a few medical procedures just because it was on the floor, and it was done without real knowledge about the machine. However, after they found out the heart was beating, he was taken to a hospital bed by wheelchair again, and the siren got louder and louder.

When he placed the boy in the bed, Martin became much more anxious, and began to ask me what the different items were in the playroom. I answered what he needed to hear, and waited for a few more lines and then asked if the doctor was ready to get the quarter yet? At first, he asked about a broken hospital bed, and he began to laugh at what he said, which clearly reduced his anxiety because he immediately said (in the voice of the doctor) that he was ready to get the quarter. He asked me if I knew how to do this? I began to say that I didn't, and he interrupted and said, "Oh, I know. I heard it before. You go in the bed, and the lights go out. Then they take it and the lights go on." I said that was helpful. So now he began his version of the operation, and he said to the little boy, "OK, now, open wide." I made the scared sounds of a preschooler saying "ahhhh." He smiled and took it out. Then he said, "OK, now you are done." I asked him again at this time whether the boy's mommy and daddy were with him, and at first he asked "Mommy? Daddy?" Then he said, "Oh yeah, oh yeah. They are there and they have to stay in the hospital with the little boy for 10 days without leaving." I said that it sounded like a good plan.

After this session, no more sessions were required. Both parents said that he was no longer oppositional, and he was compliant and very pleasant. He had worked it through because he did have PTSD after going in the ambulance to the hospital without anyone he knew. In the subsequent sessions, pieces of the play changed into more mastery, and his parents also received parent training for better support of Martin due to his anxiety.

SUMMARY AND CONCLUSIONS

RPT has been clinically used successfully with type I traumas (Terr, 1991). Type I traumas are single, sudden, and unexpected. Therefore, in selecting cases suitable for RPT, it is advisable to consider the following criteria (Levy, 1938):

1. The child should be between 2 and 10 years of age (although it can work for older children with some modifications).
2. There should be a definite reactive pattern triggered by a specific stressor (e.g., a frightening experience, divorce of parents, birth of a sibling).
3. The problem should not be long-standing.
4. The traumatic experience should be in the past, not continuing at the time of referral.
5. The child should be from a relatively normal family situation.

With the foregoing criteria met, it has been shown that children do not have to know the nature of their difficulties, or of their relationship to the therapist, in order to improve. The emotional release and positive therapeutic relationship are basic therapeutic elements leading to the resolution of the trauma.

RPT has helped children resolve psychological difficulties after experiencing a traumatic experience without the appropriate support system or when the stimulus was just too strong to psychologically manage. Children were able to work through their fears, anxieties, and sadness through playing out their perceptions of what happened to them. Within weeks and sometimes within months, many children returned to their carefree childhood experiences, although at some level they had changed for good. The same is likely to happen with the victims of any traumatic event, and it is clinically proven that RPT is the treatment of choice to relieve these children of their PTSD.

REFERENCES

Ackerman, P. T., Newton, J. E., McPherson, W. B., Jones, J. G., & Dykman, R. A. (1998). Prevalence of post traumatic stress disorder and other psychiatric diagnoses in three groups of abused children (sexual, physical, and both). *Child Abuse and Neglect, 22*(8), 759–774.

American Psychiatric Association. (1980). *Diagnostic and statistical manual of mental disorders* (3rd ed.). Washington, DC: Author.

American Psychiatric Association. (1994). *Diagnostic and statistical manual of mental disorders* (4th ed.). Washington, DC: Author.

American Psychiatric Association. (2013). *Diagnostic and statistical manual of mental disorders* (5th ed.). Arlington, VA: Author.

Berliner, L., & Saunders, B. E. (1996). Treating fear and anxiety in sexually abused children: Results of a controlled two-year follow-up study. *Child Maltreatment, 1*(4), 294–309.

Berlyne, D. E. (1960). *Conflict, arousal and curiosity.* New York: McGraw-Hill.

Caplan, G. (1981). Mastery of stress: Psychological aspects. *American Journal of Psychiatry, 138,* 413–420.

Creamer, M., & Forbes, D. (2004). Treatment of posttraumatic stress disorder in veteran and military populations. *Psychotherapy: Theory, Research, Practice, 41*(4), 388–398.

Cuffe, S. P., Addy, C. L., Garrison, C. Z., Waller, J. L., Jackson, K. L., & McKeown, R. E. (1998). Prevalence of PTSD in a community sample of older adolescents. *Journal of the American Academy of Child and Adolescent Psychiatry, 37,* 147–154.

DeWolfe, D. J. (2004). *Mental health response to mass violence and terrorism: A training manual.* Rockville, MD: U.S. Department of Health and Human Services.

Ekstein, R. (1966). *Children of time and space, of action and impulse.* New York: Appleton Century Crofts.

Eth, S., & Pynoos, R. S. (1995). Developmental perspective on psychic trauma in childhood. In C. R. Figley (Ed.), *Trauma and its wake: The study of treatment of posttraumatic stress disorder* (pp. 36–52). New York: Brunner/Mazel.

Foa, E. B., & Rothman, B. O. (1998). *Treating the trauma of rape: Cognitive-behavioral therapy for PTSD.* New York: Guilford Press.

Freud, S. (1955). Beyond the pleasure principle. In J. Strachey (Ed. & Trans.), *The standard edition of the complete psychological works of Sigmund Freud* (Vol. 18, pp. 1–64). London: Hogarth Press. (Original work published 1920)

Freud, S. (1958). Remembering, repeating and working-through. In J. Strachey (Ed. & Trans.), *The standard edition of the complete psychological works of Sigmund Freud* (Vol. 12, pp. 145–156). London: Hogarth Press. (Original work published 1914)

Giacona, R. M., Reiknherz, H. Z., Silverman, A. B., Pakiz, B., Frost, A. K., & Cohen, E. (1995). Traumas and PTSD in a community population of older adolescents. *Journal of the American Academy of Child and Adolescent Psychiatry, 34,* 1369–1380.

Hamblen, J. (2004). PTSD in children and adolescents (National Center for PTSD Fact Sheet). Available at *www.ncptsd.va.gov/facts/specific/fs_children.html.*

Hampe, E., Noble, H., Miller, L. C., & Barrett, C. L. (1973). Phobic children one and two years post-treatment. *Journal of Abnormal Psychology, 82,* 446–453.

Kaduson, H. G. (1997). Release play therapy for the treatment of sibling rivalry. In H. G. Kaduson, D. Cangelosi, & C. Schaefer (Eds.), *The playing cure* (pp. 255–273). Northvale, NJ: Jason Aronson.

Kaduson, H. G. (2006). Short-term play therapy for children with attention-deficit/hyperactivity disorder. In H. G. Kaduson & C. E. Schaefer (Eds.), *Short-term play therapy for children, second edition* (pp. 101–134). New York: Guilford Press.

Kaduson, H. G. (2011). Release play therapy. In C. E. Schaefer (Ed.), *Foundations of play therapy* (pp. 105–126). Hoboken, NJ: Wiley.

Kaduson, H., Cangelosi, D., & Schaefer, C. E. (Eds.). (1997). *The playing cure.* Northvale, NJ: Jason Aronson.

Kessler, R. C., Sonnega, A., Bromet, E., Hughes, M., & Nelson, C. B. (1995). Posttraumatic stress disorder in the National Comorbidity Study. *Archives of General Psychiatry, 52,* 1048–1060.

Kilpatrick, K. L., & Williams, L. M. (1997). Post-traumatic stress disorder in child witnesses to domestic violence. *Journal of Orthopsychiatry, 67*, 639–644.

Knell, S. M. (1993). *Cognitive-behavioral play therapy*. Northvale, NJ: Jason Aronson.

Levy, D. M. (1932). The use of play technique as experimental procedure. *American Journal of Orthopsychiatry, 3*, 266–275.

Levy, D. M. (1938). Release therapy in young children. *Psychiatry, 1*, 387–390.

MacLean, P. D. (1988). *The triune brain in evolution: Role in paleocerebal functions*. New York: Plenum Press.

Mannarino, A. P., & Cohen, J. A. (1996). Abuse-related attributions and perceptions, general attributions, and locus of control in sexually abused girls. *Journal of Interpersonal Violence, 11*, 162–180.

Mannarino, A. P., Cohen, J. A., & Berman, S. R. (1994). The Children's Attributions and Perceptions Scale: A new measure of sexual abuse-related factors. *Journal of Clinical Child Psychology, 23*, 204–211.

March, J., & Mulle, K. (1998). *OCD in children and adolescents: A cognitive-behavioral treatment manual*. New York: Guilford Press.

Margolis, G., & Gordis, E. B. (2000). The effects of family and community violence on children. *Annual Review of Psychology, 51*, 445–479.

Pfefferbaum, B., Nixon, S., Tucker, P., Tivis, R., Moore, V., Gurwitch, R., et al. (1999). Posttraumatic stress response in bereaved children after Oklahoma City bombing. *Journal of the American Academy of Child and Adolescent Psychiatry, 38*, 1372–1379.

Pfefferbaum, B., Seale, T., McDonald, N., Brandt, E., Rainwater, S., Maynard, B., et al. (2000). Posttraumatic stress two years after the Oklahoma City bombing in youths geographically distant from the explosion. *Psychiatry, 63*, 358–370.

Piaget, J. (1950). *The psychology of intelligence*. London: Routledge & Kegan Paul.

Pynoos, R., Frederick, C., Nader, K., Arroyo, W., Steinberg, A., Eth, S., et al. (1987). Life threat and posttraumatic stress in school-age children. *Archives of General Psychiatry, 44*, 1057–1063.

Pynoos, R., & Nader, K. (1988). Children who witness the sexual assaults of their mothers. *Journal of the American Academy of Child and Adolescent Psychiatry, 27*, 567–572.

Pynoos, R., & Nader, K. (1993). Issues in the treatment of posttraumatic stress in children and adolescents. In J. P. Wilson & B. Raphael (Eds.), *International handbook of traumatic stress syndromes* (pp. 535–549). New York: Plenum Press.

Schaefer, C. E. (1993). What is play and why is it therapeutic? In C. E. Schaefer (Ed.), *The therapeutic powers of play* (pp. 1–5). Northvale, NJ: Jason Aronson.

Schaefer, C. E. (1994). Play therapy for psychic trauma in children. In O'Connor, K. and Schaefer, C.E. (Eds.), *Handbook of play therapy, Volume Two: Advances and innovations* (pp. 291–318). New York: Wiley-Interscience.

Shapiro, F. (1998). *EMDR: The breakthrough therapy for overcoming anxiety, stress and trauma*. New York: Basic Books.

Shelby, J. S. (1997). Rubble, disruption, and tears: Helping young survivors of natural disaster. In H. Kaduson, D. Cangelosi, & C. E. Schaefer (Eds.), *The playing cure* (pp. 143–169). Northvale, NJ: Aronson.

Terr, L. (1991). Childhood traumas: An outline and overview. *American Journal of Psychiatry, 148*, 10–20.

van der Kolk, B. A., & Fisler, R. (1995). Dissociation and the fragmentary nature of traumatic memory: Background and experiential evidence. *Journal of Trauma Stress, 9*, 505–525.

Van Fleet, R. (2010). *Child-centered play therpay*. New York: Guilford Press.

Vernberg, E. M., & Varela, R. E. (2001). Posttraumatic stress disorder: A developmental perspective. In M. W. Vasey & M. R. Dadds (Eds.), *The developmental psychopathology of anxiety* (pp. 386–406). New York: Oxford University Press.

Wolpe, J. (1958). *Psychotherapy by reciprocal inhibition*. Stanford, CA: Stanford University Press.

Zatzick, D. F., Marmar, C. R., Weiss, D. S., Browner, W. S., Metzler, T. J., Golding, J. M., et al. (1997). Posttraumatic stress disorder and functioning and quality of life outcomes in a nationally representative sample of male Vietnam veterans. *American Journal of Psychiatry, 154*, 1690–1695.

Chapter 2

☙

Cognitive–Behavioral Play Therapy for Children with Anxiety and Phobias

Meena Dasari
Susan M. Knell

*A*nxiety disorders, which include phobias, are among the most prevalent psychiatric disorders in children and adolescents (Albano, Chorpita, & Barlow, 2003; Costello, Mustillo, Erkanli, Keeler, & Angold, 2003). The most widely accepted model for understanding fears and anxiety is the cognitive-behavioral model, which proposes that the relationship between situations, thoughts, emotions, and behaviors exists and maintains anxiety. It is based on the assumption that people's emotions and behaviors are determined largely by the way they think about the world, with these thoughts being triggered by situational cues (Beck, 1967, 1972, 1976). In other words, the perception of events, not the events themselves, guides how a person feels and acts. Cognitive-behavioral therapy (CBT) has consistently emerged as a highly effective treatment for anxiety and phobias; therefore, cognitive-behavioral play therapy (CBPT) was developed by integrating these theories and related research with play therapy approaches. This chapter (1) reviews the literature on anxiety and phobias in children, (2) discusses assessment and treatment, and (3) describes the use of CBPT for anxiety and phobias in young children.

ANXIETY DISORDERS IN CHILDHOOD

Given the prevalence of anxiety in children, it is interesting to note that pre-school children suffer from anxiety disorders at a similar rate as school-age children (Egger & Arnold, 2006; Lavigne et al., 2009). If anxiety disorders in young children are left untreated, symptoms may persist and worsen into adolescence and adulthood (Albano et al., 2003; Costello et al., 2003). Research has shown that children with untreated anxiety disorders are also at greater risk for developing depressive disorders and substance use disor-ders (Costello et al., 2003; Weissman, 1999). Therefore, early identification and intervention are crucial to prevent poor developmental and long-term outcomes.

Based on DSM-5, anxiety disorders are best understood and organized using empirical data on similarities among disorders (American Psychiatric Association, 2013). Several specific anxiety diagnoses fall under the rubric of anxiety. Separation anxiety disorder is usually diagnosed in early child-hood, and its core symptom is excessive anxiety concerning separation from home or from caregivers. Generalized anxiety disorder is character-ized by excessive and uncontrollable worry about multiple events that is present for at least 6 months. Social phobia is usually diagnosed during adolescence. The core symptom is marked and persistent anxiety about social or performance situations, which is triggered by excessive worries about embarrassment or rejection. Posttraumatic stress disorder (PTSD) is categorized under trauma and stress related disorders. The disorder includes symptoms overlapping with anxiety disorders (e.g., hyperarousal, avoidance), but considered distinct because diagnosis requires that the child experiences or witnesses a traumatic event and is currently reexperiencing the event. School refusal and somatic complaints are symptoms commonly associated with several anxiety disorders (Albano et al., 2003).

Anxiety is a normal emotional experience for children and adolescents. Anxieties about specific events are considered typical and transient at each stage of development. During the preschool years, children commonly experience anxieties about separation. School-age children often experi-ence anxieties about physical health. Adolescents typically report anxieties about social performances such as playing sports and giving presentations in front of the class. In general, most children experience normal levels of anxiety around specific events, which is considered developmentally appro-priate. Normal levels of anxiety are usually described as mild to moderate, transient, and not interfering with daily functioning (Klein & Pine, 2002).

Because anxiety is a normal emotion in children, clinicians often struggle with distinguishing clinical levels that warrant an anxiety disor-der diagnosis. Clinical anxiety differs from normal levels of anxiety on a number of dimensions. Beesdo, Knapp, and Pine (2009), a foundational article for the development of anxiety disorders in children and adolescents, outlined two dimensions: (1) intensity and (2) avoidance associated with distress or impairment.

Intensity refers to whether a child's level of distress is disproportionate, given his or her developmental stage or the object or event. A good example of a clinical level of anxiety can be seen on the first day of kindergarten, which is typically a stressful event for many children. A child who cries, complains of stomachaches, throws a tantrum, and is inconsolable when parents leave is displaying greater intensity of anxiety as compared with a child who gets tearful when separating from parents but is able to calm him- or herself in a short time period. The first child's reaction is disproportionate to the second child's, and the former child is more likely to have an anxiety disorder.

The second dimension relates to whether a child's level of avoidance leads to distress or impairment, or interferes with his or her daily life. Examples include difficulty making friends or receiving failing grades because of social anxiety or test anxiety, respectively. Both are suggestive of clinical levels of anxiety inasmuch as the anxiety interferes with the child's social and/or academic development. Thus, as compared with normal levels of anxiety, clinical anxiety is a more intense emotion than experienced by other children of the same age and leads to avoidance that impairs the child's ability to achieve developmentally appropriate tasks.

FEARS IN CHILDHOOD

Fear, as an emotion, is thought to be more biologically based as compared with anxiety (Davis & Ollendick, 2005). Fear involves a brain-based reaction that consists of the interplay of physiological responses, distorted cognitions, and behaviors designed to facilitate escape and avoidance of danger (Lang, 1979). In addition, fears are a normal part of childhood, usually presenting as mild, age-specific, and transient (Muris, Merckelbach, Gadet, & Moulaert, 2000). Some fears are even considered developmentally appropriate. During the infant years, fears seem to be concrete and centered on the immediate environment, such as a loud noises or strangers. Among 4- to 6-year-olds, imaginary creatures such as monsters and ghosts, and the dark, are common themes. Between ages 7 and 12 years, fears are usually centered on realistic events such as natural disasters and physical health.

Because fear is a normal emotion and part of child development, the criteria for specific phobia should be used to determine if clinical intervention is required. Phobias are evident in approximately 5% of the population (Davis & Ollendick, 2005). According to updates in DSM-5, specific phobia is diagnosed when fear of an event or object is (1) persistent and becomes excessive, (2) leads to undue physiological arousal, and (3) triggers distress and avoidance.

ASSESSMENT OF FEAR
AND ANXIETY IN CHILDREN

Assessment is a critical step in determining the developmental appropriateness of a child's anxiety and fears. Clinical interview with parents, behavioral rating scales, and parent monitoring forms are among the most commonly used assessment tools (Beesdo et al., 2009). More specific to CBPT, behavioral observation and play assessment with the child are used to supplement more standardized measures. Based on literature reviews, a multimethod assessment approach is recommended to obtain a comprehensive picture of symptoms across several contexts (Velting, Setzer, & Albano, 2004).

A developmental perspective is important to apply when assessing anxieties and fears in children. This is because most measures have been researched in specific age groups and may lack necessary attention to age-specific issues (Beesdo et al., 2009). For example, the Multidimensional Anxiety Scale for Children (MASC; March, Parker, Sullivan, Stallings, & Conners, 1997) was developed for ages 6–19 and lacks normative data to accurately assess anxiety in children ages 3–5. In general, most assessment techniques have been validated for use with school-age populations. Therefore, the use of clinical interview and select behavioral rating scales in conjunction with behavioral observation and parent monitoring forms are recommended for preschool and early school-age children.

Clinical Interview

The clinical interview is considered the most reliable assessment method for obtaining diagnostic accuracy with anxiety disorders. Clinical interviews may be either structured or semistructured. The most widely used instrument is the Anxiety Disorders Interview Schedule for DSM-IV: Child and Parent Version (ADIS; DiNardo, O'Brien, Barlow, Waddell, & Blanchard, 1983). Both parent and child versions are used with children ages 6–17 years. The ADIS can be completed by parents of preschool-age children; however, there is currently no information on whether the reliability and validity are the same with this age group. The ADIS typically takes a trained clinician 2–3 hours to administer. Given this length of time, the ADIS is more widely used in research than in clinical practice because of the need for diagnostic specificity in the former and the time constraints in the latter.

With younger children in clinical settings, semistructured interviews are more practical because of age and time limitations. Semistructured interviews allow clinicians to ask specific questions to obtain greater detail. When used, these interviews should be conducted with parents. In addition to assessment of symptoms, several informative questions are suggested to obtain details about intensity, impairment (both for the child and family), and general coping. These include:

- How does the child and family typically deal with the fearful object/ event?
- How have the anxiety and fear interfered with the child's and family's life?
- What efforts have the parents made to help the child, and how successful or unsuccessful have these been?
- What is the extent and nature of the child's exposure to the feared stimuli?

It is also important to assess and understand any changes in the family situation or environment that may have contributed to the child's fears. Lifestyle changes, such as a move to a new house, may prompt changes in the child's sense of safety or security and may thus contribute to changes in levels of fear. Traumatic events, such as divorce, abuse, or family illness/ death, must also be understood in terms of the effects on the child's fears. Furthermore, biological factors (temperament, medical history, family history), environmental factors (school functioning, family functioning), and developmental history should be assessed and considered in order to tailor CBPT to the child's overall functioning.

Behavioral Rating Scales

Rating scales and self-reports are considered a highly informative method for assessment of observable behaviors related to anxiety disorders (Beesdo et al., 2009). Most of the commonly used measures are designed for use with school-age children (Velting et al., 2004). To assess overall anxiety, the most commonly utilized scales are the Multidimensional Anxiety Scale for Children (MASC; March et al., 1997; ages 6–19) and the Screen for Anxiety and Related Emotional Disorders—Parent Version (SCARED; Birmaher et al. 1997, ages 8–18). However, for young children, the Spence Preschool Anxiety Scale (Spence, Rapee, McDonald, & Ingram, 2001) is recommended to distinguish clinical versus normal levels of anxiety. This is due to the normative data available for ages 3–6 and strong empirical support. Other rating scales have been developed and are administered based on symptoms specific to a disorder. Some examples include the Penn State Worry Questionnaire—Children and Adolescent (PSWQ-C; Chorpita,

Tracey, Brown, Collica, & Barlow, 1997) for generalized anxiety disorder; the Liebowitz Social Anxiety Scale (LSAS; Liebowitz, 1987) for social anxiety; and the Fear Survey Schedule for Children—Revised (FSS-R; Ollendick, 1983) for specific phobias.

Parent Monitoring Forms

Another supplemental assessment method is the use of parent monitoring forms, which are helpful in understanding the parental perceptions of the child's anxieties and fears. Self-monitoring forms, commonly used with school-age children and adolescents, are not possible for very young children. Therefore, parents complete the forms and are instructed to record anxiety-provoking situations, subsequent anxiety levels, cognitions, physical sensations, and behaviors. Parents are taught to use the "fear thermometer" (0 = no fear, 10 = extreme fear). Such a task is not reliable, but helps the parents and the younger child quantify his or her fears in a concrete, understandable format. In addition, the parent monitoring forms are likely to provide valuable information on triggers and anxiety-related behaviors (Velting et al., 2004).

Behavioral Observation

Behavioral observation during session involves watching and recording the child's reactions to situations for the purpose of understanding how the child's anxiety and/or fear is displayed and connected to the environment. Behavioral observation is considered a useful assessment method when supplemented with the clinical interview and behavior rating scales, particularly with CBPT. This assessment method can be unstructured or structured (Velting et al., 2004). The unstructured approach is more commonly utilized in clinical settings and involves clinicians noting the child's body posture, facial expressions, and reactions during the initial session. This may be also obtained in other naturalistic settings such as home or school, as well as by other people such as parents or teachers. More structured approaches include the behavioral approach tests (BATs), which involve clinicians intentionally introducing anxiety-provoking or feared stimuli (e.g., parent leaving room for child with separation anxiety disorder; showing a picture of a social situation for a child with social anxiety disorder) while subjectively assessing the child's anxiety level.

Play Assessment

When implementing CBPT, an assessment of play skills is important, as research has shown that play therapy is more effective for children with good pretend play skills (Russ, 2004). Play interviews are used when necessary and can be helpful in understanding anxiety in preschool children. Further, assessment of cognitive, emotional, social, and problem-solving abilities are important, particularly as these relate to the child's developmental level. Kaugers (2011) provides a comprehensive review of evidence-based play assessments. The author concludes that although the evidence base for many measures is promising, no one measure has consistently emerged with strong empirical support for its use.

TREATMENT OF FEAR
AND ANXIETY IN CHILDHOOD

Cognitive-Behavioral Therapy

CBT has been well established as an effective treatment for anxiety disorders and phobias in school-age children and adolescents (King, Heyne, & Ollendick, 2005; Silverman, Pina, & Viswesvaran, 2008). However, its application in young children has been questioned based on developmental abilities (Hirschfeld-Becker et al., 2008). In a recent meta-analysis, Reynolds, Wilson, Austin, and Hooper (2012) analyzed the existing studies to determine whether CBT was effective for young children. Their findings indicated that children ages 4–8 who received CBT displayed better outcomes as compared to controls (i.e., no intervention or wait list), but to a smaller degree when compared to children ages 9–18.

Yet, it has been proposed that when protocols are modified to be developmentally appropriate, CBT is likely to be effective for anxiety disorders and phobias for preschool children as well (Hirschfeld-Becker et al., 2008). In two randomized clinical trials, CBT protocols adapted for children ages 4–7 years were tested in a treatment group and compared to wait list control group, with CBT demonstrating symptom improvement. Hirschfeld-Becker et al. (2010) found that children who received CBT displayed a significant reduction in number of anxiety disorders and an increase in parent-rated coping. Similarly, the Scheeringa, Weems, Cohen, Amaya-Jackson, and Guthrie (2011) study showed that the treatment group receiving an adapted CBT protocol for PTSD showed significant decreases in the trauma symptoms as assessed by parent rating on standardized clinical interview.

Introducing more developmentally appropriate interventions, including those that are play-based, would increase the effectiveness of current CBT protocols when utilized with younger children. Play therapy interventions, which are considered distinct from CBT, have been shown to be effective in treating children's internalizing symptoms (Bratton, Ray, Rhine, & Jones, 2005; Bratton & Ray, 2000; Leblanc & Ritchie, 2001). Specifically, Bratton and colleagues (2005) conducted a meta-analysis of 93 outcome studies with children who were an average age of 7 years. Results indicated a large effect size of 0.80 for play interventions, indicating that children who received the intervention reported better outcomes than children who did not. Additionally, based on their review of the empirical research, Russ, Fiorelli, and Spannagel (2011) concluded that play relates to or facilitates adaptive coping strategies for daily problems and emotion regulation, both of which correspond to successful CBT outcomes for anxiety and phobias.

Overall, given the promising results for CBT with young children and the utility of play therapy interventions in children ages 3–8, a strong empirical foundation exists that indicates that CBPT may increase the effectiveness of CBT intervention for anxiety and fear in young children. One promising approach is trauma-focused CBT (TF-CBT), an empirically supported treatment for PTSD that has been adapted from adult-based CBT interventions for use with children ages 3–18 years (Cohen, Mannarino, Berliner, & Deblinger, 2000). Because the majority of studies have explored using the TF-CBT in school-age children and adolescents, Cavett and Drewes (2012) developed a CBPT intervention that integrated TF-CBT with play for young children, which has demonstrated promising results in several case studies. Additionally, in a school-based study of preschool children, Pearson (2007) compared three-session CBPT interventions, which incorporated play with CBT techniques, with a control group. This study used CBPT interventions, but was not technically CBPT, nor did the children have any specific presenting issues. The results showed that teachers reported significantly fewer anxiety–withdrawal symptoms in the intervention group. Although the study involved a nonclinical sample (vs. children with clinical disorders) and play with CBT techniques (vs. CBPT), it represents one of the first to empirically support CBPT interventions.

Cognitive-Behavioral Play Therapy

CBPT is designed specifically for preschool and early elementary school-age children and integrates CBT with play therapy. It emphasizes the child's involvement in therapy by addressing issues of control, mastery, and responsibility for changing one's own behavior. CBPT is designed to be developmentally appropriate and to help the child become an active participant in change (Knell, 1993a, 1994, 1997, 1998, 1999). The approach has been successfully implemented for children with anxiety disorders (e.g., separation anxiety, generalized anxiety, social anxiety) and phobias (Knell, 1993a, 2009, 2011). CBPT has also been used with children with a wide range of diagnoses, such as selective mutism (Knell, 1993a, 1993b) and encopresis (Knell & Moore, 1990; Knell, 1993a) as well as with children who have experienced traumatic life events, such as divorce (Knell, 1993a) and sexual abuse (Knell & Ruma, 1996).

Treatment Interventions

The main components of cognitive-behavioral interventions are incorporated into play therapy in creative ways, with the intent of presenting them to young children in an accessible manner to optimize treatment success. Given the limited cognitive abilities and anxieties of young children, play therapy offers anxious and/or fearful children an opportunity to express and master their feelings in a safe environment.

A variety of treatment interventions—both behavioral and cognitive— are utilized in CBPT for anxiety disorders and phobias. The most common interventions are described in the following section. Based on well-established protocols for anxiety disorders such as Coping Cat (Kendall & Hedtke, 2006), CBPT is likely to be most effective when each intervention is introduced in order. However, for young children, flexibility with interventions is critical to increase achievement of treatment goals. The order and number of sessions for each intervention may need to be modified due to variability in the child's developmental level and cognitive ability. At times, each intervention is presented later or repeated using a different play technique across several sessions. After each intervention is introduced, clinicians should determine whether the child demonstrates control, mastery, and understanding before moving on to the next intervention.

The six essential interventions considered to be critical for effective CBPT (Albano & Kendall, 2002; Hirschfeld-Becker et al., 2008) are (1) psychoeducation, (2) somatic management (relaxation), (3) cognitive restructuring, (4) exposure, (5) relapse prevention and generalization, and (6) parent involvement

PSYCHOEDUCATION

Psychoeducation often teaches an individual about his or her disorder and about the CBT model. The purpose is to (1) learn the relationship between events, thoughts, feelings, and behaviors; (2) identify his or her individual anxiety symptoms; and (3) understand how treatment will alleviate symptoms (Rapee, Wignall, Spence, Lyneham, & Cobham, 2008). Education is usually done with parents only, and incorporates teaching effective parenting strategies for reducing the child's symptoms. A discussion format is commonly used, but modeling specific parenting skills can be helpful at times (e.g., the therapist interacting with the child in a way that the parent observes). Explanations of the CBT model should be provided and adapted to preschool children as well. In CBPT, modeling is often used. For example, the therapist may educate a puppet about the puppet's worries and how thinking affects feelings and behavior.

SOMATIC MANAGEMENT (RELAXATION)

Somatic management primarily refers to relaxation training. Children are taught techniques such as deep breathing and muscle relaxation for the purpose of reducing autonomic arousal and physiological responses associated with anxiety and/or fear. Relaxation training can be part of CBPT by modeling a state of calm for the child. There are various ways in which this might be done, such as having the child observe the therapist teach a puppet muscle relaxation or deep breathing. Books and tapes are often used with young children. For example, Pincus's (2012) chapter "Accepting Physical Feelings" is an excellent resource for child-friendly relaxation scripts. Also, the book *Cool Cats, Calm Kids* (Williams, 1996) models relaxation skills through the body posture and "self-statements" of cats. In addition, at times, alternatives such as helping the child engage in relaxing activities and more calming play can be used in place of teaching specific relaxation skills. Other strategies such as self-control may also function to decrease the physical symptoms of anxiety.

COGNITIVE RESTRUCTURING

Cognitive restructuring techniques deal with teaching children skills to change their negative thinking to more positive, realistic thinking. The underlying theory for cognitive techniques is that anxiety results from maladaptive cognitions, or negative thinking about events in the environment (Kendall, 1993). Children are instructed on the techniques of "labeling thinking traps" (i.e., maladaptive thoughts) and being a "thought detective" (i.e., gathering the evidence, developing alternative explanations). The purpose of these techniques is for children to develop skills in generating adaptive thinking for daily events, which alleviates fears and anxiety.

With CBPT, these techniques are adapted to a child's developmental level. For example, before a birthday party a preschool child with maladaptive cognitions might think, "The kids won't like me" or "I'll be really bad at the party games," which leads to anxious feelings and behaviors (e.g., stomachaches, avoiding the party by hiding in the bathroom). Young children can learn more adaptive thoughts, such as "Birthday parties can be fun" or "No one will be good at *all* the party games." Thus, it is hypothesized that changes in thinking will produce changes in behavior. The therapist helps the child to identify, modify, and/or build cognitions. In addition to helping the child identify cognitive distortions and teaching the child to replace these maladaptive thoughts with more adaptive ones, the therapist also provides the child with an opportunity to test his or her new skills.

COGNITIVE CHANGE STRATEGIES AND COUNTERING MALADAPTIVE THOUGHTS

Once the child and therapist have identified maladaptive beliefs, the child can be taught to counter these beliefs using a number of different techniques. Based on the Coping Cat, techniques for cognitive change strategies usually involve a three-pronged approach: (1) identifying the maladaptive thought and its relationship to anxiety; (2) looking at the event differently; and (3) developing alternative thoughts (Kendall & Hedtke, 2006). For example, when treating a needle phobia, the child is taught that the thought "I can't handle the pain" is maladaptive and creates the fear. Then, he or she works with the therapist to consider different perspectives, which are used to develop more adaptive thoughts, such as "Shots help me fight diseases and illnesses" or "It will only hurt for a few seconds."

With CBPT, these cognitive change strategies are further adapted for preschool children given that the existing approaches, developed with older children, are typically beyond their cognitive abilities. Often, with young children, the therapist has to take a more active role in identifying the maladaptive thoughts by using the child's play, verbalizations, and information from the parents or other caregivers. Helping the child change cognitions will mean that the child will need assistance from an adult in generating alternative explanations, testing them, and changing beliefs (Cavett & Drewes, 2012; Emery, Bedrosian, & Garber, 1983). Cavett and Drewes (2012) utilize a magnetic cognitive triangle to visually represent maladaptive thoughts collected from different sources and indicate distinction from feelings and behaviors. The authors incorporate the technique within play.

In addition, to challenge one's beliefs, it is usually necessary to distance oneself from the beliefs, a task that is beyond the grasp of most young children. The child needs an "accumulated history of events" to understand the ramifications of certain situations (Kendall, 1993). Children with limited life experiences, or those who have not formed beliefs about such experiences, often have not developed such an understanding. Despite these limitations in young children, Knell (1993a, 1993b, 1994, 1997, 1998, 1999) contends that cognitive change strategies can be adapted to the developmental levels of very young children. She argues that even preschoolers can benefit from cognitive interventions if they are presented in an age-appropriate way.

POSITIVE SELF-STATEMENTS

Individuals of all ages can be helped to develop adaptive coping self-statements (Kendall, 1993). Turning praise into self-statements is not automatic, and the child must be helped to adapt positive, self-affirming comments.

Children learn the positive value of what they do through specific labeling by significant adults, with positive feedback from those adults. Positive self-statements can teach coping strategies through active control ("I can walk past the dog whenever I feel like it"), reducing aversive feelings ("I will be able to go to school whenever I am ready"), reinforcing statements ("I am brave"), and reality testing ("There really are no monsters in our house") (Schroeder & Gordon, 1991). These are commonly integrated into CBPT. However, such positive self-statements must be adapted to the age of the child. Very young children can be taught clear, self-affirming statements that are linguistically and conceptually simple (e.g., "I am brave," "I can do this"). These statements contain an element of self-reward (e.g., "I am doing a good job"). Positive self-statements can be taught in therapy, but with a young child should be modeled by the therapist and parent alike (Kendall, 1993).

In general, research suggests that cognitive interventions alone do not facilitate mastery over fear, although the combination of cognitive and behavioral interventions appear to help children cope with fearful situations and stimuli (Kendall, 1993; Schroeder & Gordon, 1991; King, Heyne, & Ollendick, 2005). Therefore, CBPT treatment includes numerous behavioral interventions in addition to cognitive restructuring.

EXPOSURE

Exposure, a critical component of CBT, involves graduated, systematic, and controlled confrontation of feared or anxiety-provoking stimuli. Exposure is conducted until habituation occurs (i.e., anxiety subsides or decreases). The technique usually occurs in two phases: (1) preparation (i.e., developing a fear hierarchy and coping skills) and (2) active exposure (i.e., completing anxiety-producing tasks according to the hierarchy). With CBPT, this component is particularly important and helpful with young children, for whom language-based cognitive restructuring is not developmentally appropriate on its own.

This intervention is based on classical conditioning theory, which proposes that the negative association resulted from previous experiences (i.e., specific stimuli repeatedly paired with a set of aversive physiological and cognitive reactions). Thus, avoidance is triggered and leads to impairment in functioning. The goal is to weaken the negative association by repeated exposure to the stimuli while building tolerance (vs. avoidance) of the distress (Davis & Ollendick, 2005).

A recent review of the research indicates that exposure is a well-established intervention, indicating greater effectiveness in reducing anxiety and fear symptoms than no treatment, verbal coping, and participant modeling alone. Both imaginal (i.e., the therapist guides the child through experiencing the object or event visually) and *in vivo* (i.e., the therapist guides the child through directly experiencing the object or event) exposures were shown to be equally efficacious (Davis & Ollendick, 2005). Therefore, it is suggested that a blend of both be used. When setting up *in vivo* exposure paradigms with a CBPT approach, it is important that the therapist has control over the feared stimulus (e.g., a cooperative dentist, an elevator that is not in a busy building and can be held at a floor for brief periods of time).

RELAPSE PREVENTION AND GENERALIZATION

An important goal when treating anxious and fearful children is for them to maintain adaptive behaviors after the treatment has ended, and to generalize these behaviors to the natural environment (Hirschfeld-Becker et al., 2008). Achievement of this goal means that if a child learns to overcome fears and anxieties during treatment, he or she will maintain this new ability after treatment ends, and that more adaptive behavior and thinking will be evident in all settings, not just the psychotherapy setting. Promoting and facilitating generalization should be part of CBPT with young children; it will not necessarily happen without such planning (Meichenbaum, 1977). Generalization can be dealt with through using real-life situations in modeling and role playing, teaching self-management skills, involving significant adults and caregivers in the treatment, and continuing with treatment past the initial acquisition of skills to ensure that adequate learning takes place. Furthermore, in CBPT and based on the theoretical principles of the "inoculation" against failure (Meichenbaum, 1985; Marlatt & Gordon, 1985), the therapist may create play scenarios similar to those the child may face in the future, and include adaptive coping skills and positive behaviors as part of the play.

PARENT INVOLVEMENT

Parents should be actively involved in the treatment of young children because when children are diagnosed with anxiety disorders or phobias, parental anxiety and lack of parental coping skills often maintain the child's symptoms (Hirschfeld-Becker et al., 2008). Parents of children with anxiety disorders are commonly diagnosed with anxiety disorders themselves (Hudson & Rapee, 2001). In addition to genetic factors, anxious parents often have difficulty helping their children manage anxious feelings. They may model maladaptive coping skills, limit their autonomy, express overly protective thoughts, and encourage the child's avoidance of feared situations (Hirschfeld-Becker et al., 2008). When parent work is provided in conjunction with individual work, it may increase the efficacy of anxiety disorder and phobic treatments with young children (Barrett, Dadds, & Rapee, 1996).

With CBPT, parent work is integrated into the assessment phase through clinical interview, behavioral rating scales, and/or behavioral observations at home. After the assessment is completed, a parent meeting is recommended to review the assessment findings and develop a treatment plan. During the intervention phase, parent involvement usually occurs in two parts: (1) psychoeducation and (2) skill building. During psychoeducation, clinicians help parents to understand their child's anxiety symptoms by defining those symptoms. In addition, parents are asked to describe their responses to their child's anxiety and then categorize the behaviors that are helpful and unhelpful.

The skill-building phase includes building parenting skills, with the goal of helping their child manage anxiety independently. Rapee et al. (2008) suggest that parents develop five strategies to accomplish this goal. First, parents are taught to communicate their empathy effectively. They are instructed to label the emotion and validate the experience (e.g., statements such as "Sounds like you are nervous about this visit" and "I can imagine that it is hard for you to face this fear"). A second strategy is teaching parents to reward coping or "brave" behavior. Once the brave behavior is defined, the therapist instructs the parents to provide consistent and meaningful reinforcement, using verbal praise and stickers. In conjunction with the second strategy, the importance of decreasing attention for anxious behaviors (e.g., ignoring whining, tearfulness, tantrums) is explained to parents. In addition, parents are taught to prompt their child to use coping strategies and problem-solving skills, using statements such as "What are some ways in which you can help yourself feel less nervous?" The parents then coach their child to come up with his or her own solutions in the moment. Finally, parents are encouraged to model brave coping behavior for their children. In general, the goals of these five strategies are to help their child (1) independently cope with anxiety or fear and (2) to use adults as a support rather than a crutch.

Parent work should also be extended to interventions involving generalization, primarily through exposure. Parents function as "coaches" at home and outside of session by learning the child's coping strategies and then prompting the application in anxiety-producing situations (Hirschfeld-Becker et al., 2008). It is common for therapists to work with parents to create a fear hierarchy to plan and implement tasks that systematically and gradually increase in anxiety rating.

In addition, therapy should be geared toward helping the parent and child maintain gains and prevent relapse. High-risk situations, which often involve new challenges and transitions, should be identified as they commonly coincide with normal developmental tasks (e.g., starting a new school year) or with the child's life situation (e.g., coping with a divorce). The child and parents should work with the therapist to develop a plan using treatment interventions to manage anxiety in such situations. Furthermore, part of relapse prevention should also include developing a plan on when to seek professional help (Hirschfeld-Becker et al., 2008). More specifically, parents collaborate with the therapist to identify both new symptoms and specific criteria related to intensity and impairment that warrant resuming therapy.

Additional Interventions

In addition to the interventions discussed above, there are other important CBT interventions that can be incorporated into CBPT.

MODELING

Modeling is well researched and used frequently with fearful and anxious children. The intervention is based on social learning theory, which proposes that learning can occur vicariously by observing a model interact with feared stimuli. Children will begin to break the negative association between the stimuli and aversive outcomes. The goals are to decrease avoidance and/or impairment as well as to disconfirm cognitive distortions. When applied to anxiety disorders and phobias through CBPT, modeling can take many forms such as (1) symbolic modeling, whereby the models, often in stories, cope with feared stimuli; and (2) participant modeling, in which the therapist directly interacts with the model guiding the child through steps to overcome fears. Since no direct experience of the aversive outcomes occurs, this intervention may be particularly useful for a child without the requisite skills to deal with his or her fears. Specifically, this is often true for young children for whom approaching tasks, and engaging in exposure or systematic desensitization, may be too difficult. In a systemic review, this intervention was shown to be well established, with studies indicating greater effectiveness than no treatment and systematic desensitization alone (Davis & Ollendick, 2005). In many ways, modeling is one of the most critical components of CBPT, since all interventions can be introduced to the child through modeling by using a wide range of toys, books, and other play materials.

SYSTEMATIC DESENSITIZATION

Systematic desensitization (SD) is the process of reducing anxiety or fear by replacing a maladaptive response with an adaptive one (Wolpe, 1958, 1982). Using classical conditioning theory, the emphasis is on breaking the association between a particular stimulus and the anxiety or fear response that it usually elicits. The stimulus is presented, but the anxiety is inhibited or prevented from occurring. SD involves a person experiencing a hierarchy of anxiety-provoking scenes, either *in vivo* or imaginal, in combination with these incompatible responses.

Relaxation is the most common incompatible response, and children over the age of 6 years can be taught modified relaxation techniques (Cautela & Groden, 1978; Davis & Ollendick, 2005), although some children may find other techniques more useful, such as calming play activities or visualization of calming scenes. Schroeder and Gordon (1991) even suggest the use of laughter, giving the example of a child imagining a feared monster dressed in red flannel underwear.

SD is a useful intervention with anxious and fearful children, especially when high levels of physiological reactivity (e.g., racing heart) and extreme avoidance are exhibited (King et al., 1988). In a systemic review, this intervention is considered probably efficacious, which means it is more effective when compared to either no treatment or relaxation alone but less effective than other interventions such as participant modeling (Davis & Ollendick, 2005). Thus, SD is likely to be more effective when implemented in conjunction with other interventions.

CONTINGENCY MANAGEMENT

Contingency management is a general term that refers to techniques that modify a behavior by controlling its consequences. Management programs can be set up within the play therapy sessions or in the natural environment. Positive reinforcement, shaping, stimulus fading, extinction, and differential reinforcement of other behavior (DRO) are all forms of contingency management, with the first two being the most commonly used in CBPT.

POSITIVE REINFORCEMENT

Positive reinforcement is an important component of almost every treatment for childhood anxieties and fears (Rapee et al., 2008). It is used by specifying a target behavior, determining a reinforcer, and making the reinforcement contingent on the occurrence of the target behavior. It often involves social reinforcers (e.g., praise) or material reinforcers (e.g., stickers), and can be direct (e.g., praising a child with separation anxiety for venturing off to school without Mom) or more subtle (e.g., reinforcing independent play, which can ultimately lead to greater confidence in the ability to be away from a parent figure). Reinforcement can come from the therapist as well as the parents and significant others, who have been trained by the therapist to use appropriate reinforcement as the child conquers his or her fears.

For many children and especially with young children, chart systems that specify the desired behavior and reward can be extremely useful as part of CBPT. Chart systems can help operationalize the target behavior and ensure that the reinforcements are given in a systematic, immediate way. For example, a girl fearful of sleeping in her own room can have a chart specifying that she will receive a sticker for going to bed within a certain time after being asked, staying in her room without constantly complaining, and staying in her bed all night. Such reinforcement also helps the child see that she can master the feared situation.

SHAPING

Shaping is a way of helping a child get progressively closer to a targeted goal. The child is given positive reinforcement for closer and closer approximations to the desired response. Eventually, the child reaches the desired behavior. One does not expect a fearful child to overcome his or her fears at once. Thus, a young boy who sleeps with his parents because he is fearful of sleeping in his own room could be shaped by providing reinforcement of his efforts in small steps (e.g., sleeping on the floor next to his parents' bed; sleeping on the floor in the hall toward his own room; sleeping on the floor in his room; sleeping in his own bed).

STIMULUS FADING, EXTINCTION, AND DIFFERENTIAL REINFORCEMENT OF OTHER BEHAVIOR

Stimulus fading is a technique designed to change behaviors by modifying their situational cues. A child may have some skills for the adaptive response, but may exhibit the behavior only in specific circumstances or with specific people (i.e., situational cues). The therapist helps the child to use positive skills in one setting, and then helps the child transfer the skills to other situations. In addition, extinction is a technique used to gradually eliminate anxiety and fear responses by eliminating reinforcing variables. With young children, parental attention is a common reinforcing variable. Anxiety and fear responses can be diminished by withholding parent reinforcement for a particular maladaptive behavior. Because extinction does not teach new behaviors, it is frequently used in conjunction with differential reinforcement of other behavior (DRO). With DRO, the parent instead reinforces the child for learning and applying adaptive behaviors that are often incompatible with the maladaptive behavior that had previously been reinforced. For example, if a child is exhibiting both brave and fearful behavior (e.g., saying she thinks that she can go in to school, while tugging on the parent to keep from entering the building), the parent should reinforce the brave, adaptive behavior, rather than focusing on the fearful behavior.

SELF-CONTROL

Self-control is really not an intervention per se. Rather, it is a strategy geared toward teaching an individual to use new behaviors and ways of thinking that enhance the person's sense of control (Kendall, 1993). Through cognitive self-control programs, children are taught to monitor, evaluate, and reinforce themselves for using more adaptive coping skills. Through self-control training and techniques such as utilization of the STOP acronym (Scared, fearful Thoughts, Other thoughts [coping], Praise), fearful children can be taught to regulate their own behavior (Eisen & Kearney, 1995). Evidence suggests that a child's control over his or her own behavior may be more efficient and more durable than interventions initiated by significant others on behalf of the child (Kendall, 1993).

BIBLIOTHERAPY

Bibliotherapy refers to the use of therapeutic books for psychoeducation and skill building, and is used increasingly as an adjunct to therapy. Recent research has shown that bibliotherapy alone can reduce anxiety symptoms but appears to be more effective when supplemented with other techniques (Silverman et al., 2008). The focus of using self-help books with children is somewhat different than with adults. Most therapeutic books for children provide a story with a child (model) who copes with a situation similar to the one the child may be facing. Such stories may model a child's reaction to a particular situation, with the hope that the listener will incorporate some of the ideas presented into his or her own approach to the problem.

At times, published materials may not be available or appropriate, and in these cases it may be desirable to create books specifically for a particular child. Often, when creating the book during treatment sessions, the therapist can model problem solving and developing positive self-statements for and with the child. The advantages of working on the book together with the child are numerous. First and foremost, through such collaboration the child becomes a more active participant in change than if a previously published or therapist-written book is brought to the therapy session. As the child actively participates in the creation of the book, it is possible to incorporate spontaneous material brought to treatment by the child. Further, as the book is written, the child is given additional practice opportunities to apply interventions such as cognitive change strategies. That is, if the child voices maladaptive thoughts, the child and the therapist can collaboratively work on more adaptive, positive self-statements to include in the book.

SETTING/MATERIALS

CBPT is usually conducted in a playroom with a wide array of play materials available. A typical play therapy room is well stocked with toys, art supplies, puppets, dolls, and other materials. The more directive and goal-oriented techniques of CBPT may require certain materials to meet the needs of a child's specific problems. Sometimes it is not necessary to buy toys for specific situations because of the child's ability to be creative and flexible with existing toys. For example, a child fearful of sitting on the toilet may be able to play with a doll on a plastic bowl that resembles a toilet. However, the child may not be able to "pretend" in this way and may have an easier time using a specifically designed dolls' play toilet.

The fearful or anxious child may need to be treated *in vivo*, in a real-life setting, rather than in a playroom. Thus, the child fearful of elevators may need to be seen in and around an elevator, the child with school refusal may need to be treated at or around the school, and a child afraid of dogs may need to be seen in a setting where dogs are allowed. Children with social anxiety may have to be treated in group situations with other children; those with separation anxiety may be better treated in situations where they can separate from a parent gradually.

Stages of Treatment

CBPT takes place as the child moves through several treatment stages, which have been described as the introductory/orientation, assessment, middle, and termination stages. After preparation for CBPT, the assessment begins. During the middle stage of CBPT, the therapist has developed a treatment plan, and the therapy is turning to focus on increasing the child's self-control, sense of accomplishment, and learning more adaptive responses to deal with specific situations. For fearful and anxious children, this will incorporate a wide array of cognitive and behavioral interventions specifically geared to helping the child with his or her specific concerns. Generalization and relapse prevention are incorporated into the middle stages, so that the child can learn to utilize new skills across a broad range of settings and begin to develop skills that will diminish the chance of setbacks after therapy is completed. During the termination phase, the child and family are prepared for the end of therapy (see Knell, 1999, for further description of these stages in CBPT).

CASE ILLUSTRATION

The case of Henry, a 4-year-old boy, illustrates the use of CBPT to treat social anxiety disorder. Henry presented with intense anxiety in new, unfamiliar social situations. These situations included playdates, birthday parties, and extracurricular activities (e.g., swim lessons, baseball). Prior to attending any of these events, Henry often said he did not want to go and would cry and throw tantrums. When his parents pushed him to attend social situations, Henry became avoidant by clinging to them and refusing to interact with others. If his comfort increased with time, he left his parents' side but was quiet and stood at a distance from other children. Henry attended a preschool in an urban area where he was well liked and accepted by children his own age, resulting in invitations to many social events. These symptoms started at age 3, so that the activities that he attended and participated in had gradually decreased in the past year. The social anxiety was starting to limit his social world.

For assessment, a clinical interview with parent, behavioral observation, and behavior rating scale were used. Based on the clinical interview with the mother, a full understanding of the social anxiety symptoms described above was obtained. Mother denied symptoms of other anxiety disorders. Henry's medical history was unremarkable and major developmental milestones were achieved within normal limits. Mother reported that parents responded inconsistently to Henry's anxiety and avoidance of social situations. At times, parents were empathic to his feelings and at other times expressed frustration and anger. Similarly, his parents pushed Henry to participate in some instances and allowed him to avoid others.

As a supplement to the clinical interview, the Spence Preschool Anxiety Rating scale—Parent Report was obtained. His mother's pretreatment ratings indicated clinical levels of overall anxiety (i.e., total score of 17 with clinical level cutoff of 14.12). Behavioral observations were also consistent with other assessment measures. Henry seemed anxious and was reluctant to engage during the initial session. When meeting the therapist, Henry was able to introduce himself and shake hands only after being prompted by his mother. But then he requested that his mother respond to the therapist's questions after he whispered the responses in his mother's ear. He was able to separate from Mom and accompany the therapist to the play therapy room where he was shown all the materials. Henry immediately selected animals, but deferred to the therapist to introduce and have the animals talk. He appeared fidgety and responded to questions with one word or short phrases.

Interventions of somatic management, cognitive restructuring, positive self-statements, exposure, modeling, and shaping were implemented to lessen anxiety symptoms and to increase social interactions. All interventions were done within the play therapy room. Materials primarily included several animal puppets that were named by the therapist given Henry's reluctance to engage. The dog puppet, "Buddy," was introduced as the character that worries about meeting new people. Other materials were used such as poster board, markers, balls, and props representing specific themes as needed (i.e., chair as treehouse).

To prepare for development of CBT skills, psychoeducation on emotions was the first intervention. Henry had difficulties acknowledging and identifying his anxiety. Therefore, emotions were introduced (1) as internal experiences that involve body sensations and thoughts and (2) as common experiences for everyone. Puppets took turns discussing different emotions by describing what they felt in their body and what they thought. In addition, YouTube clips from Henry's favorite cartoon were selected based on the main character reporting or expressing anxiety. Using the animals and the cartoon characters, body sensations and thoughts were identified, discussed, and normalized as part of his anxiety.

After these sessions, Henry was able to discuss his emotions and anxiety specifically. However, given his developmental level, anxiety was referred to as "worry" throughout treatment. He identified his worry as consisting of heart racing, stomach butterflies, and shaky legs. He was unable to identify anxiety-related thoughts common for preschool-age children, but acknowledged his maladaptive thoughts related to "Something bad will happen." To implement CBPT for emotional education, modeling interventions were used. Buddy, the dog puppet, was identified as having "worries about making friends and being in new situations."

Somatic management/relaxation was introduced. Henry learned body breathing with Buddy and other animals. Next, self-control was integrated into play as distraction, which is a strategy that uses a new behavior to increase control over anxiety. In play, Henry identified that Buddy played soccer and flew a plane to take his mind off his worries. He was able to demonstrate and to play out distraction with the other animals. Henry came up with squeezing a ball as an activity to distract him from the body sensations related to his worry outside of session.

Once relaxation and distraction were practiced for 1 week at home, cognitive restructuring was started. First, Henry was taught the concept that changing negative thoughts to more positive realistic thoughts lessens anxiety. Labels of "worry thoughts" and "calm thoughts" were used. Different play situations were created (e.g., treehouse, soccer game, pool party) and the therapist identified both types of thoughts using the animals' verbalizations. Shaping was used as Henry, over three sessions, was gradually asked to identify a worry thought and then a calm thought. Henry was able to identify calm thoughts that he practiced repeating at home. Examples included "Worry is just a feeling in my body" and "I am strong and can fight worry." We selected one calm thought as Henry's main positive self-statement, which was "I do things to make worry go away."

After Henry showed understanding and mastery of the strategies, exposure was initiated in two parts. First, Henry was asked to meet other children or to do new, unfamiliar activities. Prior to practicing at home, Henry played different scenarios with Buddy and different animals. For example, Henry brought in his favorite animal from home (Max) and practiced introducing him to Buddy and his playgroup. SD was incorporated into play and as part of exposure as the "calm-down plan." It was created as the adaptive response to replace avoidance with steps of (1) three deep breaths, (2) calm thought of "I do things to make worry go away," and (3) do something fun and distracting like squeeze ball. When Henry appeared confident and comfortable with play situations about social situations, the expectation was moved to summer activities outside of the therapy room.

The second part of exposure was meeting new adults in session. Initially, Henry was asked to practice in play with Buddy completing the task first. In addition to the calm-down plan, Henry was taught three adaptive skills for introductions to replace avoidance or withdrawal (i.e., getting quiet and withdrawn), which involved looking a person in the eye, shaking hands, and saying "Nice to meet you." Again, when he displayed mastery in play, Henry was asked to practice meeting new adults in natural settings such as the wait staff, school security guard, and parents at play or sports settings.

Parent involvement supplemented the individual session with Henry. All parent sessions were done either before Henry's session or by phone. Psychoeducation was provided related to the diagnosis. Mother was taught the CBT model (i.e., connection between events, thoughts, emotion [anxiety], and behavior) as well as about social anxiety disorder symptoms. Specifically, Mom was helped to understand that the diagnosis involves core fears about performance and about rejection from others. This resulted in distress and avoidance in unfamiliar social situations. Therefore, Henry tended to seek approval from others, which likely lead to his reluctance to share experiences that made him seem inadequate.

Mother was also integrated into Henry's practice of skills outside of session. For example, related to emotions, Mom was asked to help Henry identify body sensations and thoughts when he was anxious and to discuss her own anxiety as well (i.e., modeling acceptance of anxiety). For relaxation and the calm-down plan, Mother was taught deep breathing and asked to practice each night at home to build skills. During the exposure intervention, Mother remained in the play therapy room when Henry met new adults. The therapist modeled positive reinforcement and shaping to replace Mom's increased attention for avoidant behavior (i.e., DRO).

Henry was prepared for termination by being told therapy was ending because he did a great job and learned to manage his worry. The final session focused on relapse prevention. He was asked to create a book summarizing treatment into three corresponding chapters. The first chapter emphasized emotional identification of worry (e.g., body sensations, thoughts, behaviors). The second chapter described worry management strategies (i.e., calm-down plan). The last chapter listed all the exposure tasks that Henry completed in and outside of session. The purpose was to remind him that "doing" tasks helped him to feel a sense of control and mastery over worry.

The course of treatment was 14 individual sessions, three parent sessions via phone for psychoeducation and skill building, and one session including Mom for coaching on the exposure task. Improvements in social functioning were noted. In addition, Henry's play ability within sessions also improved, showing more organization and structure around complex themes. For example, when playing that animals were going to the park, Henry built slides out of markers and boats, made from paper, to float on a lake. This represents that Henry was better able to participate in play without fear of evaluation or rejection.

Mother's posttreatment ratings on the Spence Preschool Anxiety Rating Scale—Parent Report indicated normal levels of overall anxiety (i.e., total score of 12 with clinical-level cutoff of 14.12) as compared with clinical level score at pretreatment (i.e., total score of 17). This rating matched mother's verbal report of decreased anxiety and increased approach behavior (vs. avoidance) in social situations. Henry was social at camp and during summer activities. He expressed interest in going to social events and, prior to arriving, used the calm-down plan. He was able to greet and then play with other children when at events.

SUMMARY AND CONCLUSIONS

Anxiety disorders and phobias are among the most commonly occurring psychiatric disorders in childhood, with preschool children demonstrating similar prevalence rates as school-age children and adolescents. The cognitive behavioral model is the most widely accepted model for understanding and treating these disorders. According to the DSM-5, generalized anxiety disorder, social anxiety disorder, separation anxiety disorder, and specific phobia are categorized under anxiety disorders and are typically the focus of CBT. Since many children experience developmentally appropriate anxiety and fear, it is important to distinguish between normal and clinical anxiety. The dimensions of intensity and avoidance can help guide these decisions. Clinical assessment of anxiety and phobias is further used to understand the child, to diagnose disorders, and to individualize treatment. Assessment typically involves a combination of clinical interview, behavior rating scales, behavioral observation, play assessment, and parent monitoring forms.

CBT is a well-established treatment for anxiety disorders and phobias in childhood populations; thus, the foundations of cognitive behavioral play therapy (CBPT) were developed by adapting empirically supported techniques for use with younger children in a play setting. CBPT is designed specifically for preschool and early elementary school-age children (i.e., ages 3–6) and emphasizes the child's involvement in therapy by including the child as an active participant in the change process. CBT interventions are incorporated into play in order to make them most accessible to the child.

Six critical interventions have been identified. They include psychoeducation, somatic management, cognitive restructuring, exposure, response prevention and generalization, and parent involvement. Other intrventions, such as modeling and bibliotherapy, can be incorporated into the therapy. Recent literature suggests treatment should be implemented in two phases: (1) skill building (psychoeducation, somatic management, and cognitive restructuring) and (2) exposure, with the emphasis being to move quickly through phase one and to focus on phase two (Kendall et al., 2006).

With CBPT, a significant component of overcoming fear and anxiety appears to be the child's gaining control and mastery over negative emotions. Developing this sense of control may mean that the child learns to deal with the feared stimuli, to manage feelings associated with the fear, or to learn specific coping skills to deal with the fear. CBPT provides such learning opportunities within play, as well as the specific skills necessary to overcome fears and anxieties. By "pretending" and practicing, a child may overcome the feared stimulus and anxiety-provoking situations.

REFERENCES

Albano, A. M., Chorpita, B. F., & Barlow, D. H. (2003). Childhood anxiety disorders. In E. J. Mash & R. A. Barkley (Eds.), *Child psychopathology* (2nd ed., pp. 279–329). New York: Guilford Press.

Albano, A. M., & Kendall, P. C. (2002). Cognitive behavioral therapy for children and adolescents with anxiety disorders: Clinical research advances. *International Review of Psychiatry, 14,* 128–133.

American Psychiatric Association. (2013). *Diagnostic and statistical manual of mental disorders* (5th ed.). Arlington, VA: Author.

Barrett, P. M., Dadds, M. R., & Rapee, R. M. (1996). Family treatment of childhood anxiety: A controlled trial. *Journal of Consulting and Clinical Psychology, 64,* 333–342.

Beck, A. T. (1967). *Depression: Clinical, experimental, and theoretical aspects.* New York: Harper & Row.

Beck, A. T. (1972). *Depression: Causes and treatment.* Philadelphia: University of Pennsylvania Press.

Beck, A. T. (1976). *Cognitive therapy and the emotional disorders.* New York: International Universities Press.

Beesdo, K., Knapp, S., & Pine, D. S. (2009). Anxiety and anxiety disorders in children and adolescents: Developmental issues and implications for DSM-V. *Psychiatric Clinics of North America, 32,* 483–524.

Birmaher, B., Khertarpal, S., Brent, D., Cully, M., Balach, L., Kaufman, J., et al. (1997). The Screen for Child Anxiety Related Emotional Disorder (SCARED): Scale construction and psychometric characteristics. *Journal of the American Academy of Child and Adolescent Psychiatry, 36,* 545–553.

Bratton, S., & Ray, D. (2000). What the research shows about play therapy. *International Journal of Play Therapy, 9*(1), 47–88.

Bratton, S. C., Ray, D., Rhine, T., & Jones, L. (2005). The efficacy of play therapy with children: A meta-analytic review of treatment outcomes. *Professional Psychology: Research and Practice, 36,* 376–390.

Cautela, J. R., & Groden, J. (1978). *Relaxation: A comprehensive manual for adults, children, and children with special needs.* Champaign, IL: Research Press.

Cavett, A. M., & Drewes, A. A. (2012). Play applications of trauma-specific TF-CBT components for young children. In J. A. Cohen, A. P. Mannarino, & E. Deblinger (Eds.), *Trauma-focused CBT for children and adolescents: Treatment applications* (pp. 124–148). New York: Guilford Press.

Chorpita, B. F., Tracey, S. A., Brown, T. A., Collica, T. J., & Barlow, D. H. (1997). Assessment of worry in children and adolescents: An adaption of the Penn State Worry Questionnaire. *Behaviour Research and Therapy, 35,* 569–581.

Cohen, J. A., Mannarino, A. P., Berliner, L., & Deblinger, E. (2000). Trauma-focused cognitive behavioral therapy for children and adolescents: An empirical update. *Journal of Interpersonal Violence, 15,* 1202–1223.

Costello, E. J., Mustillo, S., Erkanli, A., Keeler, G., & Angold, A. (2003). Prevalence and development of psychiatric disorders in childhood and adolescence. *Archives of General Psychiatry, 60,* 837–844.

Davis, T. E., & Ollendick, T. H. (2005). Empirically-supported treatment for specific phobia in children: Do efficacious treatments address the components of a phobic response? *Clinical Psychology: Science and Practice, 12,* 144–160.

DiNardo, P. A., O'Brien, G. T., Barlow, D. H., Waddell, M. T., & Blanchard, E. B. (1983). Reliability of DSM anxiety disorders categories using a structured interview. *Archives of General Psychiatry, 35,* 837–844.

Egger, H. L., & Angold, A. (2006). Common emotional and behavioral disorders in preschool children: Presentation, nosology, and epidemiology. *Journal of Child Psychology and Psychiatry, 47,* 313–337.

Eisen, A. R., & Kearney, C. (1995). *Practitioners guide to treating fear and anxiety in children and adolescents.* Northvale, NJ: Jason Aronson.

Emery, G., Bedrosian, R., & Garber, J. (1983). Cognitive therapy with depressed children and adolescents. In D. P. Cantwell & G. A. Carlson (Eds.), *Affective disorders in childhood and adolescence: An update* (pp. 445–471). New York: Spectrum.

Hirschfeld-Becker, D. R., Masek, B., Henin, A., Blakely, L. R., Rettew, D. C., Dufton, L., et al. (2008). Cognitive-behavioral intervention with young anxious children. *Harvard Review of Psychiatry, 16,* 113–125.

Hirshfeld-Becker, D. R., Masek, B., Henin, B. A., Blakely, L. R., Pollock-Wurman, R.

A., McQuade, J., et al. (2010). Cognitive behavioral therapy for 4- to 7-year-old children with anxiety disorders: A randomized clinical trial. *Journal of Consulting and Clinical Psychology, 78,* 498–510.

Hudson, J. L., & Rapee, R. M. (2001). Parent–child interactions and anxiety disorders: An observational study. *Behavioral Research Therapy, 39,* 109–124.

Kaugars, A. S. (2011). Assessment of pretend play. In S. W. Russ & L. N. Niec (Eds.), *Play in clinical practice: Evidence-based approaches* (pp. 51–82). New York: Guilford Press.

Kendall, P. C. (1993). Cognitive behavioral therapies with youth: Guiding theory, current status, and emerging developments. *Journal of Consulting and Clinical Psychology, 61,* 235–247.

Kendall, P. C., & Hedtke, K. A. (2006). *Cognitive-behavioral therapy for anxious children: Therapist manual.* Ardmore, PA: Workbook.

Kendall, P. C., Robin, J. A., Hedtke, K. A., Suveg, C., Flannery-Schroeder, E., & Gosch, E. (2006). Considering CBT with anxious youth?: Think exposures. *Cognitive and Behavioral Practice, 12*(1), 136–148.

King, N. J., Hamilton, D. H., & Ollendick, T. H. (1988). *Children's phobias: A behavioral perspective.* New York: Wiley.

King, N. J., Heyne, D., & Ollendick, T. H. (2005). Cognitive-behavioral treatments for anxiety and phobic disorders in children and adolescents: A review. *Behavioral Disorders, 30*(3), 241–257.

Klein, R. G., & Pine, D. S. (2002). Anxiety disorders. In M. Rutter & E. Taylor (Eds.), *Child and adolescent psychiatry* (4th ed., pp. 486–509). Oxford, UK: Blackwell.

Knell, S. M. (1993a). *Cognitive-behavioral play therapy.* Northvale, NJ: Jason Aronson.

Knell, S. M. (1993b). To show and not tell: Cognitive-behavioral play therapy in the treatment of elective mutism. In T. Kottman & C. Schaefer (Eds.), *Play therapy in action: A casebook for practitioners* (pp. 169–208). Northvale, NJ: Jason Aronson.

Knell, S. M. (1994). Cognitive-behavioral play therapy. In K. O'Connor & C. Schaefer (Eds.), *Handbook of play therapy: Vol. 2. Advances and innovations* (pp. 111–142). New York: Wiley.

Knell, S. M. (1997). Cognitive-behavioral play therapy. In K. O'Connor & L. Mages (Eds.), *Play therapy theory and practice: A comparative presentation* (pp. 79–99). New York: Wiley.

Knell, S. M. (1998). Cognitive-behavioral play therapy. *Journal of Clinical Child Psychology, 27,* 28–33.

Knell, S. M. (1999). Cognitive behavioral play therapy. In S. W. Russ & T. Ollendick (Eds.), *Handbook of psychotherapies with children and families* (pp. 385–404). New York: Plenum Press.

Knell, S. M. (2009). Cognitive-behavioral play therapy: Theory and applications. In A. A. Drewes (Ed.), *Blending play therapy with cognitive behavioral therapy* (pp. 117–133). Hoboken, NJ: Wiley.

Knell, S. M., & Dasari, M. (2006). Cognitive-behavioral play therapy for children with anxiety and phobias. In H. G. Kaduson & C. E. Schaefer (Eds.), *Short-term play therapy for children* (2nd ed., pp. 22–50). New York: Guilford Press.

Knell, S. M., & Dasari, M. (2009). CBPT: Implementing and integrating CBPT into clinical practice. In A. A. Drewes (Ed.), *Blending play therapy with cognitive behavioral therapy* (pp. 321–352). Hoboken, NJ: Wiley.

Knell, S. M., & Dasari, M. (2011). Cognitive-behavioral play therapy. In S. W. Russ & L. N Niec (Eds.), *Play in clinical practice: Evidence-based approaches* (pp. 236–263). New York: Guilford Press.

Knell, S. M., & Moore, D. J. (1990). Cognitive-behavioral play therapy in the treatment of encopresis. *Journal of Clinical Child Psychology, 19,* 55–60.

Knell, S. M., & Ruma, C. D. (1996). Play therapy with a sexually abused child. In M. Reinecke, F. M. Dattilio, & A. Freeman (Eds.), *Casebook of cognitive-behavior therapy with children and adolescents.* (pp. 367–393). New York: Guilford Press.

Lang, P. J. (1979). A bio-informational theory of emotional imagery. *Psychophysiology, 16,* 495–512.

Lavigne, J. V., LeBailly, S. A., Hopkins, J., Gouze, K. R., & Binns, H. J. (2009). The prevalence of ADHD, ODD, depression, and anxiety in a community sample of 4–year-olds. *Journal of Clinical Child and Adolescent Psychology, 38*(3), 315–328.

LeBlanc, M., & Ritchie, M. (2001). A meta-analysis of play therapy outcomes. *Counseling Psychology Quarterly, 14,* 149–163.

Liebowitz, M. R. (1987). Social phobia. *Modern Problems in Pharmacopsychiatry, 22,* 141–173.

March, J. S., Parker, J. D., Sullivan, K., Stallings, P., & Conners, C. (1997). The Multidimensional Anxiety Scale for Children: Factor structure, reliability, and validity. *Journal of the American Academy of Child and Adolescent Psychiatry, 36,* 554–565.

Marlatt, G. A., & Gordon, J. R. (1985). *Relapse prevention: Maintenance strategies in the treatment of addictive behaviors.* New York: Guilford Press.

Meichenbaum, D. (1977). *Cognitive-behavior modification: An integrative approach.* New York: Plenum Press.

Meichenbaum, D. (1985). *Stress inoculation training.* New York: Pergamon Press.

Muris, P., Merckelbach, H., Gadet, B., & Moulaert, V. (2000). Fears, worries, and scary dreams in 4- to 12-year-old children: Their content, developmental pattern, and origins. *Journal of Clinical Child Psychology, 29,* 43–52.

Ollendick, T. H. (1983). Reliability and validity of the Revised Fear Survey Schedule for Children (FSSC-R). *Behaviour Research and Therapy, 21,* 685–692.

Pearson, B. (2007). *Effects of a cognitive behavioral play intervention on children's hope and school adjustment.* Unpublished doctoral dissertation, Case Western Reserve University.

Pincus, D. B. (2012). *Growing up brave: Expert strategies for helping your child overcome fear, stress, and anxiety.* New York: Little, Brown.

Rapee, R., Wignall, A., Spence, S., Lyneham, H., & Cobham, V. (2008). *Helping your anxious child: A step-by-step guide for parents.* Oakland, CA: New Harbinger.

Reynolds, S., Wilson, C., Austin, J., & Hooper, L. (2012). Effects of psychotherapy for children and adolescents: A meta-analytic review. *Clinical Psychology Review, 32,* 251–262.

Russ, S. W. (2004). *Play in child development and psychotherapy: Toward empirically supported practice.* Mahwah, NJ: Erlbaum.

Russ, S. W., Fiorelli, J., & Spannagel, S. C. (2011). Cognitive and affective processes in play. In S. W. Russ & L. N. Niec (Eds.), *Play in clinical practice: Evidence-based approaches* (pp. 3–22). New York: Guilford Press.

Scheeringa, M. S., Weems, C. F., Cohen, J. A., Amaya-Jackson, L., & Guthrie, D. (2011). Trauma-focused cognitive-behavioral therapy for posttraumatic stress disorder in three- through six-year-old children: A randomized clinical trial. *Journal of Child Psychology and Psychiatry, 52*(8), 853–860.

Schroeder, C. S., & Gordon, B. N. (1991). *Assessment and treatment of childhood problems.* New York: Guilford Press.

Silverman, W. K., Pina, A. A., & Viswesvaran, C. (2008). Evidence-based psychosocial treatments for phobic and anxiety disorders in children and adolescents. *Journal of Clinical Child and Adolescent Psychology, 37,* 105–130.

Spence, S. H., Rapee, R., McDonald, C., & Ingram, M. (2001). The structure of anxiety symptoms among preschoolers. *Behaviour Research and Therapy, 39,* 1293–1316.

Velting, O. N., Setzer, N. J., & Albano, A. M. (2004). Update on and advances in assessment and cognitive-behavioral treatment of anxiety disorders in children and adolescents. *Professional Psychology: Research and Practice, 35,* 42–54.

Weissman M. M. (1999). Children with pubertal-onset depressive disorder and anxiety grown up. *Archives of General Psychiatry, 56,* 794–801.

Williams, M. L. (1996). *Cool cats, calm kids: Relaxation and stress management for young people.* San Luis Obispo, CA: Impact.

Wolpe, J. (1958). *Psychotherapy by reciprocal inhibition.* Stanford, CA: Stanford University Press.

Wolpe, J. (1982). *The practice of behavior therapy* (3rd ed.). Oxford, UK: Pergamon Press.

Chapter 3

৵

Theraplay®

The Use of Structured Play to Enhance Attachment in Children

Evangeline Munns

*T*heraplay is an attachment-based model of play therapy that is characterized by playful, joyous interactions between parents and their child. In our achievement-driven world, it is refreshing to find a treatment method that puts fun and laughter back into family life. As Panksepp (2006) advocates, we need to stimulate the "joy juice" in our brains. An atmosphere is created that emphasizes the positive strengths of both child and parent. This helps the family to anticipate each session and produces comments such as an adolescent's "I never want this to end" and from a father who participated in a father–son group Theraplay program, "This is the most precious time in the week for me and my son."

HISTORY

Dr. Ann Jernberg, founder of Theraplay, and cofounder, Phyllis Booth, were strongly influenced by Austin des Laurier, who was treating schizophrenic children and those on the autism spectrum with a treatment method that was highly unusual at the time. It was nonverbal, physical, and action-oriented. des Laurier ignored the bizarre behavior of his clients and instead focused on their strengths. Dr. Jernberg adopted his method and called it

Theraplay (Booth & Jernberg, 2010; Munns, 2000). Dr. Jernberg was given a federal grant to apply her model to Head Start mothers and their children in Chicago, with a mandate to increase their attachment with each other. The program was successful, and since then it has grown in popularity around the world.

I was trained by Drs. Jernberg and Booth, and in the early 1980s I helped to make Theraplay known across Canada, the United States, and now internationally. Likewise, Ulrike Franke started Theraplay in Germany and Dr. Juka Makela initiated Theraplay in Finland, where Theraplay has a strong presence today. Both of these countries have produced a number of research studies on Theraplay (Munns, 2009). Today, Theraplay is practiced in 44 countries. Its international headquarters are located in Chicago at The Theraplay Institute.

THEORY AND PRACTICE

Theraplay is a short-term, cost-effective, structured treatment method based on attachment theory with its belief that the first relationship a child forms with its chief caregiver is the most important one of all because it forms a template for later relationships (Bowlby, 1988). Theraplay tries to replicate normal parent–child relationships. This includes meeting the child at its emotional age, and going back to where the parent–child attachment was disrupted or never formed in the first place. The therapist tries to give the child positive experiences that were missed earlier in his or her life. This means that in Theraplay the child might participate at first in activities geared for a young child. As treatment progresses, more activities are geared to the child's chronological age.

Theraplay's prime goals are to enhance the attachment between parents and child, to increase trust, self-confidence, and self-regulation. Therapists first model interactions between child and adult while parents observe for several sessions, and then participate directly with their child under the guidance of the therapist. Helping parents become more empathically attuned and responsive to their child's cues and needs is an important objective. This includes strengthening their responses appropriately to their child's arousal level: to calm and soothe the child when he or she is distressed, but also be able to share the fun and laughter in enjoyable moments without overwhelming the child. This is key in helping the child move toward self-regulation.

Theraplay is nonverbal: interpretations are not made and probing questions are not asked, although reflections of the child's feelings are sometimes given. Due to its similarity with the goals of the nondirective model of play therapy, experienced clinicians are able to combine Theraplay and

Filial play therapy (Munns, 2013). However, in Theraplay, no toys are used. The emphasis is placed on playful interactions characterized by physical contact and fun between the child, parents, and therapist. As well, these interactions are guided by the cultural traditions of families coming from a diversity of backgrounds and ethnic groups and therefore are sometimes modified accordingly (Atkinson, 2009; Perry & Sutherland, 2009).

APPROPRIATE CLIENTS

Clients appropriate for Theraplay span the whole age range—infants, preschoolers, latency-age children, adolescents, adults, and the elderly (Munns, 2000, 2008, 2009, 2011a). Theraplay is also applicable to a broad spectrum of internalizing and externalizing emotional, behavioral, and social difficulties; from the withdrawn, timid, depressed child to the acting-out aggressive, deregulated child (Booth, Lindaman, & Winstead, 2014; DiPasquale, 2009; Eyeles, Boada, & Munns, 2009). It is especially appropriate for adoptive children, foster children, stepchildren, and those on the autism spectrum. It is less appropriate for children who have recently lost a loved one and are still grieving or for those very recently traumatized where Theraplay, if used, needs to be modified (Rubin, Lender, & Mroz, 2009).

MAIN DIMENSIONS OF THERAPLAY

Dr. Jernberg made hundreds of observations of interactions between normal children and their parents. She categorized her observations under four main dimensions that form the underlying principles of Theraplay and guide every activity (Booth & Jernberg, 2010).

Structure

Every child needs some structure where the adult is in charge to provide a sense of safety, security, regulation, and predictability. Children usually have regular, structured routines for sleeping, waking, eating, bathing, and so on. In Theraplay the adult leads the activities according to a preplanned agenda that reflects the family's needs. Each session has a definite beginning and end (i.e., entrance, welcome song, checkup at the beginning and at the end, a goodbye song). There are some activities that are included in every session like powdering or lotioning of hurts and feeding.

Even the most resistant child is usually cooperative with the directions from an adult when they are incorporated into following the rules of a game. For example, stopping on the command of "red light" and moving to "green light" is inherent in the game of "Red Light/Green Light" or responding to the rules of other well-known games such as "Simon Says" or "Mother, May I?," where the adult gives directions to the child. In these games the child is learning to cooperate with the adult and to have fun doing it.

Structure is emphasized for resistant children such as those who are impulsive, aggressive, behavior-disordered, conduct-disordered, and/or deregulated.

Engagement

Ordinarily parents engage their children in hundreds of delightful ways such as the "peek-a boo" or "hide-and-seek" games of early childhood that bring pleasure to all involved. Engagement builds connections between family members and helps the child to learn about his or her body image and boundaries. In this process, the child learns that he or she can be a source of delight to his or her parents.

In Theraplay, the therapist engages the child as soon as he or she greets him or her in the waiting room—"Johnny, I have been waiting all day to see you!" An entrance such as "follow-the leader" or "stepping stones" brings the child into the center or corner of the room where everyone can sit comfortably on pillows or beanbag chairs. A welcome song is sung during which everyone holds hands and each member's name is included. Transitions between activities are kept short so the child's attention does not have much time to wander. The aim is to keep the child fully engaged throughout the session.

This dimension is particularly needed with withdrawn, depressed, or fearful children, or with those on the autism spectrum.

Nurture

Nurture is needed by all children in order to thrive (Ford, 1993; Gerhardt, 2004). Parents ordinarily express their love through their constant caring and nurturing of their child, leaving the child with a sense that he or she is valued, important, accepted, and loved. Growing within such an atmosphere is conducive to shaping the child's inner self-image or "inner working model" to be a positive one (Bowlby, 1988). Nurturing is expressed through fulfilling the child's basic needs such as feeding, caring for hurts, cradling and rocking, soothing when the child is distressed, physical affection through caressing, hugging, kissing, and the like. When this is done in an attuned, empathic way to the child's cues, it helps toward establishing a more secure attachment.

The Theraplay therapist uses many nurturing activities such as feeding the child, cradling and rocking him or her while singing a special song about the child, lotioning or powdering his or her hurts, giving manicures, and so on. Nurturing activities help to calm and soothe the child especially when he or she is deregulated. The spirit of nurturing is well described by Gaskill (2014):

> In a manner of speaking, the child is laterally encoding the neurological experience of being loved and cared for through the play with the play therapist. The child's low brain encodes warm, loving, caring associations between adult and child. What it feels like to be calm, safe and physically at peace. These associations will become the associational template for self-regulation, caring relationships for others, and parental nurturing behaviors later in the child's life. (p. 204)

Nurturing, as mentioned before, is needed by all children, especially those coming from deprived, neglectful, or abusive backgrounds. As well, behavior- or conduct-disordered children who are continually in trouble, or those who are pseudomature (parentified), or those coming from a series of foster homes or orphanages usually need a lot of basic nurturing.

Challenge

Hopefully, children are given challenging activities at home and school that are appropriate for their developmental age and skills. Sometimes they are not challenged enough (overprotected children) or pressured too much (overachieving children). Ideally, they are given the kind of challenges they can master, giving them a sense of self-confidence and competence.

In Theraplay challenging activities are geared to the child's developmental skills. The child is encouraged to take small risks (but is never forced) to expand his or her skills within the child's capabilities. Challenging activities begin with easy, simple steps leading to more complicated ones. If the child starts to fail, the task is simplified again.

Challenging activities are emphasized for timid, fearful children and also used as a means for releasing tension in aggressive children. Adolescents who are at a stage where they enjoy taking risks (Siegel, 2014) are given more challenging activities in Theraplay.

EVIDENCE OF EFFECTIVENESS

The research related to Theraplay has grown over the years from clinical anecdotes and case studies to pre–post studies using standardized measures, to those using control groups, and finally to those using randomized control groups. In 2009, Theraplay was rated by the California Evidence-Based Clearinghouse as demonstrating promising research evidence (*www.theraplay.org*).

The following is a brief review of some of the research studies pertaining to Theraplay.

1. *Pre–post evaluations using standardized measures or ratings.* Morgan (1989) found an increase in self-esteem, self-confidence, self-control, and trust in the ratings of observers evaluating children before and after Theraplay. Munns, Jensen, and Berger (1997) reported on two studies using the Achenbach Child Behavior Checklist (CBCL) and found a significant decrease in aggression scores and in externalizing scores. Bernt (2000) found significant improvement in the ratings of failure-to-thrive babies. Mahan (1999) found improved attachment scores, as did Meyer and Wardrop (2005). Lassenius-Panula and Makela (2007) found significant improvements in behavior (using the CBCL), parent–child relationships, and stress hormone levels (cortisol) in three locations in Finland. These positive results remained at a 6-month follow-up.

2. *Studies using nonrandomized control groups.* Ammen (2000) found a significant increase in empathy scores of high-risk teenage mothers in her study using Theraplay and infant massage. Hong (2004) found significantly higher scores in self-esteem ratings of her Theraplay group. Kim's (2007) Theraplay group showed significantly higher attachment scores. Kwon (2004) had significantly higher scores on preschooler's Emotional Intelligence Quotient in her Theraplay group. Ritterfeld (1990) found significantly improved expressive language scores and social–emotional scores in her group of language-disordered children who had received Theraplay compared to two control groups: one receiving speech therapy and the other receiving arts-and-crafts activities.

3. *Studies using randomized control groups.* Sui (2007) found significantly higher self-esteem scores and fewer internalizing symptoms in her Theraplay group. Sui (2014) in her second study found significant improvement in social awareness, social motivation, social communication and social cognition in her Theraplay group with developmental disabilities as compared to a control group. Higher self-esteem scores were also found in a research study by Young-Kyung (2011) in an elderly group compared to randomized controls. Weir, Lee, Canosa, Rodrigues, McWilliams, et al. (2013) combined Theraplay and family systems theory (Whole Family Therapy) to treat the parents and all the siblings within adoptive families. Significant benefits included more positive family

communication, adult interpersonal relationships, and children's behavioral functioning.

4. *Matched controls*. Wettig, Franke, and Fjordbak (2006) reported on two studies: children with language and behavior disorders were comparable to matched nonclinical controls after receiving Theraplay. These results were later repeated with a much larger sample (333 children coming from nine different clinical settings). Wettig, Coleman, and Gerder (2011) also reported on improved scores with shy, introverted children after receiving Theraplay.

For a more detailed review of Theraplay research studies see Coleman (2010), Munns (2011a), Meyer and Wardrop (2009), and Lender and Lindaman (2007). More details on research studies are also described at The Theraplay Institute's website (*www.theraplay.org*).

The above studies have shown that Theraplay has some good evidence that it helps to lower aggression, increase self-esteem, and foster parent–child attachment. More research studies are needed using randomized control groups as well as comparing Theraplay to other well-validated treatment methods. As well, more control groups should have some kind of face-to-face interactions to control for placebo effects. Finally, Theraplay needs to have more research studies published in peer-reviewed journals.

RELATED BRAIN RESEARCH

Theraplay is in harmony with some of the latest brain research, particularly the neurosequential programming originated by Dr. Bruce Perry (Perry, 2009; Perry & Szalavitz, 2006), which will be described later.

Theraplay helps to stimulate the growth of the right hemisphere which processes sensory–motor information and social–emotional experiences. (The left hemisphere processes language). The right hemisphere is dominant in the first 3 years of a child's life, which also has the greatest surge of neuronal growth and is the same period that is critical for the formation of parent–child attachment (Schore, 2005; Schore & Schore, 2008). Theraplay also helps the lower brain to become more regulated. The lower brain (brain stem, cerebellum, and diencephalon) is the first to mature. It helps control our survival systems such as breathing, digestion, body temperature, heart rate, sexual urges, and so on. It also is the seat of our instinct to flee, fight, or freeze in the face of danger. In traumatized children this instinct is often easily triggered, so such children are often hypervigilant, their breathing and heart rates are higher, their core temperature is elevated, and they are constantly ready to react (Perry & Szalavitz, 2006). Theraplay helps to soothe and calm these children, building a more secure foundation with their parents (Booth & Jernberg, 2010). One of the ways Theraplay helps to do this is through touch and rhythm that are controlled by the cerebellum of the lower brain (Levitin, 2007; Munns, 2009).

The emotional brain, or limbic system, is the next to mature. Its watchdog is the amygdala that looks for danger from the environment. It has strong, neuronal fibers connecting it to the lower brain. In children who have been chronically abused, the amygdala is overactive and easily stimulated. Theraplay tries to make the world a safer, calmer, more nurturing place for these children and to help regulate their emotional reactivity. Structured activities in Theraplay help the child to wait, take turns, and to develop self-control. Nurturing activities help the child to feel soothed, calm, and cared for.

The higher brain, or cortex, is the last to mature. It is the center for our more complex mental functions such as abstract thinking, planning, judgment, and logic. In some of the challenging activities in Theraplay, children use more of their higher brain functions, but these activities are emphasized more toward the end of treatment or with older children such as adolescents. Generally, the focus in Theraplay is more on the stimulus and organization of the lower and middle parts of the brain and on the right hemisphere, especially at the beginning of treatment.

In neurosequential programming, Dr. Perry advocates meeting the child's needs according to his or her level of brain functioning. Since the maturation of the brain is sequential, with higher parts dependent on the good organization of the preceding part, Dr. Perry starts his treatment with the optimal stimulation of the lower part (Perry, 2009; Perry & Szalavitz, 2006). Thus, if a child was traumatized in his or her early years, he would start treatment with activities designed to stimulate the lower brain such as those involving touch, rhythm, and repetition (massage, drumming, dancing, and Theraplay activities). Later on, he would stimulate the middle or emotional brain using psychodrama, sandplay, play therapy, and expressive arts. The last stage of treatment would make use of higher thinking processes such as those found in cognitive-behavioral therapy, narrative therapy, psychotherapy, and other methods of verbal treatment. Similarly, Theraplay also starts with the emotional age of the child (which is usually much younger than his or her chronological age) by using activities that would be normally used with a young child (including touch, rhythm, nursery rhymes, rocking, feeding, etc.). As Gaskill (2014) notes, "Low brain, empathic responses are functional long before cognitive, empathic functions, compelling play therapists to address low brain empathic responding in play therapy" (p. 199). As treatment progresses more activities are introduced that reflect the child's chronological age. In some more complex cases, Theraplay is combined with other therapies that use more verbal, cognitive approaches such as dyadic developmental psychotherapy (Rubin, Lender, & Mroz, 2009).

RELATED TOUCH RESEARCH

When a baby is born, its most advanced sensory system is tactile. Babies need touch to thrive (Field, 2000; Gerhardt, 2004; Makela, 2005; Nickelson & Parker, 2009; Sunderland, 2006). The way he or she is held, cuddled, and put down gives the baby its first self-image and the feeling as to whether he or she is valued, wanted, and important (Ford, 1993). The baby explores his or her world often by reaching out, grasping objects, and bringing them to his or her mouth, which is a highly tactile, sensitive area. When a baby is given physical affection by cuddling, caressing, being held, and rocked, hormones such as opioids and oxytocin are released, which help to regulate the baby's arousal system and affect the bonding process between parent and child (Gerhardt, 2004). The stress hormone cortisol, which can be damaging to the developing brain if highly and frequently activated, can be diminished with positive physical contact. In Theraplay, there is a lot of positive physical contact especially in the nurturing activities. Care is taken to never force the child to accept nurturing and can be modified so it is more acceptable to the child. This is especially true with children who have been physically or sexually abused. For example, a child may not want to have his or her "hurts" powdered or lotioned. The therapist may turn to an activity such as "powder hand prints" where the child's palm is sprinkled and rubbed with baby powder and then pressed against a piece of dark-colored paper to form a hand print. Once the child has experienced this activity, there is usually no objection to having "hurts" cared for.

In Theraplay parents are usually present and involved so a clinician's apprehension regarding possible accusations of inappropriate touching is not usually a worry. As well, Theraplay activities are often demonstrated with the parents in a session previous to treatment with their child, so the parents know beforehand what to expect (Makela & Sako, 2011).

Internationally known clinicians dealing with traumatized and abused children such as Hindman (1991) and James (1994) advocate the use of positive touch. Field (2000) has conducted well-controlled research demonstrating the significant positive effects of touch through massage therapy with premature babies (increased body weight and higher sensory motor scores), with aggressive adolescents (less aggression), and with children with attention-deficit/hyperactivity disorder (ADHD) (better concentration). Other research showing the benefits of physical contact has come from studies using "Kangeroo Care" in which the baby is carried in a pouch "skin-to-skin" against the parent's chest (Ludington-Hoe, 1993; Sunderland, 2006).

In our touch-phobic world it is important to realize how important healthy touch is to the well-being of our children. Some research suggests that if they do not receive touch in positive ways, they will seek it in a negative, aggressive manner. Thayer (1998) found that countries showing the least amount of positive touch between family members had the highest amount of violence within their country.

CHARACTERISTICS OF THERAPLAY THAT MAKE IT EFFECTIVE AS A SHORT-TERM TREATMENT METHOD

Theraplay goes to the basis or roots of attachment and replicates what the child may have missed earlier in his or her life. This starts happening right from the first session. It does not rely on words, but on action. Theraplay "walks the talk" by modeling healthy interactions with the child and then having parents directly play with their child under the guidance of the therapist.

In Theraplay, parents are fully involved from the beginning, so they can practice the techniques at home. Parental involvement is conducive to good generalization of treatment effects. Thus, changes occur not only in the clinical setting, but also at home. This creates a double impact on the child. Theraplay is intense, intimate, and often physical, which brings changes quickly. Since it is practiced through play and games, the child usually joins in easily without a lot of resistance. It involves positive touch, which every child needs in order to thrive. Making positive physical contact between people can help to make connections quickly if it is done in a sensitive manner.

Theraplay promotes laughter and fun through joyful play, which is conducive for healing and can often change negative attitudes to positive ones in a short period of time. Theraplay provides a way for children to receive essentials for their well-being: responsive, empathic attunement to their cues and needs, nurturance, and unconditional acceptance. This creates a healing atmosphere right from the first session. Theraplay also, at times, provides nurturance to parents who may need this before they can genuinely give nuturance to their children. Theraplay is simple in its theoretical underpinnings so parents can understand it easily and start using it. Theraplay replicates normal parent–child interactions so parents are already familiar with some of its activities.

CASE ILLUSTRATION

Intake History

This case illustrates using Theraplay with two young children, Johnathan, age 3 years, and Sasha, age 5 years. Both siblings had been adopted from an orphanage in Romania. Little was known about their biological parents except that they had dropped off their children at the orphanage when Johnathan was an infant and Sasha was 2 years old.

A young professional couple had adopted these two children 2 years before seeking treatment. They were struggling to maintain this adoption and were on the verge of giving up. Referral problems for both children included noncompliance, overreactions, temper tantrums, deregulation, high anxiety, and ambivalence. The older sibling, Sasha, showed other symptoms of reactive attachment disorder, was also very manipulative, controlling, often rejecting and aggressive not only to her younger brother but to the parents as well. She did not have friends at school and was often isolated. Moreover, she was disobedient and defiant with her teachers at times. Johnathan was described as being very ambivalent: sometimes he would reject affectionate approaches from his parents, while at other times he was very clinging. Both children showed strong separation anxiety if their parents tried to go away.

The parents were confused, felt helpless, were beginning to feel hopeless, and were at "their wit's end." They had been seeing a family worker weekly for several months before being referred to Theraplay. On the positive side, both parents were highly motivated, caring, sensitive, healthy physically and emotionally, and in a stable marriage. Parents were supportive with each other and had relatives who were also helpful. Their economic status was comfortable with no financial issues.

In the initial interview an in-depth developmental, emotional, and behavioral history was taken, not only of each child, but also of the family background of each parent including their marital history. Research studies have indicated that parents are highly likely to repeat the attachment patterns that they had formed with their own parents in the past with their own children in the present (De Klyen, 1996; Fonagy, 1994; Zeanah, 1994, 1996) (intergenerational transmission of attachment patterns).

The Marschak Interaction Method

Following the intake interview, a family assessment took place using the Marschak Interaction Method (MIM), designed to observe how parents and children relate to each other, particularly in how parents structure, challenge, engage, and nurture their children and how their children respond (DiPasquale, 2000). This assessment included the mother and children performing four or five simple tasks (playing together with squeaky toy animals, powdering each other's hands, assembling a puzzle, parent leaving the room for 1 minute, etc.). Similar tasks took place with father and the children. Then the whole family participated with tasks such as putting hats on each other, playing a familiar game, feeding each other, and so on. Therapists observed the parent–child interactions as well as the marital interchanges behind a one-way mirror. The whole procedure was videotaped, with previous written permission granted by the parents.

Marschak Feedback

In the next session, attended only by the parents, the MIM video was reviewed with discussion of the positive strengths as well as the trouble spots of the family. Theraplay was explained and final goals were agreed on both by the parents and the therapists. These goals included the following: to enhance the attachment between parents and children, to increase their trust of each other, to help the parents structure and regulate their children, to increase parents' attunement to their children's cues, and to raise the self-esteem and confidence of all family members. An important goal also was to have everyone enjoy each other and to just have fun!

Since both children had had little basic nurturing in their orphanage when they were very young, the therapists felt that they should emphasize trying to replicate the parent–child interactions that normally occur in the attachment process with young children. This would include rocking the children in a blanket, feeding them a lollipop while singing a special song about them, and possibly feeding them a baby bottle while in the arms of their parents.

Theraplay Treatment Sessions

Three therapists were assigned to this case—one therapist for each child and an interpreting therapist to answer questions from the parents while they observed the therapists modeling interactions with their children. This was the initial plan. However, the children started to cry and cling to their parents at the attempt to usher the latter into the observation room. So the parents were included in the Theraplay sessions right from the beginning. However, after the second session when the children were more familiar with the therapist, there was a successful attempt to have the parents observe a session behind the one-way mirror. Parents reported that this observation period was very valuable and helped them to be more objective about both children, particularly in their responses to the therapists' directions.

When the parents were in the Theraplay sessions the format varied from having each parent interact with one child while being guided by a therapist to having the whole family playing with each other. Each child had turns interacting with each parent.

Some of the sessions will be described in detail so the reader can gain a better understanding of what actually occurs in Theraplay.

The therapy room was bare except for a colorful rug on which was centered a soft blanket with pillows on it. This is where the family and therapists sat. Theraplay materials such as a bottle of baby powder and lotion, a bag of potato chips, balloons, and other items were placed on the side of the room on a shelf. An agenda of the Theraplay activities for the session was pinned to the wall.

Session 1

• *Entrance.* Follow the leader. A therapist leads the line of family members one behind the other, imitating whatever the leader does such as taking big and little steps, fast and slow steps, and so on until they reach the blanket and pillows in the center of the room. (Many therapists also use beanbag chairs in a corner of the room.)

• *Welcome song.* A simple song including everyone's name is sung— "Hello, Sasha; hello, Johnathan; hello, Mom and Dad; we're glad you came to play"—while holding hands in a circle.

• *Checkup or inventory.* A few positive things regarding each child are noted: for example, "Sasha, I see you have brought your beautiful blue eyes and blond hair. Look at that dimple in your cheek—did you know that when you smile it can really grow big!" Therapists notice things at first while in later sessions the parents do the checkups.

• *Powdering of hurts.* A therapist takes the hand of each child and finds little scratches or "boo-boos" or red marks or freckles and gently rubs powder around each one on each hand. (Sometimes the therapist will powder or lotion the hurts on the hands of a parent if that parent has come from a neglectful or abusive background.)

• *Balloon toss.* Everyone stands in a circle taking turns tossing a balloon to each other. Then several more balloons are tossed keeping them all in the air without touching the floor.

• *Motor boat.* Everyone joins hands in a circle and steps to the right singing "Motor boat, motor boat go so slow, motorboat, motorboat go so fast, motorboat, motorboat step on the gas, motor boat motorboat out of gas" Here everyone sits down.

- *Pass a funny face.* Each participant has a turn making a funny face that his or her neighbor passes on to the next person around the circle.
- *Feeding.* Each therapist takes a turn feeding everyone a potato chip including parents. About four or five rounds of feeding the chips takes place. (The therapist places a chip right into the mouth of the recipient. Later, parents take a turn feeding everyone.) The children are fed the most.
- *Goodbye song.* While holding hands in a circle a goodbye song is sung mentioning each person's name: "Goodbye, Johnathan; goodbye, Sasha; goodbye, Mom and Dad; goodbye Sally and Linda—we're glad you came today."

This first session went very well after the initial attempt at separating the parents to go into the observation room was abandoned. Both children and parents participated fully and enjoyed themselves, especially in the activity of "Pass a funny face."

The Theraplay session took about 30 to 40 minutes and was immediately followed by a parent counseling session for another half hour while the children and a therapist went into another play room where there were books, puzzles, and toys. In good weather, the children were taken outside to play on the grounds while their parents remained for the counseling session for debriefing and for checking progress at home and school. This was a time that also allowed parents to revisit their own childhood experiences and to relate them to their present family. (Note that in classical Theraplay the parent counseling session takes place after two or three Theraplay sessions where the parents come in alone for a separate session. Sometimes this debriefing of previous sessions is done by phone.)

Session 2

- *Entrance.* Stepping stones: stepping stones (colored sheets of construction paper) are placed on the floor from the door to the center of the room to the blanket and pillows. Under a few of the sheets of paper a small candy is placed on top of a tissue, which the child can discover and eat as he or she continues walking toward the center of the room.
- *Welcome song.* Same as previously described.
- *Checkup.* Dad notices positive things about one child and Mom notices things about the other child.
- *Lotioning of hurts.* The therapist takes care of the hurts on one hand of a child and the parent attends to the hurts of the other hand.
- *Slippery slip.* The therapist rubs lots of lotion on the hands of a child who then places his or her hand between the hands of the therapist. The

child tries to slip his or her hand out and away while the therapist tries to hang on to his or her hand. A parent sits behind the child so if he or she falls backward he or she will fall safely into the arms of the parent.

- *Motor boat.* Same as previously described.

- *Copying clapping patterns.* A therapist demonstrates a simple clap pattern by clapping his or her hands together, for example, clap, clap (fast), then clap, clap (slow). The group imitates this sequence of claps. The complexity of the sequence increases gradually and touching your neighbor is included—for example, clap, clap (pause) clap, clap, clap, clap, touch your neighbor's shoulder on the final clap. If someone fails to remember the sequence, the leader goes back to a simpler sequence so everyone succeeds.

- *Feeding.* Everyone gets fed pieces of apple with most of the pieces going to the children.

- *Goodbye song.* Same as previously described.

In this session, both children continued to cooperate, although Sasha initially refused "slippery slip." Her refusal was accepted by the therapist, who reflected "You don't feel comfortable doing that?" However, as Sasha watched her brother enjoying this activity, she decided to join in.

Session 3

In this session the parents were able to stay behind the one-way mirror in the observation room in order to watch the therapists model interactions with their children. Since the children were more familiar with the therapists, and they knew their parents were observing them, they did not display separation anxiety.

- *Entrance, welcome song, checkup, lotioning of hurts.* Similar to previous sessions. This was followed by "Play Doh trophies" (Play Doh casts are made of a child's fingers, toes, ears, and so on . Each time the cast is examined and compared to the child's real body part. This activity help the children to gain a clearer and more positive body image.)

- *Blowing soap bubbles and catching them.*

- *Red Light/Green Light.* Everyone formed a line on the other side of the room, facing the leader who explained the game. "When I say 'green light' you may move forward, but when I say 'red light' you must stop. If you don't stop and I catch you moving, then you will need to go back to the beginning of the line. Whoever gets to touch me first is the next leader." The leader then turned her back and called out the instructions—"red light" or "green light." On "red light" she would turn her head quickly to see if she could catch anyone moving.

- *Feeding of pretzels.*
- *Goodbye song.*

Both children did very well in this session considering that their parents were not in the room. In the parent counseling session the parents said it was very insightful to see how their children reacted, especially Sasha and her pouting and controlling behavior. The therapist who usually managed to cheerfully divert Sasha's attention to something else and to get her engaged in the activity also noticed this behavior. It was important to have one activity flow into the next with short transition times in order to keep the children's attention, interest, and cooperation.

Parents were starting to realize that it was important to notice early on what triggered their children's resistance and how to manage it, without allowing resistance to escalate into a full-blown temper tantrum.

Session 4

Parents observed for the first 10 minutes and then came into the Theraplay room for the remainder of the session.

- *Entrance, welcome song, checkup, lotioning of hurts.* Similar to previous sessions.
- *Hiding under the blanket.* The children hide under the blanket and when the parents enter the room they pretend to hunt for them. When they find them, they give the children a hug.
- *Ring around a rosy.* Everyone holds hands in a circle and sings the song as they move around: "Ring around a rosy, pockets full of posies, husha, husha, we all fall down."
- *Bean Bag Hug.* A bean bag is passed around to each person sitting in a circle while everyone chants: "One potato, two potato, three potato, four, five potato, six potato, seven potato, more." Whoever gets the bean bag on the word "more" gets a hug from his or her neighbors on either side. This sequence is repeated until everyone gets a turn being hugged.
- *Blanket rock.* Each child receives a turn being swung in a blanket while everyone sings a special song including the child's name: "Rock-a-bye our Sasha, in the tree tops. When the wind blows the cradle will rock. When the wind stops, the cradle won't fall. And up will come Sasha, cradle and all." At this point the child was placed in a parent's arms, who then

walked to and sat on a pillow against a wall, in preparation for the next activity

- *Cradling and feeding a lollipop.* The children are cradled in each parent's arms while sucking on a lollipop of their choice. Each therapist sits alongside a parent–child dyad while singing a special song about the child to the tune of "Twinkle, twinkle, little star." The song went something like this: "Twinkle, twinkle, little star, / what a special girl/boy you are. / Shiny hair and rosy cheeks, / sparkling eyes from which you peek. / Twinkle, twinkle, little star, / what a special girl/boy you are."

- *Feeding of potato chips.*

- *Goodbye song.*

This was a special session. The parents felt very moved as they cradled and rocked their child and helped to sing a special song. In later sessions other verses were added and sometimes the song was just hummed. As well, sometimes parents talked about their positive baby memories when their children were first adopted as they cradled them.

The children got quite excited and giggled while hiding under the blanket before the parents came in. One of the therapists hid under the blanket with them in case they got frightened at being covered up.

Parents were asked to do homework, which consisted of trying a few of their favorite Theraplay activities at home with their children.

Session 5

Parents again observed for the first 10 minutes and then came into the room for powder hand prints.

- *Entrance, welcome song, checkup, lotioning of hurts.* Similar to previous sessions.

- *Powder Hand Prints.* Baby powder is sprinkled and rubbed on the palms of the children and parents and then pressed onto a dark-colored piece of construction paper to form hand prints. Everyone compares their hand prints with each other, noticing similarities and differences.

- *Mother, May I?* Everyone lines up in a straight line on one side of the room while the leader faces this line on the other side of the room. The objective of the game is to see who will reach the leader first. Each member takes turns asking the leader questions like: "Mother, may I take three steps forward?" (or two jumps forward, or five baby steps, etc.). Each member must preface his or her request with "Mother may I," or he or she will lose his or her turn. The leader answers "Yes, you may" or "No, you may not" or changes it to something else like "You may take one giant step instead." At the beginning of the game, the leader is usually one of the therapists; however, a parent is soon asked to be the leader so the children learn to take directions from the parent, which is the real objective of this game.

• *Row, row, row your boat.* Two sitting rows are formed with a child, parent, and therapist, one behind the other, in one row facing a second row with the second child, other parent, and other therapist. The children who are facing each other join hands while everyone else holds on to the waist of the person in front of them. Everyone sings "Row, row, row your boat, gently down the stream, merrily, merrily, merrily, merrily, life is but a dream" as they sway back and forth to the song. The tempo varies from slow to fast to turbulent (sideways movement) as a pretend storm approaches, and then back to slow and calmness.

• *Blanket rock.* Each child takes a turn being rocked in the blanket while the group holds on to each corner of the blanket while singing to him or her. At the end, the child is scooped up in the blanket into the arms of one of the parents who then sits down against a wall ready for the next activity

• *Feeding and cradling the child.* The parent cradles and rocks the child in his or her arms while a special song is sung about the child and a juice box or baby bottle with juice in it is fed to the child with the parent holding one end of the bottle. (Both Sasha and Johnathan were fed a baby bottle of juice in the arms of each parent.)

• *Feeding potato chips to everybody.*

• *Goodbye song.*

This was a turning point for this family and a profound experience for the parents. The parents felt truly close to their children when they cradled and fed the baby bottle to their children. They felt that their children were "our babies." (In the past they had not felt this so strongly.) Both children snuggled into their parent's arms and took the bottle without hesitation. Dr. Gaskill (2014), who practices neurosequential programing notes that in "developmentally regressed play where the child may regress to infantile behavior, baby talk, sucking on the bottle, wanting to be rocked or held, put to bed with a lullaby, etc.—the child and therapist have become neurologically attuned through eye contact, face-to-face gaze, soft tones and gentle touch" (p. 204).

The children cooperated with all of the activities, although Sasha had some trouble initially with the game "Mother, may I." She said she did not like it and did not want to play it. The leader reflected her feelings and said she could still stay in the line and just watch—which she did. A little later she was ready to join in and received a round of applause from everyone for doing so. Her initial reluctance to play the game may have been more a fear of not fully understanding what was required of her, resulting in her fear of failure.

The parents reported that the children were more obedient at home and their tantrums had significantly diminished. Their homework of doing Theraplay activities at home was working out well and they were lotioning hurts and doing checkups of positive features of their children every night at bedtime.

Sessions 6, 7, 8, and 9

The format for these sessions remained the same as in previous sessions, but increasingly the parents were asked to lead the activities. The therapists tried to make certain that each child was paired with a parent equally. For example, in a previous session Sasha had been cradled and fed by her mother and Johnathan by his father. In the next session, this was switched to Sasha being cradled by her father, and Johnathan cradled by his mother. The cradling and bottle feeding continued except for the last session. Parents reported that at home they had found that if the children got overexcited or out of control, then cradling and bottle feeding was very effective in bringing them into a calm, contented state.

The parents had started to arrange for playdates with other children. This was going well, whereas previously the children would cling to their parents and would remain outside the playgroup. Both children were starting up friendships with a neighboring child and his friends.

In the seventh session termination of treatment was discussed. The parents felt much more confident and closer to their children. They were enjoying and taking delight in them. The idea of giving up the adoption had disappeared. They were practicing Theraplay activities at home every day. The children seemed more regulated in their emotions, their tantrums were rare, they were more trusting and secure in their relationships with their parents, they were more open to new experiences, were less anxious, were more obedient, accepted physical affection from their parents easily, and laughed and smiled more often. They were happier children.

In the seventh session the children were told that there would be only two more sessions and they would not be coming every week anymore, but there would be a party at the last session and we would include their favorite activities. This party was planned with the family's favorite activities and the parents were asked to bring special food (like cake, cookies, etc.). The therapists were to provide the drinks and party hats.

In the ninth and last session, a special party took place with the usual beginning format of entrance, welcome song, checkup, and lotioning of hurts, followed by the family's favorite activities. The session ended with everyone exchanging hats and sitting down to eat the special food, cake and popcorn. Photos were taken of everyone and presents were given to the children (small inexpensive presents bought by the therapists) as well as mementos from the Theraplay sessions (i.e., family hand prints).

Checkups

Four checkups were planned for the coming year. The first one was dated 6 weeks after treatment, the second one 2 months later, then 3 months later, and finally 4 months later. These checkups were like regular Theraplay sessions. The parents were encouraged to keep practicing the Theraplay activities and principles at home.

During these checkups the family continued to show positive gains in their attachments with each other, the children had friends, their cooperation with adult direction at home and school continued to improve, and parents felt stronger and more confident in their parenting skills. They were a happier family.

SUMMARY AND CONCLUSIONS

Sasha and Johnathan were two young children adopted from an orphanage that had proved such a challenge to their young, inexperienced parents that their adoption was in danger of being terminated. A big factor in the rapid progress of this family was the high motivation of the parents, their openness, and their good physical and mental health. Their growing sensitivity to their children's cues and needs played an important part. In spite of their children's difficult past, the family's progress was rapid in a short period of time (nine weekly Theraplay sessions). The children's explosive temper tantrums, high anxiety, defiance, rejection, ambivalence, and separation anxiety significantly decreased. Moreover, the parents and children were closer in their attachment to each other, and they could truly enjoy each other. The playful Theraplay activities helped to promote this. As well, the children, whose self-confidence was growing, were starting to make friends with neighboring children and at school. At the end of therapy the parents stated that all adoptive parents should take a course in Theraplay.

Theraplay is a structured, short-term model of play therapy that seeks to replicate the interactions that normally occur between parents and their young child. It goes to the roots of attachment formation in an effort to give to the child the kind of experiences he or she may have missed in early childhood. It is increasingly research-based and is in harmony with some of the latest brain and touch research.

Theraplay is based on attachment theory and its main goals are to enhance parent–child attachment, to increase the trust and self-esteem of all family members, to guide the parents to more attuned, empathic responsiveness to their child's needs, and to increase the child's self-regulation. Four main principles underlie Theraplay activities:

1. *Structure,* where the adult chooses and leads the activities, thus creating an atmosphere of safety, security, and predictability.
2. *Engagement,* which increases parent–child connections in an enjoyable, fun way.
3. *Challenge,* where the child learns to take age-appropriate risks and gains mastery with self-confidence.
4. *Nurture,* leaving the child to feel valued, cared for, accepted, and loved.

Having the parents involved from the beginning, first as observers to the modeling interactions between therapist and their child, and later with their direct participation is an important factor in this process. Parents practice Theraplay activities at home, as well as in the clinical setting, during the treatment period and in four checkups throughout the year.

Theraplay includes a lot of positive touch, which research has shown is essential for children to thrive. This is done in a playful, safe atmosphere that often brings laughter and joy to all involved.

REFERENCES

Ammen, S. (2000). A play-based teen parenting program to facilitate parent/child attachment. In H. Kaduson & C. Schaefer (Eds.), *Short term play therapy for children* (pp. 345–369). New York: Guilford Press.

Atkinson, N. (2009). Theraplay used in a multicultural environment. In E. Munns (Ed.), *Applications of family and group Theraplay* (pp. 131–157). Lanham, MD: Jason Aronson.

Berndt, C. (2000). Theraplay with failure-to-thrive infants and mothers. In E. Munns (Ed.), *Theraplay: Innovations in attachment enhancing play therapy* (pp. 117–138). Northvale, NJ: Jason Aronson.

Booth, P., & Jernberg, A. (2010). *Theraplay: Helping parents and children build better relationships through attachment-based play* (3rd ed.). San Francisco: Jossey-Bass.

Booth, P., Lindaman, S., & Winstead, M. (2014). Theraplay in re-unification following relational trauma. In. C. Malchiodi & D. Crenshaw (Eds.), *Creatve arts and play therapy for attachment problems.* New York: Guilford Press.

Bowlby, J. (1988). *A secure base: Parent–child attachment and healthy human development.* New York: Basic Books.

Coleman, R. (2010). Research findings that support the effectiveness of Theraplay. In P. Booth & A. Jernberg (Eds.), *Theraplay: Helping parents and children build better relationships through attachment-based play* (3rd ed., pp. 85–97). San Francisco: Jossey-Bass.

De Klyen, M. (1996). Disruptive behavior disorder and intergenerational attachment patterns: A comparison of clinic-referred and normally functioning preschoolers and their mothers. *Journal of Consulting and Clinical Psychology, 64*(2), 357–365.

DiPasquale, L. (2000). The Marschak Interaction Method. In E. Munns (Ed.), *Theraplay: Innovations in attachment enhancing play therapy* (pp. 27–51). Northvale, NJ: Jason Aronson.

DiPasquale, L. (2009). The dysregulated child. In E. Munns (Ed.), *Applications of family and group Theraplay* (pp. 27–44). Lanham, MD: Jason Aronson.

Eyles, S., Boada, M., & Munns, C. (2009). Theraplay with overtly and passively resistant children. In E. Munns (Ed.), *Applications of family and group Theraplay* (pp. 45–55). Lanham, MD: Jason Aronson.

Field, T. (2000). *Touch therapy.* New York: Churchill Livingstone.

Fonagy, P. (1994, October). *Crime and punishment: Representations of attachment relationship in a severly personality disordered prisoner group.* Paper presented at the International Conference on Attachment and Psychopathology, Toronto, Ontario, Canada.

Ford, C. (1993). *Compassionate touch: The role of human touch in healing and recovery.* New York: Simon & Schuster.

Gaskill, R. (2014). Empathy. In C. Schaefer & A. Drewes (Eds.), *The therapeutic powers of play* (2nd ed., pp. 195–209). Hoboken, NJ: Wiley.

Gerhardt, S. (2004). *Why love matters: How affection shapes a baby's brain.* New York: Brunner-Routledge.

Hindman, J. (1991). *The morning breaks: 101 "proactive" treatment strategies breaking the trauma bonds of sexual abuse.* Ontario, OR: Alexandria Associates.

Hong, J. (2004). *The effects of a family resilience promotion program applying family Theraplay.* Presentation at Sookmyung Women's University Seoul, Korea.

James, B. (1994). *Handbook for the treatment of attachment-trauma related problems in children.* New York: Lexington Books.

Kim, Y. (2007). Development and evaluation of a group Theraplay program to enhance attachment of infants. In D. Lender & S. Lindaman (Eds.), *Research supporting the effectiveness of Theraplay and the Marschak Interaction Method* (pp. 20–23). Chicago: Theraplay Institute.

Kim, Y. (2011). The effect of goup Theraplay on self-esteem and depression of the elderly in a day care center. *Korean Journal of Counselling, 12*(5), 1413–1430.

Kwon, E. (2004). The effect of group Theraplay on the development of preschoolers' emotional intelligence quotient. In D. Lender & S. Lindaman (Eds.), *Research supporting the effectiveness of Theraplay and the Marschak Interaction Method.* Chicago: Theraplay Institute.

Lassenius-Panula, L., & Makela, J. (2007). *Effectiveness of Theraplay with symptomatic children ages 2–6: Changes in symptoms, parent–child relationships and stress hormone levels of children referred for psychiatric care in three university hospital districts in Finland.* Paper presented at the Third International Theraplay Conference, Chicago, IL.

Lender, D., & Lindeman, S. (2007). *Research supporting the effectiveness of Theraplay and Marschak Interaction Method.* Paper presented at the Third International Theraplay Conference, Chicago, IL.

Levitin, D. (2007). *This is your brain on music.* New York: Plume.

Ludington-Hoe, S. (1993). *Kangeroo care: The best you can do to help your pre-term infant.* New York: Bantam.

Mahan, M. (1999). *Theraplay as an intervention with previously institutionalized twins having attachment difficulties.* Unpublished doctoral dissertation, Chicago School of Professional Psychology, Chicago, IL.

Makela, J. (2005). The importance of touch in the development of children. *Finnish Medical Journal, 60,* 1543–1549.

Makela, J., & Sako, S. (2011). Theraplay—vanhenmen ja lapsen volinenvuorovaiku-tushoito lasten mielenterveysonggelmissa. [Theraplay—parent–child interactions treatment for children with mental health problems]. *Duodeclm, 127,* 29–39.

Meyer, L., & Wardrop, J. (2009). Research on Theraplay effectiveness. In E. Munns (Ed.), *Applications of family and group Theraplay* (pp. 171–182). Lanham, MD: Jason Aronson.

Meyer, L., & Wardrop, J. (2005). *Research on Theraplay.* Paper presented at the Second International Theraplay Conference, Chicago, IL.

Morgan, C. (1989). *Theraplay: An evaluation of the effect of short-term structural play on self-confidence, self-esteem, trust and self-control.* Unpublished research, York Center for Children, Youth and Families, Richmond Hill, Ontario, Canada.

Munns, E. (2013). Filial therapy and Theraplay. In N. Biddel-Bowers (Ed.), *Play therapy with families* (pp. 147–160). Lanham, MD: Jason Aronson.

Munns, E. (Ed.). (2011a). Theraplay: Attachment enhancing play therapy. In C. Schaefer (Ed.), *Foundations of play therapy* (2nd ed., pp. 275–296). Hoboken, NJ: Wiley.

Munns, E. (2011b). Integration of child-centered play therapy and Theraplay. In A. Drewes, S. Bratton, & C. Schaefer (Eds.), *Integrative play therapy* (pp. 325–340). Hoboken, NJ: Wiley.

Munns, E. (Ed.). (2009). *Applications of family and group Theraplay.* Lanham, MD: Jason Aronson.

Munns, E. (2008). Theraplay with zero to 3 year olds. In C. Schaefer, S. Kelly-Zion, J. McCormick, & A. Odnogi (Eds.), *Play therapy for very young children* (pp. 157–170). New York: Jason Aronson.

Munns, E. (Ed.). (2000). *Theraplay: Innovations in attachment enhancing play therapy.* Northvale, NJ: Jason Aronson.

Munns, E., Jensen, D., & Berger, L. (1997). *Theraplay and the reduction of aggression.* Unpublished research, Blue Hills Child and Family Services, Aurora, Ontario, Canada.

Nickelson, B., & Parker, L. (2009). *Attached at the heart.* New York: Universe.

Panksepp, J. (2007). Can play diminish ADHD and facilitate the construction of the social brain? *Journal of the Canadian Academy of Child & Adolescent Psychiatry, 16*(2), 57–66.

Perry, B. (2009). Examining child maltreatment through a neurodevelopmental lens: Clinical applications of the neurosequential model of therapeutics. *Journal of Loss and Trauma, 4*(4), 240–255.

Perry, B., & Szalavitz, M. (2006). *The boy who was raised as a dog and other stories from a child psychiatrist's notebook: What traumatized children can teach us about loss, love, and healing.* New York: Basic Books.

Perry, L., & Sutherland, P. (2009). Theraplay and aboriginal peoples. In E. Munns (Ed.), *Applications of family and group Theraplay* (pp. 97–114). Lanham, MD: Jason Aronson.

Ritterfeld, U. (1990). Theraplay auf dem Prufsland: Bewertung des Therapieerfolgs am Beispiel sprachauffalliger Vorsehulkinder [Putting Theraplay to the test:

Evaluation of therapeutic outcome with language-delayed preschool children]. *Theraplay Journal, 2,* 22–25.

Rubin, P., Lender, D., & Mroz, J. (2009). Theraplay and dyadic developmental psychotherapy. In E. Munns (Ed.), *Applications of family and group Theraplay* (pp. 171–182). Lanham, MD: Jason Aronson.

Schaefer, C., & Drewes, A. (Eds.). (2014). *The therapeutic powers of play* (2nd ed.). Hoboken, NJ: Wiley.

Schore, A. (2005). Attachment, affect and the developing right brain: linking developmental neuroscience to pediatrics. *Pediatrics Review, 26*(6), 204–217.

Schore, J., & Schore, A. (2008). Modern attachment theory: The central role of affect regulation in development and treatment. *Clinical Social Work Journal, 36*(1), 9–20.

Siegel, D. (2014). *Brain storm.* New York: Torcher/Putman.

Sui, A. (2009). Theraplay in the Chinese world: An intervention program for Hong Kong children with internalizing problems. *International Journal of Play Therapy, 18*(1), 1–12.

Sui, A. (2014). Effectiveness of group Theraplay on enhancing social skills among children with developmental disabilities. *International Journal of Play Therapy, 23*(4), 187–203.

Sunderland, M. (2006). *The science of parenting.* New York: Dorling Kindersley.

Thayer, T. (1998, March). March encounters. *Psychology Today,* pp. 31–36.

Weir, K. N., Lee, S., Canosa, P., Rodrigues, N., McWilliams, M., & Parker, L. (2013). Whole Family Theraplay: Integrating Family Systems Theory and Theraplay to treat adoptive families. *Adoption Quarterly, 16*(3–4), 175–200.

Wettig, H. G., Coleman, R., & Gerder, F. (2011). Evaluating the effectiveness of Theraplay in treating shy, socially withdrawn children. *International Journal of Play Therapy, 20*(1), 26–37.

Wettig, H., Franke, U., & Fjordbak, B. (2006). Evaluating the effectiveness of Theraplay. In C. Schaefer & H. Kaduson (Eds.), *Contemporary play therapy: Theory, research, and practice* (pp. 103–235). New York: Guilford Press.

Yoon, J. (2007). *Effects of family group Theraplay to enhance interaction between child and mother in low-income families.* Paper presented at the Third International Theraplay Conference, Chicago, IL.

Young-Kyung, K. (2011). The effect of group Theraplay on self-esteem and depression of the elderly in a day care center. *Korean Journal of Counseling, 12*(5), 1413–1430.

Zeanah, C. H. (1994). *Intergenerational transmission of relationship psychopathology: A mother–infant case study.* Paper presented at the International Conference on Attachment and Psychopathology, Toronto, Ontario, Canada.

Zeanah, C. H. (1996). Beyond insecurity: A reconceptualization of attachment disorders of infancy. *Journal of Consulting and Clinical Psychology, 64*(1), 42–52.

Chapter 4

☙

Short-Term Play Therapy for Children with Disruptive Behavior Disorders

Scott Riviere

*W*ith all of the changes in the fifth edition of the *Diagnostic and Statistical Manual of Mental Disorders* (American Psychiatric Association, 2013), the entire classification system of disruptive behaviors has evolved. Oppositional defiant disorder (ODD), conduct disorder (CD), and intermittent explosive disorder (IED), as well as a few other diagnoses, are classified in the disruptive, impulse-control, and conduct disorders, whereas attention-deficit/hyperactivity disorder (ADHD) is classified in the neurodevelopmental chapter of DSM-5. Regardless of the classification and diagnostic changes, the essential features of these conditions remain the same. These children often have moderate to severe emotional, behavioral, and psychological consequences resulting from these conditions and are a frequent referral to mental health professionals. ODD, ADHD, and CD can affect anywhere between 2 and 16% of school-age children (Dickstein, 2010; Hinshaw & Lee, 2003; Rader, McCauley, & Callen, 2009). If we deduct that number from 100%, it can mean that 84–98% of school-age kids in the United States do not meet the criteria for these disorders. There can also be children who do not meet the clinical symptoms of these disorders but share similar temperament traits. For example, strong-willed, anxious–nervous, and negative–pessimistic temperaments can also share similar disruptive behaviors (Flick, 1996).

77

In my experience, all children misbehave (as do most adults adults as well!). However, most kids can acknowledge their mistakes, apologize, and learn alternative ways of coping with life. In contrast, children with disruptive behaviors and temperaments often struggle with these very things and blame others for their mistakes. In all of my years of practice, children exhibiting disruptive behaviors have always been a love of mine. I know many therapists who would rather refer a child with disruptive or impulsive behavior than treat him or her. I believe this is because so many of the behavior interventions that are "supposed to work" seem ineffective with these children.

In this chapter I hope to educate you on a *method* of working with these children that focuses on their strengths, builds their competencies, and makes a positive impact on their sense of self. Techniques will come and go, but having a solid method to operate from gives mental health professionals some parameters to design their own creative interventions to help such children. The method's primary function is to help parents, teachers, and mental health professionals get a glimpse of how these children see the world, as well as how their behavior affects the adults in their life. I have found that this method can be applied to a variety of activities, games, and therapeutic interventions, as well as to parenting skills. It can be equally effective in one session or over a period of time. Because most of the attention is given to the behavioral effects of these disorders, this chapter is primarily designed to assist mental health professionals in understanding the *emotional* effects of these conditions. By understanding the dynamics of how these children see their world, you will better be able to help them. The cornerstones of this method consist of three important concepts:

1. Buttons
2. Punishment versus reward-based theory
3. Self-confidence bucket

As you consider these concepts, it is important to remember that these children see the world very differently. Although the techniques can be effective for all types of children, the concepts presented in this chapter are predominantly for children with ODD and ADHD. However, I have also found that this method is effective for children who are anxious and/ or depressive–pessimistic. The interventions discussed in the upcoming sections are most effective for children ages 5–12.

BUTTONS

The first concept to be considered is buttons (see Figure 4.1). You have probably heard or said the phrase "Boy, that kid really knows how to press

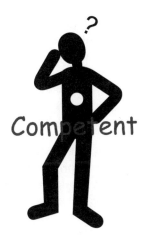

FIGURE 4.1. Disruptive behavior disorder button.

my buttons." If you have children, you know full well that as early as age 2 they know how to press your buttons. So, how do humans react whenever their buttons are pressed?

The first thing most people do when their buttons are pressed is become defensive, and the first thing most of us do when we become defensive is to point the finger and blame somebody else. This is called *externalizing blame*, and children are generally experts at it. A child may be asked, "Who left the toys on the floor?," with the child quickly responding, "Not me!" Maybe you ask your teenager, "Did you bring your permission slip home?," only to hear "You were supposed to remind me!" So, what is the button for these children? For them, the button is a *fear* of incompetence or of not being "good." Thus, anything that points out that they did something incorrectly or that they are not "the best" at something is going to press their buttons. For example, if they come in at second place in a game, that is just as bad as being in last place, because second indicates not being the best. Therefore, the first thing these children tend to do is become defensive and blame somebody else: "Well, it's not my fault! Somebody tripped me up," or "So-and-so doesn't like me," or "They picked me last." Because the child does not take responsibility for his or her own behavior, the child feels there is nothing that has to change.

When a child makes a mistake, most parents and teachers want the child to accept responsibility for what he or she has done and to try to figure out how to do things differently. But, as long as the child is defensive, he or she will not take responsibility and tends to believe that it is the other person who needs to change. So, as we work with these children in a helping environment, we design techniques and interventions to help them to avoid becoming defensive. If we can develop interventions that don't press the child's button, then the child will be better able to accept responsibility for his or her behavior and make the necessary changes. Therefore, by limiting the number of times we press the child's button, the child can spend more time learning about how to behave better.

Key Points 1

- Due to their fear of being incompetent, anything that points out children's mistakes is going to press their buttons.
- Pressing their buttons makes children defensive.
- When people are defensive, they blame others for their mistakes; because the child believes the misbehavior was not his or her fault, there is nothing for him or her to change.

PUNISHMENT- VERSUS REWARD-BASED SYSTEMS

The two main behavior modification theories can be categorized as either punishment-based systems or reward-based systems. How were most of us raised? What methods do we use in schools? What methods do we use in society? Punishment-based behavior modification principles are widely used and can be effective for most people. Often, parents associate "punishment" with spanking. However, spanking is a technique. More modern techniques include conduct cards, color-coded levels (green, yellow, red), and restricting access to privileges. Think about what these two systems symbolize for a child. I use the chart shown in Figure 4.2 to help parents explore the expectations of each system and what the child "gets" from the adults.

In a punishment-based system, what do you think the expectation is— that the child will behave or that the child will not behave? In a punishment-based system, the expectation tends to be that the child will behave. The reason this is known to be true is that the only time the adult has to intervene is when the child misbehaves. So if I expect a child to pick up his or her shoes, if I expect a child to eat his or her dinner, or if I expect a child to follow what I say in class, the odds are that I am going to leave the child alone, because the child is doing what I expect him or her to do. The only reason I would need to intervene in a punishment-based system is if the child misbehaves. In other words, if a parent says, "Go pick up your toys," and the child picks up eight out of 10, in a punishment-based system the parent would say, "Why did you leave those two out?" Now assume in a punishment-based system that the expectation is that a child is going to do everything she is told to do that day. However, the child performs only

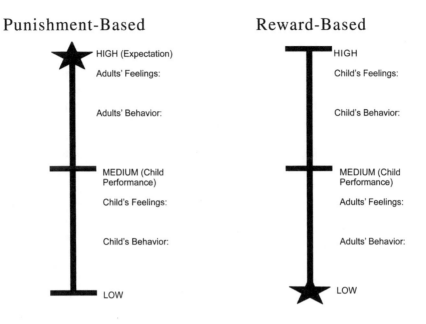

FIGURE 4.2. Punishment- versus reward-based systems.

half-way up to those expectations. As an adult, how are you going to feel? Most parents say, "Well, I get frustrated, I get angry, and I start getting hopeless and more pessimistic about the future." If a parent is feeling that way, he or she is much more likely to be irritable with the child and point out more things that the child is doing wrong. Imagine implementing this approach for 1–2 years, with the child not living up to expectations and possibly misbehaving more. Most adults admit to beginning to feel incompetent in managing the child's behavior. Consider the same system from the child's point of view. If a child is fearful that she is not good, then what is her expectation of herself? High or low? If you said low, then ask yourself this question: What place do such children want to be in at the end of a game? Because of their insecurity about their performance, these children often need to win and expect themselves to be the best. Therefore, what we find is that children experience the same emotions as adults. Most children, believe it or not, want approval from the adults in their lives. So, if a child wants to impress parents or a teacher and is not able to, he or she is going to feel increasingly frustrated and angry. Even the child's own motivation to perform is going to drop. In time, the child may begin to feel incompetent, which, as mentioned earlier, decreases the child's inner desire to perform.

To help you remember the needs of children with disruptive behaviors, I have developed what I call the "three-*A* model." More than anything else, these children seek *approval*. Approval helps to counterbalance a child's fear of incompetence. If the child cannot get approval, then he or she will work for *attention*. Attention is always negative. In other words: "If I can't show you I am good, I will show you I can be really bad." The final *A* is *alone*. Being ignored or left alone is very aversive for these children because to them it confirms their inadequacies. Parents often report that when they ignore a child, the disruptive behavior escalates to a point where they can't ignore it and they have to intervene. Therefore, any system that is not designed to meet children's primary need for approval is not going to be effective.

Punishment-based systems are primarily designed to give the child adult attention—that is, the parent steps in when the child has not done what was expected. Because the child perceives that he or she cannot gain approval, the motivation to perform continues to drop and the behavior worsens. In contrast, a reward-based system is almost the exact opposite. In that system, the parent practically expects the child to misbehave the entire day. The parent wakes up in the morning thinking, "Today is going to be a nightmare. My child is not going to get up when he is supposed to. He is going to fight me about getting out of bed. He is not going to eat breakfast. He is really not going to want to get dressed or brush his teeth and comb his hair. He is going to miss the bus, and I am going to have to drive him to school. I am probably going to have three or four phone calls from the school, and when he gets home, it is going to be another fight to do his homework." These expectations are not spoken out loud, just built into the parent's mind for that day.

In a reward-based system, if the adult's expectations are quite low, and the child complies with some of the parents' requests (as on a punishment-based day), how is the parent going to feel? More optimistic, hopeful, empowered, and confident in his or her own ability as a parent? Because the parent feels that way, he or she is much more likely to be optimistic with the child, and ideally, points out those positive things to the child. This approach also tends to increase the parent's motivation to reengage in parenting, and be more diligent in finding the good things the child is doing. However, if I am a child in this system, imagine what it is like for me when I have my mom or my dad, or maybe even my teacher, pointing out all the great things I am doing. I am much more likely to want to perform for them because I have found a way to receive my primary need for approval and my internal motivation to perform also increases.

Key Points 2

- These children are fearful that they are not good. Therefore, they want to be the "best" at what they do.
- Punishment-based systems point out what the child is not doing, thus only giving them attention.

- Pointing out the child's mistakes makes the child defensive and causes him or her to blame others.
- Reward-based systems point out the good things the child is doing, thus giving the child approval.
- In reward-based systems, because the child is not defensive, he or she is more likely to see what he or she missed and want to correct it.

SELF-CONFIDENCE BUCKET

The final concept considered here is the child's self-confidence. Most children have a healthy degree of self-confidence. However, children with disruptive behaviors tend to be very insecure in their abilities. In order to visualize self-confidence, I use the image of a bucket (Figure 4.3). If you fill up the bucket of a typical child with praise, the child's confidence will rise and he or she will feel empowered. However, for a child with a disruptive temperament, the bucket is much different. This child's bucket is filled with holes. According to Hallowell and Ratey (1994) in their book *Driven to Distraction,* a primary symptom of adult ADHD is "a sense of underachievement regardless of how much one has actually accomplished." This symptom is very descriptive of the level of self-confidence of children with chronic disruptive behavior. Regardless of how well they perform, if they do not win, they do not feel successful. One way to deal with this "bucket full of holes" is to constantly praise the child. Therefore, if a parent gives the child a consistent stream of praise, the bucket will fill, but the minute the parent stops praising, the child's bucket empties and his or her confidence fades. Numerous parents have reported, "I just can't praise him enough! As long as I am praising him, staying on him, and telling him all the great things he is doing, he does fine, but occasionally, I need a break." This approach is ineffective and often leads to parent burnout.

To better illustrate this point consider the analogy of two boys playing baseball: one child is temperamentally disruptive and the other child is a typical laid-back, go-with-the-flow child. Both children go up to bat, and they both hit home runs. Both boys feel great. The next time they go to bat, the laid-back child strikes out, and although he may be disappointed, he still has confidence left over from the previous home run. However, if the child with a disruptive temperament strikes out, most parents indicate the child breaks down emotionally and behaviorally, saying, "I hate this game," "I am never playing again," or "That was not a strike." Therefore, when designing an intervention, the primary goal is to show the child that he or she is successful. If the child feels competent, this will help to "plug up" those holes. When the child's self-confidence is higher, it should be apparent in the child's behavior. For example, when that child strikes out,

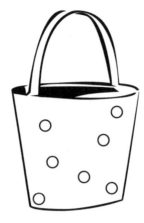

FIGURE 4.3. Self-confidence bucket.

he may still be upset but will not, it is hoped, have a melt-down. That child may even come in second place and not have a temper tantrum.

Key Points 3

- Children may or may not show that they feel insecure.
- The strong-willed or oppositional defiant child tends not to show that he or she feels insecure or incompetent on the inside.
- Occasionally, children with ADHD have their melt-downs and show their inadequacies.
- Generally, anxious/worry-type children frequently show that they feel insecure about their abilities.
- Because these traits are personality characteristics, for the most part these children will probably have them for the rest of their lives.

WORKING WITH PARENTS

When working with children with disruptive temperaments, it is very important not to neglect their parents. Most parents report that they bring many issues into the child's treatment (Harborne, Wolpert, & Claire, 2004). The child may be the identified patient, but the parents often struggle with raising the child.

Kaduson (2000) identifies seven issues that parents bring to their children's treatment. It is important for parents to understand that it is common to struggle in parenting these children. To increase their awareness, parents can simply identify which of the following issues they may be bringing to their child's treatment.

Denial and Vain Hopes

The first thing parents tend to bring to their child's treatment is a combination of denial and vain hopes. Clinicians are familiar with the parent who says, "Oh, I was like that when I was a kid. He's just a little bit hyper. He is going to grow out of it." This attitude can be an obstacle to treatment, just as much as the attitude of the parent who says, "All we have to do is this behavior plan, and he is going to be fine." There is no "magic" pill or technique that will always work. Parenting is a tough job and being a responsible parent is even more difficult. Odds are that such parents are going to struggle with their children's behavior well into adulthood.

Guilt and Inadequacy

Because of their inability to help improve a child's behavior, parents often bring guilt and inadequacy to treatment. These are the parents who blame themselves for their children's behavior problems. They feel badly. They wish they had never had children. They do not know why God gave them a child because they are just such incompetent parents. In time, these parents can become very permissive in their parenting, owing to their lack of self-confidence and self-defeating guilt.

Overinvolvement

Parents who are overinvolved in their child's life are easy to spot. These parents often blame others for the child's behavior and generally feel victimized. However, overinvolvement tends to have a good motive at its source. The parents' desire to shield the child from any kind of hurt tends to be the motive for overinvolvement. Consequently, in shielding a child from hurt, what the parent is also shielding him or her from is the valuable learning of lessons they get when they experience hurt or painful feelings. This can also signal to the child that he or she cannot solve the problem on his or her own and needs outside help. Involvement in the child's life is a great thing, overinvolvement not so much.

Fears and Worries

Fears and worries are often expressed by parents, which can also become an obstacle to progress. If parents have mapped out the next 10 or 15 years of their child's life, and it involves juvenile detention, failing, teenage pregnancy, or runaways, the parents may note such fears and worries to be discussed in their child's treatment. The problem with parenting out of fear is that the parent usually gets the very thing that he or she feared the most! Reassurance on the part of the therapist and seeing that the techniques are effective are great allies against fears and worries.

Emotional Bankruptcy

Emotional bankruptcy is very common. Many of the parents whom I work with often initially report that they are completely drained, they just do not have anything left in them to give to the child. This difficulty is similar to burnout, but is specific to the child and directly affects parenting.

Feeling Attacked and Not Understood

The next thing that parents tend to bring to treatment is a sense of being attacked and not understood by others, such as school personnel and in-laws. When a child is having a behavior problem, teachers may ask a parent, "Is there something going on at home?," and in-laws may be ready to step in: "You give him to me for one weekend, and I'll straighten him out." The reality is that most people do not understand how difficult it is to manage these types of children.

Anger and Resentment

Anger and resentment tend to be the end of the road for most parents. They may be angry at God for giving them a child like this, angry at professionals for not being able to help, angry at teachers for not being able to teach their child, and generally angry at the child for being the way he or she is. Hopelessness and waiting too long to seek treatment tend to be contributors to these emotions. These issues make it very difficult for a parent to find the motivation to enter treatment or to gain tools in parent training.

THE MAIN REASONS WHY CHILDREN MISBEHAVE

When parents bring their child to treatment, I have found that they often ask, "Why does he (or she) act that way?" There are several factors that can influence a child's behavior. Kaduson (2000) offers several dynamics (as listed in Figure 4.4) for parents to evaluate in order to better understand

1. Child characteristics
   a. Activity level   1 2 3 4 5 6 7 8 9 10
   b. Attention span   1 2 3 4 5 6 7 8 9 10
   c. Impulse control   1 2 3 4 5 6 7 8 9 10
   d. Emotionality   1 2 3 4 5 6 7 8 9 10
   e. Sociability   1 2 3 4 5 6 7 8 9 10
   f. Response to stimulation   1 2 3 4 5 6 7 8 9 10
   g. Habit regularity   1 2 3 4 5 6 7 8 9 10
   h. Physical characteristics   1 2 3 4 5 6 7 8 9 10
   i. Developmental abilities   1 2 3 4 5 6 7 8 9 10

2. Parental characteristics

3. Family stress
   a. Parents' emotional control   1 2 3 4 5 6 7 8 9 10
   b. Parental perceptions   1 2 3 4 5 6 7 8 9 10
   c. Direct effects on child   1 2 3 4 5 6 7 8 9 10

4. Learning history

FIGURE 4.4. The main reasons why children misbehave.

what motivates children's behavior. It may also be helpful for both parents to score independently, as the child may behave differently with each parent. I usually review each characteristic with the parent(s) and ask each one to evaluate every trait on a scale of 1–10, rating their child in general.

Child Characteristics

This section covers several factors that can influence a child's behavior. When reviewing these with parents, I explain each factor independently and give the parent(s) time to score from 1–10.

Activity Level

Activity level is the general level of physical energy or activity that the child demonstrates. Thus, a low number on this scale (1, 2, or 3) may indicate a child who is not active at all. This is a child whom you really have to get started because he or she does not have energy derived from the motivation to do things. A 9–10 on this scale may indicate a child who is incredibly active. From the moment of waking until the child goes to bed, he or she is always on the go.

Attention Span

Attention span reflects the child's ability to concentrate regardless of interest level. A low number on this scale suggests a child who is very easily distracted, even from things that he or she enjoys. A high number on this scale indicates a child who, regardless of what he or she is doing, even if it is something boring, can maintain concentration.

Impulse Control

Impulse control consists of the child's ability to manage and control his or her behavior. A high number on this scale indicates a child who thinks before he or she acts. This child learns quickly from consequences and typically does not need to be told more than once not to do something. A low number on this scale is typical of a child who tends not to learn from consequences and frequently does things without thinking about them (even when consequences have consistently been applied).

Emotionality

Emotionality basically reflects the child's ability to regulate and express emotions. A low number on this scale indicates a child who really does not show any emotions or does not express them. This is a child who is very flat in affect, and it is difficult to tell when the child is happy, sad, or mad. A high number on this scale indicates an unduly hypersensitive child, when he or she is angry, everybody knows it, and when the child is happy, everybody knows it as well.

Sociability

Sociability reflects how social the child is. Thus, a low number on this scale indicates a child who prefers to be by him- or herself, does not like being in groups, and tends not to feel comfortable when he or she is around people. The high end of this scale suggests a child who regards no one as a stranger, loves being in large crowds, and whose batteries are charged when he or she is around others.

Response to Stimulation

A low number on response to stimulation (1, 2, or 3) indicates a child whom you almost have to "crank start." This child does not get excited easily, even for something he or she seems to enjoy; the child drags on and has to build up momentum. A high number on this scale suggests that all you have to do is say the word, and this child is ready to go.

Habit Regularity

Habit regularity reflects the child's need for a routine or schedule. A low number on this scale indicates a child who does not need a routine, does not need a ritual, is very flexible, and will go with the flow. A high number on this scale is typical of a child who needs ritual, who does not like it when things change, even something as simple as a departure from, "We always have chicken nuggets every Monday." Even moving the furniture may upset this child.

Physical Characteristics

Physical characteristics include anything, whether it is an advance or a delay, that distinguishes the child physically from other children. There may be nothing to score in this area, but it would include things like "My child has a hearing aid" or "He's overweight for his age" or, perhaps, "She's taller (or shorter) than the majority of kids in her class."

Developmental Abilities

Developmental abilities include advances, as well as developmental delays, that make the child different from other children his or her age. Maybe the child is better coordinated or less coordinated. Maybe he or she is a better reader or a worse reader. This trait includes anything in the child's development that you would say separates this child from other children of the same age.

Parental Characteristics

The second section of the chart is parental characteristics. Reviewing parental characteristics allows parents to develop some insight into their parenting styles. I typically ask parents, "Take a few moments to write down words that you would say best describe your parenting style. Remember, do this for yourself and not for your spouse." It is usually a lot easier for a husband or wife to describe the other parent, but I want each of the parents to think about how he or she manages the children and what words would best describe his or her own style. Words that some parents have used include "permissive," "drill sergeant," "strict," "rigid," "absent parent," and "parenting out of guilt or fear."

Family Stress

Family stress, the third contributor to children's behavior, consists of three subcategories.

Parents' Emotional Control

A low number on this scale indicates parents who do not have much control over their emotions and may feel that their emotions are in control of them. So, if such a parent is angry or is sad or is happy, everybody knows it. Even when it is best to show a little restraint, these parents have a hard time. A high-end number on this scale indicates parents who have almost too much control over their emotions. You never know how they feel because they tend to be so flat in their affect.

Parental Perceptions

The next item on the chart is the parents' true perceptions of the child. It is important that parents are given permission to put negative items in this section. Most parents report, "My child is a joy," "She is a blessing," or "I am so fortunate to have him." But it is also OK to admit that, at times, the child can be frustrating and annoying. Ask parents to take a few moments to write down their true perceptions of their child.

Direct Effects on the Child

The last subcategory consists of things that have happened within the family that the parents think have had a direct effect on the child. These can be both positive and negative events. An example of a positive thing may be eating dinner as a family every night. An example of a negative event may be the separation of the child's parents or their divorce. Negative events can also include deaths in the family or frequent moves. The parents should include all the things that they believe have had a direct effect on the child.

Learning History

The final contributor to the child's behavior is learning history. This includes anything the child has learned within the home (such as on television), or outside the home, that the parent did not necessarily want him or her to learn. It can include things like the meaning of the "middle finger," inappropriate websites, and curse words. Obviously, parents are not going to be able to write down everything because there are too many examples.

Children have learned all kinds of things at home and in the larger world that we may or may not have wanted them to learn. So, in this section, parents are to write down a few examples of these behaviors.

Of the four items on the list, which two would parents say are the main reasons why children naturally misbehave? Most parents pick item 2, parental characteristics, and item 3, family stress. However, the main reasons why children *naturally* misbehave are item 1, the child's natural temperament, and item 4, the child's learning history. Most parents do not teach their children bad things, but a child's natural temperament can lend itself to behavioral problems. If the child ranks at 10 on activity level, that child is naturally going to misbehave because he or she is so active. If the child ranks very low on attention span, that child is naturally going to misbehave because he or she cannot concentrate. If the child ranks very low on impulse control, the child is naturally going to misbehave because he or she does not stop and think and tends not to learn from consequences. So the parent can breathe a sigh of relief learning that the predominant reason why the child misbehaves is usually a combination of the child's natural temperament with his or her learning history.

Therefore, if 1 and 4 are the main contributors to why children misbehave, 2 and 3 must be the main contributors to why children can behave. This is really good news because on this list, 2 and 3 are the only things we can truly change. A child's natural temperament is what he or she was born with, and parents are not allowed to lock their children in the basement and shield them from the effects of society. But a parent can change his or her parenting style, and a parent can change the family stress, which can have a powerful impact on modifying a child's behavior.

Thus, a child who is naturally a 10 will probably never, barring some kind of brain injury, go to being a 1 or 2. However, parents can shape a child's behavior to the point at which they may rate the child as a 6 or a 7. Most parents say, "I can handle a 6. I just can't handle a 10." Or, "I can handle a 5. I just can't handle a 1."

GOALS OF TREATMENT

When designing a treatment program for a child with a disruptive temperament, the goals of treatment should be clear. Because such children have an inward sense of insecurity and incompetence, the first goal of any treatment plan should be to help the child succeed. Kaduson (2000) offers the following components to a successful treatment plan. After each component, I have included an intervention that the mental health professional can implement to greatly improve the effectiveness of treatment.

Have the Child Succeed

As you devise interventions, the primary goal is to make sure that those interventions are success-oriented. Fortunately, reward-based behavior modification systems can meet this need.

Intervention: Reward-Based Play Therapy

The primary "reward" for children with disruptive behaviors is approval. Therefore, during their time together the therapist points out specific behaviors of the child that are acceptable. Pointing out specific behaviors, such as "You hit the center of that target" versus indiscriminate praise like "Great job" can be more beneficial for enhancing the child's self-concept. For young children, it can be helpful to provide tangible "proof" of approval throughout the session; examples are small tokens, tickets, or stickers. The therapist gives these out frequently as a sign to the child that he or she was successful. I typically do not recommend allowing children to "turn in" their stickers or tickets for secondary rewards, but suggest allowing them to simply brag to parents or others about how many tickets they receive. You can also keep track of the number of stickers by placing them on a chart so that a child can see his or her improvement. I also recommend that parents be taught similar techniques to use at home so that the child can get their approval as well.

Build Self-Esteem

The second goal of a treatment program is to build the child's self-esteem. Some research indicates that the psychological, educational, and behavioral impacts of these conditions lead to long-term impacts on self-confidence (Molina et al., 2009). So any treatment program needs to focus on the fact that these children need to have their self-esteem enhanced. The best way to do that is to point out the good things they do. In my opinion, simply praising a child in the absence of good behavior does little to impact self-confidence. Having the child see that he or she can *do* good things seems to impact his or her confidence more that verbal encouragement alone.

Intervention: Punch Cards

The use of punch cards can be an effective technique in a variety of settings. Both parents and teachers have reported that this simple intervention has proven effective with individuals and in group settings. The therapist simply draws graphics on 3 × 5 index cards and gives a card to the child.

Graphics typically include smiley faces, stars, or circles. A punch card can have as many graphics on it as the therapist deems appropriate. Typically, each card includes at least 10 graphics. Either in session or at home, the adult punches out one of the graphics for each good behavior. Once the child has received all of his or her punches, the child can hang up the card where people can see it. A tip that I learned early on is for the adult to obtain a specialty hole punch so that children are not able to punch out the graphics themselves with a standard hole punch. It is not uncommon for a child to lose a punch card. Simply give the child another one, but do not punch out the punches obtained previously. This holds the child accountable for losing the card and gives him or her an immediate opportunity to earn approval.

Teach On-Task Behavior

The next area to be addressed is teaching on-task behavior. Children with disruptive temperaments are notoriously off-track. Whether a task is something they enjoy or something they are somewhat bored with, they tend to be distracted very easily. Helping a child to build impulse control skills so that he or she can focus and concentrate is beneficial.

Intervention: Therapeutic Game Playing

Therapeutic game playing can be effective for a variety of treatment conditions. The first thing you need to decide is what skill to teach. For instance, suppose you want to teach a young boy impulse control. Then simply select a game that requires that particular skill in order to win. Examples include "Pick-Up Sticks" and "Red Light/Green Light." Next invite the child to play. Because children with disruptive temperaments are naturally competitive and enjoy winning, they often respond favorably. Prior to initiating this technique, prepare for the child to win, *but* keep the game competitive so that the child stays engaged. As the game begins, invite the child to go first in order to engage him in the intervention and lower his defenses. Observe the child's play and pay close attention to any incidents of being off-task. Once the child's turn is over, imitate the child's behavior that has caused him to lose a turn (or to be otherwise penalized) and simply announce the mistake out loud, using a casual tone—for example, "Oh man, I lost track of what I was doing," "I got too excited." Continue playing the game in this manner while imitating the child's off-task behavior, announcing the behavior out loud. However, also begin to demonstrate positive coping strategies and express these out loud as well—for example, saying to yourself, "OK, Scott, pay attention, pay attention." The primary thing you are looking for is the child's beginning to imitate your behavior. By using this technique, you are indirectly teaching the child the skill without having to point out his mistakes in the game. The reason this technique is very effective is that young children learn easily through observation and imitation. Remember to keep game competitive so that the child remains engaged. Examples of games that can be used are "Concentration," card games, and board games involving taking turns.

Teach Self-Control

The fourth goal of a treatment program should be self-control. As discussed earlier, a child may be rated very low in the impulse control skill area. A treatment program can provide ways to help the child learn to stop and think and learn self-discipline.

Intervention: Therapeutic Game Playing

See description above. Examples of games to play are "Pick-Up Sticks," "Jenga," and "Red Light/Green Light," and "Simon Says."

Channel Aggression Appropriately

Another aim of a treatment program should be helping the child channel aggression appropriately. The reason that children with disruptive behaviors get very frustrated really makes sense. For instance, if all a little girl really wants to do is show Mom and Dad and her teacher that she is a good person, but she is in a punishment-based system that points out the things she does not do well, then in time that child is going to become frustrated and aggravated because she is not able to reach her goal. Frustration and aggravation often lead to aggression in young children.

Intervention: "Shake 'Em Up"

The "Shake 'Em Up" intervention is very helpful for children who externalize their anger and are generally aggressive. The supplies needed for this activity include an empty clear water bottle, children's paint, marbles, and superglue. Begin the activity by explaining to the child that anger is a normal emotion and that some children find that letting that anger out of their bodies helps them to feel better. Fill up the bottle three-quarters of the way with water, and then ask the child to pick a paint color that reminds her either of anger or of being relaxed. Once the child selects the color, allow her to pour a small amount of her color selection into the bottle. Next ask the child to pick between five and ten marbles, and encourage her to place the marbles into the bottle as well. After the paint and marbles are placed in the bottle, carefully put a small amount of superglue on the inside of the cap and tighten the cap onto the bottle; this helps to ensure that the contents stay in the bottle (and that parents stay happy). The game that can be played with this activity is called "Shake 'Em Up." Set a timer for 1 minute, and challenge the child to shake the bottle as hard as she can until the buzzer goes off. Once the buzzer goes off, I find that the child is exhausted and smiling—all at the same time. This activity helps the child to externalize his or her anger in an appropriate manner, as well as to metabolize the adrenaline produced when the child becomes angry. I have also found that the majority of school counselors are very receptive to keeping shake 'em up bottles in their offices for children to use when necessary.

Allow Expression of Anger through Play

The next thing a treatment program should do is help the child channel his or her anger. As discussed earlier, these children often become annoyed when they do not come in at first place. Unfortunately, always coming in first place is not a reality for most children. There will be times when they lose or are not as successful as they want to be. Therefore, designing a program to help a child channel this anger and frustration can be beneficial, especially if it utilizes the child's natural language, which is play.

Intervention: Being the Boss

In this intervention, inform the child that he can "be the boss" for the entire session. My primary training is in cognitive-behavioral theory so I use the overt intervention of "Being the Boss" to remind myself to switch my skill sets to those of child-centered play therapy. Use basic, nondirective play therapy skills (Axline, 1974) such as tracking and attending, and encourage the child to express him- or herself openly during this time. The only limits set are those that ensure the safety of both child and therapist. For example, "We can do pretty much whatever you want to do as long as it is not dangerous or destructive." Define these words, but allow some latitude in your definition. Common experiences I have had during this "boss time" include being given time-outs, being fired, and playing the indentured servant. This intervention allows the child an opportunity to express his or her anger within predefined limits that help to ensure the safety of both parties. I frequently teach this intervention to parents and encourage them to give their child 5 minutes of boss time every other day. This helps the child to see that he or she does not have to fight his or her parents for "the power," because it will be given to him or her a few times a week. It also helps the child to work out his or her emotions toward a parent, *with* that parent.

Practice Patience

The next part of treatment is helping children to practice patience. Most young children find it difficult to delay gratification. They want what they want, when they want it, and what color they want it in. What I have tried to do is design a program that helps the children learn the value of delaying gratification or to save up now for something better later on.

Intervention: Domino Stacking

I have always been fascinated by those contests that encourage an individual to stack a sequence of dominoes that will fall in a specific order once the first one is knocked down. This intervention not only helps a child to develop patience but also improves the child's self-control. Suppose you are working with a 6-year-old girl. Divide a standard pack of dominoes between the players (you and the little girl), and follow the rules of the game as outlined here: Each player is given 14 or more dominoes; the child is given the opportunity to go first and stack one of her dominoes on the table vertically. The therapist then has to place a domino either in front or behind the domino that the child placed, making sure that it is close enough to make the other one fall. The child then places another one of her dominoes either in front or behind one of the dominoes that are already in place. If at any time during the game the dominoes fall, the game starts over. Once both players have placed all their dominoes, the child is given the opportunity to knock down the first domino on either end. If all the dominoes do not fall, the game starts over. The purpose of this intervention is to help the child to develop the impulse control that is necessary to be successful, and to teach patience in a frustrating activity. You can model positive self-talk during the game, as well as offer frequent praise and encouragement.

Help Problem–Solve through Play

The final aim of any treatment program is to help children develop problem-solving skills. Schaefer and Drewes (2011) indicate one of the inherent qualities of play is to help children learn problem-solving skills. Children with attention and impulse-control issues can be very creative problem solvers, but they may not be very functional. A story of one of the children I have worked with in the past can help illustrate this point. This was a child whose parents had given him a key to let himself into the house when he got home every day after school. Within a year of doing this, the child had lost three or four keys because he had forgotten them or misplaced them. Of course, it was somebody else's fault. One day, the child got home and realized that he had once again lost the key. The last thing he wanted to do was to call his parents because he knew he was going to hear a lecture about his having screwed up again. He remembered that his father had recently used a glass cutter to cut some glass, so he went into the garage and found his dad's tool chest. He took the glass cutter, went to his bedroom window, and cut out a little half-moon above the lock. He poked it through with his knuckle, turned the lock, and let himself into the house. He was so excited about what he had done that he could not wait for Mom and Dad to come home. He greeted them at the door with, "I've got good news and bad news. The bad news is I've lost the key, but the good news is I've found a way to let myself in the house without having to call you." He excitedly took his mom and dad into his bedroom and showed them how he did it. Unfortunately, Mom and Dad thought it was not a great plan, because not only had he let himself into the house, but he had left the window open for other people to get in as well! Any treatment program should consist of helping a child to develop functional problem-solving skills. A great opportunity for this is within their play.

Intervention: Ask the Expert

I have found that most people are effective at solving other people's problems but often get stuck when they are in similar situations. In the "Ask the Expert" activity, a young boy, for example, is given an opportunity to explore his current dilemma from "the expert" perspective. To set up this activity, write the child's problem on an index card and place it in the center of the room. Then help the child to figure out his current perspective on the problem and write that on the card—for example, "I don't know what to do." Then place that card on the floor a few feet away from the problem card. Direct the child to either stand or sit behind his current perspective card and help the child to explore his thoughts, feelings, and options. Once the child has explored this perspective, invite the child to explore his problem from another perspective. Then write "The Expert" on a card and place that card a few feet away from the center card, but on the other side of the room. Direct the child to stand or sit behind the expert card. The therapist may provide costumes or props to help the child to dress or act the part so that he can fully embrace this perspective. Then encourage the child to explore his thoughts, feelings, and options from this perspective. Next, write on a card all of the options the child expresses, helping him to brainstorm as much as possible. Once the child has identified several options, ask him to select the one or two options he is willing to implement. After the child has selected his choice(s), explore ways to build in accountability for completion—for example, e-mailing the therapist when completed, behavior charting, or leaving a voicemail.

SUMMARY AND CONCLUSIONS

Although dealing with children who have disruptive temperaments can be challenging, using the method described here can bring about positive change in a child's life. In a perfect world the therapist would also train the child's parents and teacher in this method, so that all of the adults are on the same page. Techniques will have to be modified for each setting, so I encourage you to develop your own interventions that focus on acknowledging the child's successes. However, if you are unable to engage parents and/or teachers in this method, do not get discouraged. Even one person in the child's life who gives him or her a place where he or she is acknowledged and accepted can have a profound impact on that child's future. I hope that this information has given you some insight into how these children see the world. In applying this method, I hope you find the success and fulfillment you are looking for in your work with children.

REFERENCES

American Psychiatric Association. (2013). *Diagnostic and statistical manual of mental disorders* (5th ed.). Arlington, VA: Author.

Axline, V. M. (1974). *Play therapy*. New York: Ballantine Books.

Dickstein, D. P. (2010, May). Oppositional defiant disorder. *Journal of the American Academy of Child and Adolescent Psychiatry, 49*(5), 435–436.

Flick, G. L. (1996). *Power parenting for children with ADD/ADHD*. West Nyack, NY: Center for Applied Research in Education.

Hallowell, E. M., & Ratey, J. (1994). *Driven to distraction*. New York: Pantheon Books.

Harborne, A., Wolpert, M., & Clare, L. (2004). Making sense of ADHD: A battle for understanding parents' views of their children being diagnosed with ADHD. *Clinical Child Psychology and Psychiatry, 9*(3), 327–339.

Hinshaw, S. P., & Lee, S. S. (2003). Conduct and oppositional defiant disorders. In E. J. Mash & R. A. Barkley (Eds.), *Child psychopathology* (pp. 144–198). New York: Guilford Press.

Kaduson, H. (2000). *Play therapy for children with ADHD*. Workshop presented in New Orleans, LA.

Molina, B. S., Hinshaw, S. P., Swanson, J. M., Arnold, L. E., Vitiello, B., Jensen, P. S., et al. (2009, May). The MTA at 8 years: Prospective follow-up of children treated for combined-type ADHD in a multisite study. *Journal of the American Academy of Child and Adolescent Psychiatry, 48*(5), 484–500.

Rader, R., McCauley, L., & Callen, E. C. (2009, April 15). Current strategies in the diagnosis and treatment of childhood attention-deficit/hyperactivity disorder. *American Family Physician, 79*(8), 657–665.

Schaefer, C. E., & Drewes, A. A. (2011). The therapeutic powers of play and play therapy. In C. E. Schaefer (Ed.), *Foundations of play therapy* (2nd ed., pp. 15–26). Hoboken, NJ: Wiley.

Chapter 5

&

Short-Term Trauma Resolution by Combining Art and Play Therapy for Children

Terry Pifalo
Sarah Hamil

*T*he combined modalities of art and play therapy create a unique treatment option for short-term trauma resolution for children. In young children imaginal representation dominates thought, determines affect, influences behavior, contributes to cognition, and promotes the assimilation of traumatic material (Lusebrink, 1990). When the imagery inspired by art therapy is paired with the power of expressive play therapy, where objects provide a concrete means for manipulation, role play, and kinesthetic movement, a powerful catalytic bond is formed. The interaction between the two therapies creates a synergistic pairing that has multiple benefits.

Drawings, painting, sculptures, and other art expressions depict the child's understanding of life events and experiences in a way that is visual and tangible (Hamil, 2011; Pifalo, 2009). The trauma can be portrayed in the images, and then the art product can serve as a reference in constructing a coherent narrative. The use of both art and play therapy in conjunction provides an opportunity for the child to explore his or her traumatic experience through creative expression. Through the art, the child has "the opportunity to step back and evaluate the meaning of his subjective art expressions" (Linesch, 1993, p. 26).

It has become clear in the 20-plus years since trauma-focused cognitive-behavioral therapy was developed (Cohen, Mannarino, & Deblinger, 2006; Deblinger, McLeer, & Henry, 1990) that children respond very differently to therapy than adults do. The element of play has become a crucial ingredient in engaging children in the therapy process (Briggs, Runyon, & Deblinger, 2011, p. 169). Combining play and play-based techniques such as art therapy can help the child digest difficult and emotion-laden trauma material more easily. In fact, the two modalities can become a sort of "enzyme" (Goodyear-Brown, 2010) that serves to dissolve the painful connection to traumatic memories, thereby easing the discomfort and increasing the control and confidence within the child. This pairing of art and play therapy creates an atmosphere where laughter, playful competition, pride, and feelings of connection with others can thrive, paving the way for effective and efficient trauma-focused treatment.

GETTING THE BIG PICTURE

The experience of childhood trauma has the potential to interrupt the child's ability to function in all developmental domains. When the child's understanding of physical and emotional safety has been shattered, the turmoil may be safely expressed in the art he or she creates. This expression of trauma through imagery then provides a base upon which to construct therapeutic objectives. There is enhanced potential for positive outcomes for trauma victims when play therapists integrate art modalities into the therapeutic process. One of the core features of trauma occurs in the reexperiencing of the traumatic event. Reexperiencing or flashbacks often take the form of chaotic and fragmented memories that are confusing and disorienting for the child. The trauma victim has problems orienting him- or herself in time and space, which may lead him or her to respond to his or her environment with high levels of anxiety, exhibiting hypervigilance, and an exaggerated hyperstartle reaction. The visual nature of traumatic memories invites the use of art in the creative process, allowing children to "speak" about the trauma without having to use words, thus reducing their anxiety.

Although many children experience stressful situations such as divorce or the death of a beloved relative, these stressors generally do not rise to the level of a traumatic event. Features that comprise a traumatic event include sudden and unexpected events that are of a shocking nature—for example, death and/or a threat to life or bodily integrity. These traumatic events engender subjective feelings of intense terror, horror, or helplessness (American Psychiatric Association, 2013). Events associated with childhood trauma would include physical or sexual abuse; witnessing or being a victim of domestic violence; community or school violence; severe motor vehicle or other accidents; potentially life-threatening illnesses such as cancer, burns, or organ transplantation; exposure to natural disasters; the sudden death of a parent, sibling, or peer; and exposure to war or terrorism.

Not all children, of course, develop traumatic symptoms even after experiencing such events. Many factors, including the child's developmental level at the time of the trauma, his or her inherent or learned resiliency, and his or her external sources of support, also impact which children will develop difficulties, and to what degree these difficulties will impact his or her future. Each child's constitution, temperament, strengths, sensitivities, attachments, abilities, and the reactions of his or her significant family members—all contribute to how the child experiences and manages a potentially traumatizing event. Trauma symptoms in children refer to the behavioral, cognitive, physical, and emotional difficulties that are directly related to the traumatic experience.

Trauma symptoms directly related to the trauma experience are generally divided into the following categories: emotional, cognitive, behavioral, and physical. Dividing the symptoms in this way is consistent with the "cognitive coping triangle" (Deblinger & Heflin, 1996), a model that helps the child to see the critical relationship between feelings, thoughts, and behaviors, and more importantly, understand how changing thoughts can lead to changing feelings, thoughts, and behaviors. For the purpose of this design, the therapeutic goals and tasks in each session also strive to reinforce this connection.

THE VISUAL NATURE
OF ENCODING TRAUMATIC EXPERIENCES

Due to the dissociation of the memories of traumatic experiences and the resulting disruption of the traumatized child's ability to translate feeling states into words—a state referred to as "alexithymia"—gaining access to traumatic events is exceedingly difficult. According to research, this difficulty may be due not only to psychological defenses, but also to the neurological processes responsible for the actual coding of such events (Johnson, 1987). Much evidence suggests that humans have two forms of memory encoding: one is a primitive, visually based memory that records an event as a whole in its exact detail; the second form of memory is based on coding experience according to a hierarchical system of constituent parts, so that each memory is really a reconstruction derived from common elements (Penfield & Perot, 1963).

In times of overwhelming stimulation, the more highly developed cognitive system is temporarily by-passed and traumatic events are recorded in a "photographic" form. This global record is unlikely to be integrated conceptually with other memories through normal, associative links. For these reasons the child's memory of the trauma may not be available to be processed, worked through, or transformed, as are other aspects of memory. Therefore, art and play therapy are uniquely suited to gain access to traumatic images and memories. Because the encoding of traumatic memories are of a photographic nature, a visual modality and a kinesthetic approach such as art and play therapy may offer a more efficient and nonthreatening means of bringing traumatic information into the child's consciousness. In fact, there is precedent for using drawings and play to obtain this type of information (Greenberg & van der Kolk, 1987). Kaduson and Schaefer (2009) asserted "because play is the language of the child, it allows the child to 'speak' to us without words" (p. 10). When the child engages in play therapy infinite possibilities emerge to develop skills in communication, problem solving, and functional coping for life challenges (Kaduson & Schaefer, 2009; Drewes, Bratton, & Schaefer, 2011). The child uses art and play to "speak" about the memory fragments through drawings, role play, and any number of creative expressions.

As previously mentioned, trauma symptoms may include the following: affective, behavioral, cognitive, complex posttraumatic stress disorder (PTSD), and psychological symptoms. (Cohen, Mannarino, & Deblinger, 2006, p. 6). Common affective trauma symptoms may include fear, depression, anger, and rapid mood changes. Depressive feelings after a trauma may arise from a sudden loss of trust in other people and the world in general. Also, because children typically have an egocentric view of the world, they may blame themselves for the traumatic event, and this self-blame has the potential to create further negative affect such as guilt, shame, low self-esteem, and feelings of worthlessness.

When children originally attempt to ameliorate these kinds of painful feelings, they may develop maladaptive behaviors such as avoidance of thoughts, people, places, or situations that trigger memories of the initial trauma. Although avoidance is initially used as a coping mechanism to escape uncomfortable feelings, the dependency on this effect can lead to a constriction of appropriate positive activities. When the strategy of avoidance eventually becomes less successful, a child may develop emotional numbing and in severe cases dissociation—a form of psychological adaptation employed by the child to wall off the trauma from conscious awareness and memory, as if it never happened.

Childhood trauma can also result in maladaptive thinking and distorted cognitions such as "I am worthless," "I am a bad person," "I will never be OK," and/or "This is all my fault." In a misguided attempt to find a cause for what has happened to him, the child may fall into a pattern of irrational thinking. Using this maladaptive strategy, the child may conclude that he or she in fact "deserved" the trauma to occur, thus allowing his or her external world to remain a safe and predictable place. The child sees him- or herself as "bad," not the world, as he or she must create somewhere, however inaccurate, that is safe and secure. Dhaese (2011) discussed the cognitive distortions associated with repeated or long-term trauma: "The child is left with destructive messages, such as that he is not good enough, or if he were perfect there would be no problem and he would be safe" (p. 79).

Childhood trauma may also result in psychological ramifications. Children's brains and bodies are intricately involved in the development of emotions, cognitions, and behaviors. Therefore traumatic events, especially those of long-term duration, have the potential to alter actual brain function (Cohen et al., 2006, p. 14). Combating self-destructive thoughts and behaviors requires interventions that engage the child on multiple sensory levels such as the use of art in play therapy. Hass-Cohen and Carr (2008) asserted: "The artwork can be an expression of several types of memories as it engages multiple cognitive and perceptual neural pathways processes. The serious play of the art process updates memories, and supports a broader and more flexible personal agency" (p. 172).

Because the long- and short-term effects of childhood trauma are so prevalent, and the funds available to combat them are increasingly limited, it is imperative that mental health professionals devise an effective and efficient method for delivering quality treatment to this population. The design of this treatment model must be systematic, theoretically driven, empirically grounded, and relatively brief.

SHORT-TERM TRAUMA TREATMENT IN CHILDHOOD

Combining the unique properties of art therapy and play therapy creates a dynamic, synergistic pairing—a powerful antidote with which to combat the varied and insidious effects of childhood trauma and its collateral consequences. The proposed design described in this chapter outlines a 10-week cycle of group therapy for children ages 6–12 who have experienced some type of traumatic event (see Table 5.1). Each of the weekly segments has a clear therapeutic goal. The trauma symptoms—affective, behavioral, cognitive, physical, or emotional—dictate the directives. Art and play therapy interventions then combine or work as "co-catalysts" to facilitate the accomplishment of these goals. Furthermore, the art and play from each session can be integrated into concurrent family therapy or separated into individual interactions outside of session.

TABLE 5.1. Design Model for Short-Term Trauma Resolution by Combining Art in Play Therapy

Week	Treatment objective	Therapeutic goal	Art and play Interventions
1	Introduction to group	Establish cohesion in a safe therapeutic environment	• Puzzle play • Puzzle mandala
2	Affective identification	Establish emotional literacy	• Play Feeling Detectives • Create Feelings Folder
3	Affective processing	Develop skills in self-expression	• Create Feelings Boxes • Play My Move
4	Developing coping skills	Practice focused breathing and relaxation	• Belly breathing • Play Flying Feathers
5	Parent–caregiver collaboration; including caregivers in group	Take beginning steps in sharing trauma experiences	• Role play and self-soothing puppet play
6	Practicing the trauma narrative	Lay the groundwork for mapping trauma	• Mapping practice and Chalk Walk
7	Creating the trauma narrative	Map the trauma experience	• Trauma Map • Lost and Found
8	Processing the trauma narrative	Share the trauma experience	• Trauma Narrative • Hidden Treasures
9	Identifying sources of support	Name personal resources	• Create Strings of Strength and Role Play
10	Risk reduction and termination; including caregivers in group	Establish personal boundaries and safety as group ends	• Draw a Safe Space and Play Hula Hoops

The use of art in play therapy accommodates all of the child's physical and psychological systems generally impacted by trauma. Through the use of this combined treatment model, the child has the opportunity to process his or her trauma on multiple levels and address his or her complex array of symptoms. Childhood trauma requires that treatment begin with attention to safety and support. This first task must address the fear and ambivalence in the child and family regarding the potential for recovery and the recovery of a coherent sense of self. Through the creative processes in art and play therapy, the child and family gradually rediscover that positive experiences in life are possible. The primary objective of integrating art into play therapy is to provide strategies for coping through personal imagery and "gently moving the client's narrative into more cognitive and less emotionally intense aspects of whatever is under discussion" (Briere & Scott, 2006, p. 96).

Week 1: Introduction to Group—Establishing a Safe Therapeutic Environment and Group Cohesion

The goal of the first session is to establish rapport and create a safe and trusting therapeutic environment—a kind of sanctuary that will provide a safe space where the traumatized child can begin to regain and maintain his or her emotional equilibrium. Following a traumatic event, the child may feel vulnerable and see the world now as an unsafe place. Herman (1992) pointed out that "sharing the traumatic experience with others is a precondition for restitution of a sense of a meaningful world" (p. 70). The child becomes a member of a productive, creative group with other children who have experienced a traumatic event, providing an opportunity for the child to begin the healing process in connection with others.

Using art materials always contains an element of play, so an art and play therapy group has the potential to incorporate the fun aspect of play to quickly create a child-friendly atmosphere. Children tend to feel at home in a play setting, and they readily relate to toys and art materials. Another essential component of the art imagery and the play behavior is the potential for very personal creative expression in the healing process. The child is invited to manipulate or manage the play, which prompts the development of individualized problem-solving skills and the ability to cope with challenges throughout the treatment cycle.

To foster rapid engagement in the first session, putting a colorful, age-appropriate puzzle in the hands of a child makes perfect sense. This familiar toy serves as a metaphor for the entire therapeutic process. Puzzles are available in limitless formats, but the clinician should chose one based on the developmental and emotional needs of the child. A purposeful strategy is to include images of baby animals such as puppies, kittens, fawns, and foals to establish a sense of relatedness and empathy. The rule of thumb for this Week 1 task is to select a puzzle with enough pieces for each member of the group to have one or more pieces. The group leader should also have at least one piece of the puzzle, establishing a collaborative role in describing each of the individual pieces and the connection of these pieces into a cohesive picture. To begin the group, the therapist presents the puzzle as a whole with all the pieces assembled. The group then discusses the imagery in the puzzle. The leader then explains to the group that the puzzle will be taken apart, and then put back together with each member taking part in the reassembly.

As the puzzle is taken apart, the therapist gains insight into each child's style of interaction—important information for informing future treatment goals. For example, more impulsive children may grab extra pieces, preventing other children from having enough, or withdrawn and anxious children may become emotional during the disassembly. Regardless of the group dynamics, the children have the opportunity to work therapeutically using the puzzle pieces, and at the same time to learn to negotiate and accept each other's styles. Then each child has an opportunity to describe his or her own piece of the puzzle, and to place it where it connects with the whole picture. Each group member takes his or her turn putting his or her pieces into the puzzle until the whole picture emerges—a concrete representation of each child and the entire group as a connected unit.

From interacting with an actual puzzle, it is a natural progression to engaging the group in creating a puzzle mandala, with each child having his or her own unique piece with collage elements that illustrate "things about me that I am willing to share with the group." Each group member is given an opportunity to draw and cut out a puzzle shape and then add precut pictures, giving each participant a chance to own a unique space within the group in a concrete visual way.

During the search for appealing pictures and the common sharing of art materials, the initial group encounter passes in a flurry of activity. Focused on the task at hand, the first sometimes awkward moments of meeting in a group go by without engendering undue anxiety. All the children are busy, so that no child feels unduly scrutinized or "looked at." Both art and play engage the child in a nonthreatening way and encourage expression of needs, concerns, and strengths. Engagement with the puzzles provides a concrete way to establish cohesion and a less stressful way to meet and literally connect with others. The metaphor of the puzzle allows the child to understand the "whole" picture, and when the puzzle pieces are disconnected or scattered, a link is established to represent what happens when pieces of the whole are torn away or taken away, as in childhood trauma. Dhaese (2011) asserted:

> In situations where the traumas have controlled the child's thinking, feeling, impulses, and behaviors for a long time, release alone is not sufficient. One must be able to help the child channel this new energy into constructive patterns, while retraining old habitual destructive and/or self-destructive ways of being. It is important at this stage to engage the ego, to strengthen it, and to allow it to grow in a healthy way. (p. 81)

Through the art and play the child physically connects his or her piece to another group member's piece of the puzzle, creating a reparative synergy to combat the disorientation, isolation, and confusion of the trauma experience. Group members feel empowered as they experience self-worth, and they gain a feeling of accomplishment for creating their part of the whole group puzzle. Consequently, as the puzzle pieces are reassembled each child can see him- or herself as an integral part of the whole.

Week 2: Identifying Affect—Recognizing and Naming Internal and External Feelings

One of the distinct features of trauma in childhood is the profound sense of disorientation that is experience by the child physically, socially, and emotionally (Hass-Cohen & Carr, 2008; Herman, 1992). The child needs guidance in establishing skills that will reorient him or her to feel a sense of confidence within him- or herself and with the world around him or her. Goodyear-Brown (2010) described the necessary skills of "emotional literacy" as "a child's vocabulary of feelings" (p. 168). The task of affect regulation begins with establishing emotional literacy, which includes the process of recognizing and naming what is felt internally and externally by the child.

For this task the group is invited to play a game of "Feeling Detectives." The group engages in free play outside in a safe space or engages in blowing bubbles. The children are asked to carefully note and discuss what they see in their surrounding environment. Is it hot and sunny? Are birds chirping or motors running? Is it breezy or calm? As the children blow bubbles, they are encouraged to describe the inside and outside of the bubbles. Are they shiny? Are the bubbles bursting with energy on the inside, or light and airy?

Children enjoy playing the game of detective and looking for "clues" about the environment. The child or therapist makes notes of the "clues," and what each child observes "outside." When the children notice different aspects of the environment, a dialogue begins about what is being experienced. As this dialogue develops, the child learns to identify what he or she senses both internally and externally. While the group continues to engage in free play outside, the therapist also asks the children to name the sensations that they feel "inside." Each child then has an opportunity to discuss a wide range feeling states such as calm, warm, nervous, happy, hungry, excited, and the like. The inside sensations are also written down as words or phrases. The group continues to play detective with inside and outside feelings, and identify similarities or differences in feelings. The therapist prompts the detectives to "report the clues" or to use the list of words or phrases that were generated in the play in stating "I feel _____ outside, and I feel _____ inside."

   This play activity supports the next step in personalizing the child's trauma-affective identification. The therapist begins by using a piece of paper folded in half or a plain folder. The child's hands are traced on the outside of the folded paper or folder. Then the paper or folder is opened to expose two sides. Using a variety of art materials (crayons, pens, markers, colored pencils, etc.) the child is asked to make two lists of feelings. The first feelings list contains phrases or words describing feelings and emotions any child could have experienced. The second list contains phrases or words describing traumatic feelings related to "the bad thing that happened." The lists are made side by side and colors or images may be added to foster more personal associations. Also the folded paper or folder may be opened and closed to allow the child to practice skills in "opening up" feelings safely, and "closing up" feelings when necessary. While the child safely "opens up," an important dialogue emerges through colors and imagery. This visually represents how he or she chooses to express his or her feelings on the outside (smiles/frowns, words/silence, or sharing/aggression), and how he or she shows feelings on the inside (happiness/sadness, calmness/ irritability, or confidence/confusion). The child is then invited to color or design the traced hand on the outside any way he or she would like; he or she may also use the back of the folder for free play with the art materials. The folder provides the child an opportunity to safely practice sorting through a range of feeling states, and containing them in a way that engenders power and safety.

Week 3: Processing Affect—Developing Skills in Self-Expression

After the goal of identifying feelings is achieved, the next logical step in trauma-focused treatment is to help the child express the powerful emotions that have been engendered by the trauma. Since a traumatized child can barely describe his or her experience, it is not surprising that he or she is unable to mobilize the capacity to process it. By its very definition, trauma overwhelms the child's ability to cope with a "flood of stimuli that disrupts his fragile resources" (Finkelhor, 1994). For this reason, young children often enter treatment with masses of negative feelings that they are unable to name and are even less equipped to process or "work through." It is because of this disturbed emotional and cognitive state that a combined modality such as art and play therapy is needed.

   During the third week, the therapeutic goal is to aid the child in delineating and expressing multiple feelings without having to rely strictly on words. Art and play therapy combine to create an effective intervention for children because they often prefer to communicate in ways other than talking (Malchiodi, 1998). Engaging in play and using art materials is as natural to children as breathing. Combining these two child-friendly modalities makes sense because they both harness the child's innate response to play and create. In tandem, they create a powerful tool to help the child express and modulate the negative affects associated with trauma (Golomb & Galasso, 1995).

An art therapy intervention at this juncture makes use of transforming an ordinary shoebox into a "Feelings Box." The inside/outside aspect of the box provides a concrete vehicle for separating and expressing emotions that are appropriate for sharing with the world in general on the outside of the box, and on the inside of the box those feelings that are only shared with someone who is trusted. Children are free to use precut pictures, drawings, or words to indicate their feelings.

This three-dimensional representation of feelings provides a structured framework within which to safely express potentially explosive and volatile emotions. The Feelings Boxes do not disappear like spoken words; they remain as a frame of reference to which the child may return as therapy progresses toward the development of coping skills needed to manage the identified affects. According to Deblinger and Heflin (1996), this may be particularly useful with young children, who think concretely, do not have fully developed verbalization skills, and cannot tolerate lengthy discussions.

Pifalo (2007) discussed how the experience of childhood trauma includes an embodied response in the child, which may also be addressed through physical expression and in movement during play. Pifalo stated that "this discharge of energy and tension may clear the way for therapy to begin" (p. 171). Active creative expression in play therapy engages the child in dance and/or physical activity. A game of "My Move" provides the child with a physical outlet in affective processing of traumatic experiences. The therapist begins the game by inviting the group members to try a variety of movements such as hopping, clapping, dancing, or twirling. The child selects a movement and states "This is my move." Another strategic option for this game is to include instruments like drums, shakers, horns, or tambourines as an expressive tool. After each child demonstrates "my move" in movement and/or music, the group takes turns to imitate the move of each other group member as the child's name is called. The game is meant to be energetic and spontaneous, allowing group participation in playful interactions with the understanding that "playing together this way reinforces the common pulse and builds group momentum and support for each child" (McNiff, 2009, p. 75).

Week 4: Development of Coping Skills— Demonstration of Focused Breathing and Relaxation

Once the "Feelings Detectives" have discovered multiple emotions and sorted them into the "inside/outside" aspect of their Feelings Boxes, it is a strategic time to use the combined modalities of art and play therapy to create an effective mechanism for the problem-solving and coping skills needed to manage these identified feelings. One of the first skills taught should focus on breathing. Teaching children to control their breathing patterns gives them the power to calm themselves. This skill disrupts negative patterns, helps the child learn to relax at will, and experience mastery in the process. Focused breathing, mindfulness, and meditation are practices that produce the "relaxation response" (Benson, 1975). The relaxation response has been proven to reverse the adverse physiological and psychological response to stress in both adults and children (Kabat-Zinn, 1990). Relaxation training is introduced early in treatment, so that the children and caregivers can use this technique to manage daily stressors as well as any that they may face in the context of processing traumatic memories in future sessions.

Fortunately, focused breathing is easily mastered and can be used in any context. The therapist may demonstrate the difference between "belly breathing" and shallow breathing by lying in a horizontal position with a rubber duck on his or her lower abdomen. When the duck rises "like on a big wave," then deep breathing is happening. If the duck does not rise, then shallow or chest breathing is what is occurring. Children can then be playfully engaged in practicing with their own rubber ducks, trying to "help the duck swim BIG." Later in the practice, the therapist can help the children count slowly to 5 as they inhale and exhale their breath.

This scenario can be adapted for all ages of children, who usually appear to enjoy the process of mastering this important skill in a playful manner. Children can then be told that they can use this anytime that they are having "big" feelings of being overwhelmed or scared, giving them a helpful tool with which to empower themselves and gain mastery over disruptive affects.

Progressive muscle relaxation is another beneficial coping skill that is easily taught and mastered, and can be adapted for all ages of children. Young children often enjoy the analogy of a piece of spaghetti before it is cooked (stiff) and after it is cooked (soft/ wiggly) or a tin soldier (tense/rigid) and a Raggedy Anne doll (loose/floppy). The therapist can lead the children through a variety of scripts to help them learn the benefits of reducing tension in all body parts. This skill of relaxing specific muscle groups will be especially helpful when treatment moves to focusing on actual traumatic events.

Playing a game of "Flying Feathers" combines playful exercise to enhance both focused breathing and progressive muscle relaxation. The therapist provides the group with an assortment of ordinary plastic drinking straws and colorful, light-weight feathers. The children are instructed to place one or more feathers partially into one end of the straw. Next the child is guided to "Take a big breath and blow!" The feathers fly into the air, and as the feathers float the group practices releasing tension held in the body. For example, the children tense and squeeze their shoulders as they take the breath, and purposely release the tightness as the feather floats to the ground. The feather on the ground can be used as a metaphor to teach finding balance, grounding oneself in the moment, and the concept of a safe landing. Each child then selects a feather to take with him or her as a reminder of his or her coping abilities.

Week 5: Parent–Caregiver Collaboration— Partnering to Share Trauma Experiences

A critical part of the work of recovery requires recounting the trauma in depth and detail, a process that is usually referred to as the "trauma narrative" (Deblinger & Heflin, 1996). The work of reconstructing the trauma is done in an effort to transform the traumatic memory through the process of desensitization that gradually exposes the child to thoughts, memories, and reminders of the traumatic experience until these can be tolerated without significant emotional distress (Pifalo, 2007).

Because the trauma narrative is a key component in the successful resolution of trauma, it is important that the appropriate groundwork be laid prior to the actual retelling of the traumatic experience. Care should be taken at this juncture of treatment to involve both child and parent in a detailed explanation of the reasons for discussing the specific events of the trauma. In fact, it is at this point in the treatment design that a conjoint and/or parallel therapy session should take place to more fully inform and involve both child and caregiver.

Painful and upsetting events are difficult to talk about, so it is perfectly natural to expect that both parent and child often wish to avoid this segment of treatment entirely. One may hear from caregivers such things as "Let sleeping dogs lie" or "We just want to forget about the whole thing." Mental health professionals understand that the desire to distance oneself, or dissociate, from the traumatic event is a natural form of defense that may have originally arisen out of a need to survive the actual trauma. At some point, however, the cost of maintaining the defense mechanism of avoidance will outweigh the benefits. A child who feels he or she must continue to employ his or her defenses to survive does so at great cost: it takes an enormous amount of energy to deny reality, to block emotions, or to distort the truth of what has actually occurred. Furthermore, the exaggerated efforts to defend and block childhood trauma can indeed distort the child's development and may negatively affect a person's life through adulthood.

The clinician's role in the Week 5 session is to provide brief, sensible explanations and emotional security, so that the both the parent and the child understand the purpose for moving forward through this difficult phase in treatment. At this point the therapist lends essential ego strength to the group, conveying the restorative benefits of retelling the trauma in imagery, play, and story form. The therapist discusses and demonstrates self-soothing strategies and reminds the group of the coping skills established in Week 4. Colorful feathers are kept on-hand for the parents and child to use as a soothing reminder of what they previously learned about how to calm themselves.

During the Week 5 group the caregivers and children are introduced to the "cut metaphor" (Cohen, Mannarino, & Deblinger, 2012) as a helpful way to launch into the introduction to the trauma narrative. The therapist explains that the trauma is like at cut or a wound that needs special care to get better and heal. Also, the cut or wound may need careful attention and treatment with bandages, so that the cut doesn't get worse. The therapist supports the parents and reminds them of their important role in the restorative process. The therapist provides guidance so that the caregiver can assist with the healing by being empathetic and nurturing during this process. The Week 5 group allows the adults and children to demonstrate coping strategies and the opportunity to share group resources to aid in the healing process.

To illustrate the cut metaphor the group is given an opportunity to choose among an assortment of toys to use in the restoration process. Band-Aids, bandages, soft blankets, babydolls, stuffed animals, or puppets are available for each caregiver and child to facilitate the play therapy. The children can be encouraged to practice soothing and nurturing the toys, and to rehearse what it actually means to be restored and healed. This role play fosters personal associations for healing, and serves as a bridge to self-expression. The child and parents establish words and terms to express their own feelings about the trauma, and to describe a time when they felt "hurt."

Week 6: Practice for Trauma Narrative— Establishing the Groundwork for Mapping the Trauma

As explained when setting the stage to inform both parent and child regarding the rationale for revisiting the crisis in all its detail, the work of reconstructing the trauma is done to transform the traumatic memory through the process of desensitization. This happens as the child is gradually exposed to thoughts, memories, and reminders ("triggers") until they can be managed without creating sufficient stress to interfere with his or her normal functioning. Children deserve to be free to use their energy to grow and develop, not to maintain defenses that no longer serve them. Gradually as the trauma narrative unfolds, the child takes the first steps to disconnect his or her thoughts and feelings from the overwhelming negative emotions such as terror, rage, and shame that he or she may have felt at the time the trauma occurred.

As the child moves forward in therapy, his or her initial need to dissociate from these powerful emotions gradually decreases, and he or she begins to carefully examine the trauma experience. When the narrative unfolds the child can realize a semblance of order in the traumatic situation. At this point the child begins to carefully examine the details of what has happened to him or her, and the first steps are taken toward restoring order to the chaos that is typical of trauma. During the actual process of creating his or her own personal narrative, the child has the opportunity to incorporate the traumatic experience into the fabric of his or her life. Thus the trauma becomes one part of his or her life, *not* his or her whole life. The goal of integration is to assimilate the trauma so that it no longer exists as a "split-off" piece, which requires the child to continuously summon the energy to either disown or minimize the trauma. Without fully engaging and successfully completing this process, the child may remain immobilized by the trauma.

Because the therapeutic goals of the trauma narrative are so critical for creating a positive outcome for the child, it is imperative to employ the most powerful modalities available to accomplish them: a combination of art and play therapy. By definition, the traumatized child may suffer both mental and emotional impairment—his or her cognitions have been disrupted and disordered. Since these two treatment components do not, at least initially, require the child to use cognitive skills that may not be immediately available to him or her, a new mode of self-expression is accessible in the art and play. The integration of art and play therapy creates a combined treatment model, and may offer the best choice for the most effective and efficient treatment design for brief therapy.

The use of imagery directly contributes to cognition by increasing concentration on trauma-specific issues and promotes quicker access to the processing of this information—a critical issue in brief trauma-focused therapy (Lusebrink, 1990). Children have limitations in their mental capacities to construct a coherent, verbal narrative regarding their trauma. Art and play therapy offer alternative forms of communication. Such nonverbal approaches that do not rely exclusively on words are child-friendly and highly effective tools with which to create, reenact, and rewrite the trauma narrative.

To foster success in this segment of treatment, the children are given an opportunity to practice the skills needed to create the actual trauma map in Week 7. Fortunately, the task of mapping can be readily adapted to the appropriate developmental age of each child. The therapist first demonstrates simple line drawings. Using varied papers and drawing utensils the therapist engages the group in creating a variety of lines and shapes—straight, circular, broken, jagged, or maze-like. The lines and shapes are used as symbols to represent everyday events. To demonstrate how this works, the therapist begins by using the symbols to visually narrate the sequence of events in his or her day. The next step involves the child using the symbols in a timeline to portray the events of his or her day. The group takes turns sharing their timeline with peers and/or caregivers, so that they remain engaged in the process. It is important to encourage discussion about the timelines and teach the strategy for mapping or narrating a sequence of events. This task leads to an exchange of ideas about what it feels like to have a pleasant day, and what is experienced when the day does not go as planned or is full of frustrations. Once again, the therapist is there to lend perspective for events that haunt the child and caregiver, keeping the focus on the restoration process and at the same time encouraging a meaningful integration of the traumatic events into the fabric of life.

The therapist enhances the mapping concept for the child by expanding the symbol list and vocabulary to include well-known weather conditions such as sunny, cold, hot, rainy, windy, stormy, and mild, or more intense weather situations such as hurricanes, tornados, earthquakes, and volcanoes. Simple weather symbols such as sunshine, clouds, and raindrops can be added to the child's practice map to illustrate what he or she was feeling at that particular time of his or her day. At this point in treatment, the children are making the first connections between events and feelings in a simple, child-friendly manner. For example, a child might choose a circular path with a rain cloud over it to represent a part of his or her day when he or she could not find his or her bookbag, and was consequently late for school. An ascending straight line with a bright sun may be used over the occasion of receiving stickers for a job well done. Weather symbols are a strategic component of the groundwork for connecting emotions with events in mapping the trauma. The lines, shapes, and symbols are used to illustrate and communicate events and the affects experienced by the children of all ages.

This type of self-expression is an integral part of narrating the sequence of trauma within a structured framework. The choices of imagery allow the child to develop symbolic terms to later pair with his or her traumatic material, which can be used to symbolize intensity and degree of affect. A rainy day is certainly less traumatic than a hurricane—which may be sorted into categories of intensity from 1 to 5—and a sunny day at the beach represents a completely different experience.

The group then expands the use of symbolic communication and mapping with a game of "Chalk Walk." The therapist introduces the game with sidewalk chalk for outdoor play or ordinary chalk and large sheets of brown paper for indoor play. Group members select from a variety of colored chalk to create a map of a day they consider memorable. The therapist encourages the group to use imagery and symbols to depict easy or fun parts of the map as well as personal symbols to represent obstacles or difficulties. The child then walks through the day describing the events along the path on the "Chalk Walk." The children are given an opportunity to share their "day" with the group in the form of a map or to role-play it as the "Chalk Walk" to foster trust and create connection with others. The skills learned in making and sharing the practice maps will be used in Week 7 to create the actual map of the trauma that brought the child into treatment.

Week 7: Creating the Trauma Narrative— Mapping the Trauma Experience

Deblinger and Heflin (1996) and Goodyear-Brown (2010) stated that therapists should work in a structured and prescriptive manner to aid children in reexperiencing and processing their thoughts related to trauma. The art therapy technique of creating a map is a highly structured intervention that, even in a very simple form adapted for young children, is especially effective for organizing traumatic events into a preliminary chronological order. The framework of the map imposes order on what the child may have previously viewed as an array of chaotic, confusing, and fragmenting experiences. The map becomes a visual tool to identify, organize, and restructure these events.

Using the skills acquired in making the practice maps and the kinesthetic movements from the play therapy task of making a "Chalk Walk," the children are prepared to begin to map the series of events that brought them into treatment. At this point the child is asked to name a toy or a person he or she would like to be with him or her or "by his or her side" while he or she maps his or her story. The child may request another group member or the entire group. It is possible that the child is satisfied with only the therapist as the support, or he or she may choose a stuffed animal, doll, or another item as a source of comfort. The child may also decline assistance, and this choice is honored. Regardless of the option taken, the child experiences making a choice about the support needed to move ahead on his or her journey.

The first steps include each child thinking about and recalling as many situations as possible related to his or her traumatic experience. These events are then placed into a simple list either by the child, or by the therapist acting as "secretary." The therapist facilitates this process by gently encouraging the child to use the established coping skills to present the set of images and sensations associated with the trauma event. The child is prompted to start by expressing the first thing that comes to mind when thinking about the trauma. The therapist then guides the child to continue to link associated thoughts or memories into recalling his or her story. Since the memories and sensations are often fragmented and out of order, the child's story may initially appear with gaps or missing pieces. However, as the child expresses the different parts of his or her story, connections are made and coherence emerges in the narrative. This process is possible because of the essential safety and structure built into previous sessions. Because each child chooses which experiences to include on his or her map, the trauma narrative he or she creates is both personal and accurate—validating his or her own reality and reflecting his or her perception of what happened. Each child is encouraged to place the events into a roughly chronological order and the child begins to "connect the dots" by adding simple weather symbols learned in the practice map segment of Week 6. This step is critical as it paves the way to pair traumatic events with associated feelings, thoughts, and behaviors while working within the "cognitive coping triangle" (Deblinger & Heflin, 1996).

Based on the age and skills of the children and at the discretion of the therapist, other segments can be added. The additions can include a map key using colored lines to further express affect, and ordinary road signs such as Caution, Stop, and Detour can be placed wherever the child thinks they would be helpful. Also, simple stick figures can be added along the way for those people the child views as being supportive at that particular section of his or her map. The road map is tangible; it does not disappear like the words in regular talk therapy, so it can be "walked" as often as necessary to reduce the stress associated with the events. To deepen the experience, the child may choose a particular section to explore more fully through play. A game of "Lost and Found" is helpful in supporting a wider exploration process. Hamil (2008) suggested that the therapist begin the game by stating:

> When something is lost, we have a terrible feeling. We look everywhere we can think of for what is lost. Usually we get as many people as possible to help us look for what we are missing. When we are not able to find what was lost, we have a hard time accepting the loss and we may continue looking for days, weeks, or even months. This is a very sad feeling, and it takes time to feel better after a loss. Often we are able to find what we thought was lost, and this feeling is wonderful. We are relieved and very happy. (p. 89)

After introducing "Lost and Found," the therapist invites the group to respond to the following questions:

"Have you ever lost something?"
"What did you lose?"

"Were you able to find it?"
"How did you feel?"

Each child is asked to tell the story of how he or she lost something and whether the lost item was found. The narration can be supported with a variety of expressive modalities including role play, puppets, music, movement, miniatures, and sandplay. The task for playing "Lost and Found" is to provide an opportunity for the child to practice narrating his or her experience and to demonstrate the problem-solving skills he or she used in the process. The toys and art materials are available to share his or her experience in the form of an active and personal journey. The expression of shared experiences with loss and restoration enhances a feeling of safety and fosters deeper connections with others. The act of performing provides an embodied response to his or her experience affirming a more coherent sense of self. Improvisation in "Lost and Found" supports the child's strengths and invites creative expression of thoughts, emotions, and personal gestures.

Week 8: Processing the Trauma Map—
Sharing the Trauma Experience

At the beginning of Week 8, the children will begin the most important task in resolving their own personal trauma narrative: integration of their traumatic experience. Each child will take the first steps toward assimilating the traumatic memories and affects into the larger fabric of his or her life. In this way, the traumatic material becomes a *part* of his or her life, not his or her *whole* life. The goal of integration is to transform the traumatic aspects, so that they no longer exist as a "split-off" piece that the child must continually summon the energy to either disown or minimize. Successful integration leads to the child being able to acknowledge and validate his or her history rather than waste his or her energy attempting to distort it because he or she is feeling afraid or ashamed.

In Week 7, when the children chose specific events to include on their own trauma maps, they began to bring traumatic memories to the surface where they are available to be addressed. "The very act of creating a map tends to 'jog' memories and aid cognition by providing added information and details" (Pifalo, 2007). This technique of mapping is in keeping with what is known about how children "talk" about a traumatic experience (Finkelhor, 1994). Imagery contributes to cognition in that it increases one's attention and concentration, provides for quicker processing of information, and increases one's reflective distance (Lusebrink, 1990).

The trauma map, the art product personally created by each child in Week 7, protects his or her vulnerability by allowing him or her to control the level of exposure with which he or she is able to cope at any particular time. The child may make the choice to name his or her events "just a picture," or he or she may choose to fully verbalize his or her traumatic experience by sharing the message in the art product with his or her peers and caregivers. It is critical that this choice remains in the control of the creator, so that he or she may take this step when he or she is ready. In this way, the art serves as a kind of buffer or safety valve between what the child has drawn and the reality of his or her traumatic experience. This time, however, the child is in a position of power and control in a situation where he or she may previously have felt powerless.

There is no reason to rush this process—the tangible nature of the trauma map makes it possible for the child to "walk" his or her path as many times as needed and to return to certain portions at will, because now the events and their connection with related affects are in graphic form; they will not disappear like words in traditional talk therapy do. The trauma has been transformed into a visual, concretized continuum that allows the child to gain perspective regarding his or her experience. The map's creator now literally sees that his or her life existed *before* the trauma occurred, and more importantly, that his or her life will continue *after* the trauma, thus putting the trauma into perspective in a way that verbal discussion cannot.

At this point, the children have narrated the trauma experiences with unique and personal imagery. Representing or telling the trauma in this form allows the child's experience to be seen and heard by peers and caregivers in a way that is affirming of his or her strengths and newly acquired coping skills. Opportunities abound for authentic interactions to support the child in sharing the trauma narrative using additional forms of creative expression.

Since the concept of mapping is familiar to the child, he or she will be ready to recognize other aspects within his or her map that contain hidden treasures of hope, strength, and resiliency. Validation and empathy are essential ingredients to the successful integration of the trauma map. After the trauma narrative is created in the form of a map, the therapist guides the child in finding the hidden treasures buried in his or her map. Each group member is prompted to identify the personal strengths that helped him or her get to this point. Perhaps the child had a relative, friend, or teacher who was supportive and caring. The child may choose a place (school or a friend's house) or an activity (songs, playing with siblings, watching favorite programs) that gave him or her solace and refuge. The group members are given images of love, strength, care, and laughter to further construct or reconstruct the narrative. Numerous toys, miniatures, or art materials are available to assist in this endeavor. For example, heart-shaped beads or paper hearts may symbolize love, and shiny stars, shells, and feathers could represent internal strengths or support from significant others. Gold stars or smiley faces convey hope and laughter. The group works together to find the hidden treasure in each child's map. The treasures emerge in unexpected and spontaneous expressions. Finding hidden treasures serves to balance the child's narrative within his or her fluid and dynamic life experience. In this way, the child gains a more manageable perspective of his or her experience and a positive vision of future.

Small heart-shaped boxes or other containers such as envelopes or draw-string bags are provided to each of the children for "Treasure Chests." Each group member identifies one or more of the items that they have previously chosen like beads, heart-shaped paper, feathers, or shells to represent self-care and self-worth. The child's treasure is placed in the treasure chest as a reminder of his or her inner strength and resiliency. The treasure chest metaphor may be expanded into a game that includes pirates and adventures on the high seas. The therapist guides the group to play with the idea of protecting the treasures to reflect personal strengths for future reference.

Week 9: Identifying Internal and External Sources of Support—Naming Personal Resources

The need for children to have sufficient support following a traumatic event and throughout the course of treatment for that crisis cannot be overemphasized. The dedicated involvement of parents and caregivers may be the single most critical influence on the child's ability to heal from trauma (Cohen et al., 2012). Since traumatic events have the potential to damage relationships, it is clear that the level of positive support from significant people surrounding the child may have the power to mitigate any negative effects. In the aftermath of a trauma, children are highly vulnerable. "The victim's sense of self may have been shattered, and it can only be rebuilt only as it was initially, in connection with others" (Herman, 1992). For these reasons, it is important that both types of support—external and internal—be identified and documented before the children leave the safety of the group.

The sources of external support include those persons whom the child thinks have helped him or her survive the trauma that he or she has just experienced. These people may include any or all of the following: parents, caregivers, other significant relatives, peers, counselors, law enforcement officers, clergy, teachers, therapists, animal companions, and even fantasy "helpers" such as Judge Judy and Spiderman, depending on the age and developmental level of the child. The key factor in empowering the child in this segment is that he or she is given the opportunity to choose. In addition, because children are concrete thinkers, these choices need to be documented in a creative, visual art product upon which they can depend to serve as a reminder that they do, in fact, have others who will be there in the future when they need them.

One art therapy intervention uniquely suited to accomplishing this task is the creation of "Strings of Strength" (Pifalo, 2007). Using beads of various colors, shapes, and materials, each child chooses one to symbolically represent "the person or persons who helped me." These beads can then be made into bracelets, necklaces, or tags for backpacks, depending on the age and gender of the child, making them both personal and portable.

Next, the child is encouraged to "look inward" to name his or her own coping skills and strengths that helped him or her survive the traumatic experience. These could include a sense of humor, ability to ask for help when needed, skill at self-calming techniques such as focused breathing and progressive muscle relaxation, and the willingness to reach out to others when necessary. The child then adds his or her own helpful characteristics to the art product in the symbolic form of a bead. The "Strings of Strength" now contain visual representations for both external and internal support, and they serve as transitional objects to remind children that these support systems are firmly in place as they move toward termination.

The game of "Hey, Listen Up!" is introduced to the child to practice assertively expressing the strengths and special qualities that he or she has just identified. Each child is given a microphone or megaphone, and takes center stage to perform the "Strings of Strength" by announcing to the group his unique skills learned in the group. For example, the group members may use terms about themselves such as smart, strong, calm, friendly, and so on to describe their strengths. The therapist guides the child to speak up about his or her strengths and coping skills. The child is asked to say "Hey, listen up. I am _____!" for each of the identified qualities on the Strings of Strength. The child is reassured if he or she feels silly or awkward at first, and reminded that with practice he or she will feel confident about assertive self-expression. This game is a wonderful opportunity for embodied role play and supportive group interactions. In reality the group provides an important witness to reflect each member's progress and personal growth.

Week 10: Risk Reduction and "Open-Door" Termination—Establishing Personal Boundaries and Safety

Trauma resolution occurs in stages and progress is made gradually. As the child takes the steps in self-repair the establishment of a reasonable degree of safety is paramount. Recovery from trauma is a process—much like the journey seen in the children's maps, its path is more spiral-like than linear, more turbulent than calm, and more complex than simple. In general, children who have experienced trauma are much more likely to feel an increased sense of vulnerability. Of course, it is impossible to protect children from any and all future traumatic situations; it is prudent for therapists and caregivers to avoid making promises that they will not be able to keep. Children are quick to recognize these as false assurances, and this can actually cause them to feel even less secure as a result.

To create focus on the child's perception of which people and what things he or she needs to feel safe at this time, the children are given an opportunity to use art materials to illustrate their own personal "Safe Spaces" (Pifalo, 2002). Each child is asked to envision a place where he or she has the people and resources he or she needs to feel safe and secure. The group is then given art materials to create images of the identified safe spaces. This open-ended directive allows the child the freedom to identify his or her fears and find someone or something to help alleviate them. Because each child individually composes his or her safe space drawing, its content can form the foundation of a personal safety plan for each family. Attention to the details of the drawing can alert parents and caregivers to possible modifications in the child's environment that could serve to increase his or her degree of safety. Also, the encouragement of relevant safety skills at this juncture can enhance the child's sense of mastery and self-efficacy for possible stressors and trauma in the future. This session is a perfect opportunity for therapists and caregivers to praise and congratulate the children for already having used the most important safety skill of all: telling a trusted adult about the trauma.

The final session integrates the components of each of the previous weeks to once again affirm the child's autonomy and integrity. Each group member is engaged in a role play that illustrates the concept of his or her own personal safe space. For this task the therapist uses a hula-hoop to demonstrate the concept of personal space and invites the group to play with the idea of boundaries and limits. The hula-hoop provides a physical boundary for the child to practice establishing a safe space, and others must ask permission to enter another's space. The group members are given terms to use to identify what feels comfortable or "OK" within the safe space and what is "not OK." The group proceeds to discuss and enact different types of appropriate interactions using the hula-hoop as a literal boundary. The group is encouraged to rehearse terms such as "I feel safe now" and "I don't feel safe when . . . " to communicate when a person or situation is not "OK," or appropriate. Each group member is encouraged to speak up about his or her personal ideas about interactions that include showing affection and fear. This type of play empowers the child to identify and assert his or her level of comfort about affection and touch and communicate that to others.

SUMMARY AND CONCLUSIONS

Integrating art modalities and art materials into short-term trauma resolution in play therapy has numerous benefits. The use of art serves as a bridge between therapeutic play and self-expression. Through art the child shares significant personal ideas and concerns in the imagery. The symbols and the artwork created by the child allow access to traumatic material that may not be available any other way. The child can then portray his or her experience in an entirely unique format. Using art in short-term trauma resolution augments the play therapy process by providing added dimensions in communication. As the child portrays his or her trauma experience, the impact of the event becomes evident, informing more focused treatment and accurate safety planning.

The child's symbolic communication offers opportunity for fluid and dynamic assessment of the child's strengths, needs, and concerns. The combination of modalities in each of the weekly sessions provides an intentional therapeutic progression for trauma resolution. The treatment goals and objectives support the child's ability to establish emotional literacy, hone his or her innate creative expressions, develop coping skills, and master the ability to construct a coherent trauma narrative.

The therapist is available throughout the course of this treatment to guide and support the child and the caregiver to safely share the trauma narrative and to assert their needs for safety and self-expression. Integrating art and play therapy within the structure of a trauma-focused cognitive-behavioral approach creates an individualized and efficient treatment model for short-term trauma resolution in childhood.

REFERENCES

American Psychiatric Association. (2013). *Diagnostic and statistical manual of mental disorders* (5th ed.). Arlington, VA: Author.

Benson, H. (1975). *The relaxation response*. New York: Avon Books.

Briere, J., & Scott, A. (2006). *Principles of trauma therapy: A guide to symptoms, evaluation, and treatment*. Thousand Oaks, CA: Sage Publications.

Briggs, K. M., Runyon, M. K., & Deblinger, E. (2011). The use of play in cognitive behavioral therapy. In S. W. Russ & L. N. Niec (Eds.), *Play in clinical practice: Evidence-based approaches* (pp. 169–200). New York: Guilford Press.

Cohen, J. A., Mannarino, A. P., & Deblinger, E. (2006). *Treating trauma and traumatic grief in children and adolescents: Treatment applications*. New York: Guilford Press.

Cohen, J. A., Mannarino, A. P., & Deblinger, E. (2012). *Trauma-focused CBT for children and adolescents*. New York: Guilford Press.

Deblinger, E., McLeer, S. V., & Henry, D. E. (1990). Cognitive behavioral therapy for sexually abused children suffering post-traumatic stress: Preliminary findings. *Journal of the American Academy of Child and Adolescent Psychiatry, 29*, 747–752.

Deblinger, E., & Heflin, A. (1996). *Treating sexually abused children and their nonoffending parents: A cognitive behavioral approach.* Thousand Oaks, CA: Sage.

Dhaese, M. J. (2011). An integrative approach to helping maltreated children. In A. A. Drewes, S. C. Bratton, & C. E. Schaefer (Eds.), *Integrative play therapy.* Hoboken, NJ: Wiley.

Drewes, A. A., Bratton, S. C., & Schaefer, C. E. (Eds.). (2011). *Integrative play therapy.* New York: Wiley.

Finkelhor, D. (1994). The international epidemiology of child sexual abuse. *Child Abuse and Neglect, 18*(5), 409–417.

Golomb, C., & Galasso, L. (1995). Make believe and reality: Explorations of the imaginary realm. *Developmental Psychology, 31,* 800–810.

Goodyear-Brown, P. (2010). *Play therapy with traumatized children: A prescriptive approach.* Hoboken, NJ: Wiley.

Greenberg, M. S., & van der Kolk, B. A. (1987). Retrieval and integration of traumatic memories with the "painting cure." In B. A. van der Kolk (Ed.), *Psychological trauma* (pp. 191–216). Washington, DC: American Psychiatric Press.

Hamil, S. (2008). *My feeling better workbook: Help for kids who are sad and depressed.* Oakland, CA: Instant Help Books.

Hamil, S. (2011). Integrating art into play therapy for children with mood disorders. In A. A. Drewes, S. C. Bratton, & C. E. Schaefer (Eds.), *Integrative play therapy* (pp. 177–194). Hoboken, NJ: Wiley.

Hass-Cohen, N., & Carr, R. (Eds.). (2008). *Art therapy and clinical neuroscience.* Philadelphia: Jessica Kingsley.

Herman, J. L. (1992). *Trauma and recovery.* New York: Basic Books.

Johnson, D. (1987). The role of creative arts therapies in the diagnosis and treatment of psychological trauma. *The Arts in Psychotherapy, 14,* 7–13.

Kabat-Zinn, J. (1990). *Full catastrophe living: Using the wisdom of the body and mind to face stress, pain, and illness.* New York: Delta.

Kaduson, H. G., & Schaefer, C. E. (Eds.). (2009). *Short-term play therapy for children.* New York: Guilford Press.

Linesch, D. (Ed.). (1993). *Art therapy with families in crisis: Overcoming resistance through nonverbal expression.* New York: Brunner/Mazel.

Lusebrink, V. B. (1990). *Imagery and visual expression in therapy.* New York: Plenum Press.

Malchiodi, C. A. (1998). *Breaking the silence: Art with children from violent homes* (2nd ed.). New York: Brunner/Mazel.

McNiff, S. (2009). *Integrating the arts in therapy: History, theory, and practice.* Springfield, IL: Charles C Thomas.

Penfield, W., & Perot, P. (1963). The brain's record of auditory and visual experience: A final summary and discussion. *Brain, 86,* 595–696.

Pifalo, T. A. (2002). Pulling out the thorns: Art therapy with sexually abused children and adolescents. *Art Therapy: Journal of the American Art Therapy Association, 19*(1), 12–22.

Pifalo, T. A. (2007). Jogging the cogs: Trauma-focused art therapy and cognitive behavioral therapy with sexually abused children. *Art Therapy: Journal of the American Art Therapy Association, 24*(4), 170–175.

Pifalo, T. A. (2009). Mapping the maze: An art therapy intervention following disclosure of sexual abuse. *Art Therapy: Journal of the American Art Therapy Association, 26*(1), 12–18.

Chapter 6

☙

Short-Term Gestalt Play Therapy for Grieving Children

Violet Oaklander

Gestalt therapy is a process-oriented mode of therapy that focuses attention on the healthy, integrated functioning of the total organism, comprised of the senses, the body, the emotions, and the intellect. Gestalt therapy was originally developed by Drs. Frederick (Fritz) and Laura Perls and has at its base principles from psychoanalytic theory, Gestalt psychology, various humanistic theories, as well as aspects of phenomenology, existentialism, and Reichian body therapy. From these sources, a large body of theoretical concepts and principles have evolved underlying the practice of Gestalt therapy (Perls, Hefferline, & Goodman, 1951; Perls, 1969; Latner, 1986). A few of the most salient principles of Gestalt therapy that are pertinent to working with children are discussed in this chapter.

THE I–THOU RELATIONSHIP

This is a particular type of relationship based on the philosophical writings of Martin Buber (1958). Some of the pertinent fundamental principles of this relationship are highly significant in work with children. The therapist is cognizant of the fact that, despite differences in age, experience, and education, he or she is not superior to the client; both are equally entitled.

It is a relationship in which two people come together in a dialogical stance. The therapist meets the child however he or she presents the self, without judgment, and with respect and honor.

The therapist is congruent and genuine, while at the same time respecting his or her own limits and boundaries, never losing him- or herself to the child, but willing to be affected by the child. The therapist holds no expectations, yet maintains an attitude that supports the full, healthy potential of the child. The therapist is involved, contactful, and often interactive. He or she creates an environment of safety and never pushes the child beyond his or her capabilities or consent. The relationship itself is therapeutic; often it provides an experience for the child that is new and unique.

CONTACT AND RESISTANCE

"Contact" involves the ability to be fully present in a particular situation, with all the aspects of the organism vital and available. "Healthy contact" involves the use of the senses (looking, listening, touching, tasting, and smelling), awareness and appropriate use of aspects of the body, the ability to express emotions healthfully, and the use of the intellect in its various forms such as learning, expressing ideas, thoughts, curiosities, wants, needs, and resentments. When any one of these aspects are inhibited, restricted, or blocked, good contact suffers. Fragmentation, rather than integration, occurs. Children who have troubles, who are grieving, worried, anxious, frightened, or angry, will armor and restrict themselves, pull themselves in, inhibit themselves, and block healthful expression. Healthy contact involves a feeling of security within oneself, a fearlessness about standing alone. We make good contact with others from the edge of ourselves—from the boundary of the self. "The contact boundary is the point at which one experiences the 'me' in relation to that which is 'not me' and through this contact, both are more clearly experienced" (Polster & Polster, 1973). If the self is weak and undefined, the boundary is fuzzy and contact suffers. Good contact is fluid and involves a rhythm of withdrawal. The child who maintains a fixed contact posture, requires constant attention, is never able to play alone, or talks constantly shows evidence of a fragile sense of self (Oaklander, 1988).

Most children will be resistant and self-protecting to a degree. Resistance is actually a healthy response, and good contact involves some level of resistance. It is difficult to engage in good contact with someone who does not have a clear boundary, but a high degree of resistance makes achieving satisfying contact impossible. The therapist expects some resistance and recognizes it as the child's ally. He or she is respectful of the resistance. As the child begins to feel safe in the sessions, the resistance will soften.

However, resistance comes up over and over again. When the child has experienced or divulged as much as he or she can handle or has inside support for, the resistance will come up again and must be honored. It is the child's signal that he or she has reached his or her limit of capability at this particular time. Resistance can be viewed as a manifestation of energy as well as an indication of the contact level of the child. When the energy fades and the contact shifts, this is evidence of resistance. Some children indicate the resistance in passive ways—ignoring, acting distracted, or appearing not to be listening. The child who can say "I don't want to go any further with this" is making a contactful statement.

The issue of resistance is implicated in the success of brief therapy with children. The child's resistance involves his or her very core—his or her way of coping with and surviving his or her problematic world. His or her resistance is an indication of his or her state of being. The therapist cannot push through this resistance quickly, forcefully, or mechanically. If the relationship is strong, the therapist can use all of his or her skill to gently override some of the resistance. It is a tenuous matter.

Inappropriate behaviors are often viewed as resistances or contact–boundary disturbances. As the child struggles to grow up, survive, and cope with life, he or she may manifest a variety of inappropriate behaviors and symptoms that serve to avoid contact and protect the self. He or she does not have the inner support, cognitive ability, or emotional maturity to directly express deep feelings. These symptoms and behaviors, the very ones that bring children into therapy, are actually the organism's way of attempting to achieve homeostasis, albeit unsuccessfully. The quest for equilibrium is unrelenting; the child has little awareness of cause and effect in his or her attempts to cope, get his or her needs met, and protect him- or herself. The child has a powerful thrust for life and growth, and will do anything he or she can to grow up. Paradoxically, in the service of this quest, he or she will restrict, inhibit, block, and actually cut off aspects of the self. He or she will desensitize him- or herself, restrict the body, block emotions, and inhibit the intellect. The consequence of this process is an increased diminishing of the self and impairment of his or her contact abilities, often manifesting as troublesome behaviors or symptoms.

SENSE OF SELF

Helping the child develop a strong sense of self is a prelude to emotional expression, an important step in the healing process. When children restrict and inhibit an aspect of the organism, the self is diminished. Strengthening the skills of contact play is an important part in this process. These skills—looking; listening; smelling; tasting; touching; moving in the environment; expressing thoughts, ideas, opinions; and defining the self—give the support necessary for expressing deep emotions that block healthy functioning and integration. A variety of experiences introduced by the therapist are used to strengthen the child's self, which in turn provides the self-support required for emotional expression. This is not a linear process—the therapist presents these activities as needed.

AWARENESS AND EXPERIENCE

Gestalt therapy is considered to be a process therapy: attention is paid to the "what" and the "how" of behavior rather than the "why." When the therapist can help the client become more aware of what he or she is doing that causes dissatisfaction, the client then has the choice to make changes. Awareness encompasses many aspects of life. One can become aware of one's process, sensations, feelings, wants, needs, thought processes, and actions. As the child moves through the therapy experience, he or she becomes more aware of who he or she is, what he or she feels, what he or she needs, what he or she wants, and so on (Oaklander, 1982). Some older children as well as adolescents often become cognizant of unsatisfactory ways of being, experience them fully with the guidance of the therapist, and begin to make conscious choices for new behaviors. This is beyond the scope of younger children. For these children, experience is the key to awareness. Providing varied experiences for children is an essential component of the therapeutic process. These experiences may be with aspects of themselves that are blocked, such as one or more of their sensory modalities. They might be experiences that experiment with parts of the self that have been kept dormant. All of these experiences serve to strengthen the child's self and promote good contact functioning, culminating in healing emotional expression, and, in general, facilitating new, more satisfying ways of being-in-the-world.

Many creative, expressive, and projective techniques are used to further the therapeutic experience. These techniques serve as bridges to the child's inner self and often provide the means to discover, renew, or strengthen aspects of the self. The techniques include the use of graphic arts in many forms, such as drawing, painting, and collage, as well as pottery clay, puppets, music in many forms, creative dramatics, sensory and body experiences, various games, books and storytelling, the sandtray, fantasy and imagery, and the use of metaphors. These techniques are very powerful in the context of Gestalt therapy and the relationship that develops with the therapist.

SHORT-TERM GESTALT
PLAY THERAPY APPROACH

Gestalt therapy can be an ideal discipline for short-term work with grieving children since it is directive and focusing. In longer term situations, the sessions become a sort of dance: sometimes the child leads, and at other times the therapist does. In short-term work, the therapist becomes, for the most part, the leader. He or she must assess what will best serve the child's therapeutic needs to provide the best experience in the few sessions available, while being heedful of the child's developmental level, capability, responsiveness, and resistance level. He or she must not be forceful or intrude upon the child's boundary—he or she must tread lightly, without any expectation.

The vitality and potency of these techniques make them particularly effective for short-term work, since they are so dynamic and particularly effective in cutting to the core of a situation.

Prior to doing short-term work with grieving children, the therapist must have an understanding of the issues involving loss and grief, as well as some general pointers that facilitate short-term work.

Stages of Grief

Elizabeth Kübler-Ross (1973) postulated five stages related to the reaction of the death of a loved one: denial and isolation, anger, bargaining, depression, and, finally, acceptance. Most therapists have generalized these stages to fit many kinds of loss situations. Lenore Terr, in her excellent book *Too Scared to Cry* (1990), discusses the process of mourning, as presented by John Bowlby (1973–1983) in his three-volume work, *Attachment, Separation, and Loss,* as four phases particularly relating to children: denial, protest, despair, and resolution. Children, she argues, can become stuck in any one phase for long periods of time. The therapist cannot push the client through any of these stages. However, as specific issues are dealt with, movement begins to take place. Another look at grief stages is presented by J. William Worden (2001, 2008). He describes the stages as alarm, numbness, pining (searching), depression, and finally recovery and reorganization. He presents what he calls four tasks of mourning. The first is to accept the reality of the loss. The second is to work through the pain of grief. The third is to adjust to an environment in which the deceased is missing. And finally, the fourth is to emotionally relocate the deceased and move on with life.

Issues of Loss

There are numerous possible issues involved that the therapist must be aware of when a child suffers a loss. Some of these issues include confusion, abandonment, loss of self, blaming the self, guilt, fear, loss of control, feelings of betrayal, feeling the need to take care of parents, unexpressed feelings of sadness, anger, shame, and misconceptions. The therapist must make an assessment regarding the issues besetting the child so that he or she can provide a focus to the therapy. Certain issues are particularly prevalent at various development levels. For example, the 4-year-old who loses a parent will feel responsible for that loss, since he or she is basically an egocentric individual. Generally, it can be assumed that every child is troubled by most of the issues mentioned.

Children suffer many different kinds of loss throughout their development. These losses affect the child deeply: the loss of a favorite toy, a friend, a neighborhood, a loved teacher, a pet, a parent through divorce, and the loss that comes about through some kind of physical impairment—all impact the child. The death of a parent, sibling, friend, or grandparent is certainly a traumatic loss. As children grow, the accumulation of these losses, without appropriate expression of grief, causes havoc to healthy development. It is not unusual for the child to develop worrisome symptoms and behaviors months, or even years, after a particular loss. The child certainly has the capacity to go through the grieving process naturally. However, he or she generally has introjected many messages regarding the expressions necessary for this work: It is not OK to cry. It is certainly not OK to be angry about the loss. The child feels responsible for the well-being of the adults in his or her life. He or she may be holding a secret fear that he or she is responsible for the loss.

In short, the child needs much support and guidance through the grieving process. When the process is encouraged, and any issues that impede his or her grief are addressed, the child often responds rapidly.

SHORT-TERM WORK

Often combined with the task of helping children through the grieving process is the therapist's mandate to do it quickly, a seemingly impossible task when working with children. The therapist may feel pressured to achieve results quickly. This pressure can be a detriment to the work, and the therapist must find a way to shed this burden and trust the process, even if he or she is not successful. When the child suffering the loss has functioned well prior to the loss and appears to have a fairly strong sense of self, with good support in his or her environment, only a few sessions can help him or her move through his or her grief. Furthermore, if the therapist can feel the thread of a relationship and the child can sustain contact when working with the therapist, good results can be achieved. Contact must be assessed periodically, since the child will cut him- or herself off and break contact if the work becomes too intense for him or her—if he or she lacks the self-support to deal with the task at hand. The therapist must be sensitive to this phenomenon, and when it happens, he or she must honor this resistance and perhaps suggest that the remaining time be filled with some nonthreatening activity, such as a game of the child's choosing.

When the relationship and contact are prevalent, the therapist must then make some determinations that will best fit the model of short-term work. In spite of the goals the therapist may have, he or she must be vigilant in avoiding expectations. He or she will set the framework for each session and present the activity, but to anticipate results is a breeding ground for failure. Every child is highly sensitive to expectations that may be present; this attitude can severely affect and cloud the session. Expectations present a dynamic that becomes a living part of the encounter. The therapist must take an existential stance: Whatever will happen will happen.

Several points involving short-term work need to be considered and may be helpful:

1. See the situation as "crisis intervention." Tell the child you only have a few sessions to make things better.

2. Look at the number of sessions there are and plan what you will do (without expectation that what is planned will happen.) For example, the first session would be used to establish the relationship by getting to know the child, engaging in nonthreatening activities, and providing safety for the child. When the therapist is respectful, genuine, congruent, accepts the child however he or she presents the self, and is him- or herself contactful, relationship and safety will be established.

3. Do not become enmeshed with the child. Often, when dealing with a child's loss, the therapist can feel he or she must take care of the child, make things better, feel emotional, or feel so sorry for the child that he or she allows him or her to do whatever he or she wants, even going beyond limits. If the therapist cannot maintain his or her own boundaries and have the child adhere to the limits by which he or she operates, the child becomes confused and anxious.

4. List the issues you determine are involved with this particular child and set priorities. Cut right to the core of the issues and feelings (examples are given in the next section). Depending on the age of the child, the therapist can share some of these items with the child, giving the child the choice to decide what he or she wants to work on.

5. Include parents in some of the sessions if possible. Explain to them the process of your work. Assess the communication level regarding the loss. For example, a child whose father lost his job felt he needed to cheer

up his parents, reassure himself, and look at the "bright side" of things, totally cutting off his fears. Other symptoms, such as falling grades and inability to concentrate, cropped up. In family sessions he admitted he was terrified about what was going to happen to the family. The parents admitted that they never showed their own fear, much less discussed it with the child, thinking that this disclosure would be detrimental. As they began to talk to each other about what they all were feeling, the child's symptoms faded away.

6. Therapy is intermittent with children. Termination is generally temporary. At each developmental level, new issues arise. The child can only work at his or her particular developmental level. Parents need to understand this reality.

7. Be honest and clear with the child about the reason he or she is having sessions with you. Even a very young child can understand if the therapist uses appropriate developmental language.

CASE ILLUSTRATIONS

The following are condensed accounts of work with grieving children on a short-term basis.

Case 1: Jack

Twelve-year-old Jack lost his mother to cancer when he was 7. His parents had been divorced for some time and his father had remarried. After the divorce Jack had a good relationship with both his parents, who had joint custody; did well in school; had friends; and appeared to be fairly well adjusted to life in general. When his mother died, he moved in with his father and stepmother, whom he liked very much. His father reported that there had been no problems with Jack since his mother's death. When the therapist asked how Jack had handled his grief, his father realized that actually Jack had shown very little affect outside of some brief crying when he was first told of her death.

At his present age of 12, certainly a crucial developmental age, various symptoms appeared. Jack's grades began to fall, he preferred to stay at home rather than play with his friends, he was upset when his father was not at home, and he began to have trouble sleeping. His parents did not associate his symptoms with the death of his mother years earlier. However, the therapist saw this traumatic event as a red flag, particularly since the parents reported that he handled her death "so well."

Session 1

At the first session, Jack came in with his parents. It is during this session that the therapist learns the child's "story" and the concerns of the parents. It is important that the child be present at this session to know what his parents tell the therapist. Jack agreed that he would like to work on sleeping better, since he saw himself as somewhat of an athlete and admitted feeling too tired to do anything, presumably due to lack of sleep.

Session 2

At the second session, the therapist evaluated Jack's ability to make a relationship and observed his contact skills. Jack was a bright, friendly child who quickly related to the therapist and appeared to be quite contactful. From all appearances, he was a good candidate for short-term work. The first session with Jack alone was primarily a time to help him feel comfortable and to promote the relationship. After some conversation, the therapist asked Jack to draw a safe place—a place where he felt safe. Jack drew a camping scene and talked about how much he enjoyed camping outings with his dad and stepmother. He said that he liked being with them and doing things together, and that the stresses from the regular world did not get in the way. The therapist made a list of some of these stresses as Jack dictated them. The session concluded with a game of "Uno," Jack's choice from several easy, fun games.

Session 3

At the next session, the therapist asked Jack to close his eyes and think about his mother to see what memory might come to the fore. He was invited to draw the memory or just share it. He reported that he had very few memories of his mother but proceeded to draw a beach scene. When finished, he talked about how he remembered going to the beach with her when he was little. The therapist asked Jack to give the little boy in the scene a voice. She immediately began a dialogue with the boy, saying "What are you doing?," and Jack, in spite of his initial resistance to such a silly request, answered "I'm building a sand castle." The therapist encouraged Jack to dialogue with his mother in the picture as the little boy. At the conclusion of this little exercise, Jack stated with a smile, "That was fun." Again the session was concluded with "Uno."

Session 4

Pottery clay had been set out on two boards on the table, along with a rubber mallet and some other tools. As Jack and the therapist played with the clay, she casually asked him to tell her more about his mother and some things he remembered about her. Clay has a powerful quality of providing a nurturing, sensorial experience, along with promoting expression. Jack was surprised that he actually had numerous memories. The therapist shared with him that she believed his sleeping problems and difficulty separating from his dad were related to the loss of his mother at age 7. Jack was astonished and startled at this information. She asked Jack to make a figure of a 7-year-old boy out of clay and to imagine what it was like for this little boy to lose his mother. The therapist engaged the "7-year-old" in a dialogue, again inviting Jack to be the voice of the little boy. The therapist encouraged Jack to "make up" what he imagined a little boy would say.

THERAPIST: Were you scared when your mother got sick?

JACK: When she went to the hospital I was very scared.

THERAPIST: Yes! That's a very scary thing for a little kid.

Much to his own surprise, Jack offered lots of information in answer to the therapist's casually stated questions. The therapist told him that children at that age have difficulty grieving and need help to know how to go through the grief stages. Jack was fascinated by the various stages, and more memories of that time began to flood back for him: "I remember that I was mad when my dad said she died! I was sure he was lying and I ran from the room and wouldn't talk to him. That's like denial, I guess. My dad seemed mad at me for that. I guess he didn't know about the stages."

And Jack talked about his anger, which seemed to get him into a lot of trouble. So he suppressed it, assuming that he was very bad to feel such an emotion. The therapist placed a large lump of clay in front of Jack and invited him to pound it with the rubber mallet. Jack did this with much gusto. When the therapist asked him to put words to his pounding, Jack stood up and hit the clay with tremendous force. He began to cry as he shouted, "Why did you leave me?," obviously now talking to his mother. The therapist articulated encouraging words, such as "Yes, tell her!" She knew that if she remained silent, Jack would suddenly realize what he was doing and stop his noisy outburst. Jack continued for a while and finally sat down. Quickly, the therapist praised him for being able to allow his anger to come out. The therapist fashioned a little figure that she labeled 7-year-old Jack.

THERAPIST: Jack, this is your 7-year-old self. Imagine you could go back in a time machine and talk to him. What would you say?

JACK: I don't know.

THERAPIST: Try saying "I'm sorry you lost your mother."

JACK: Yeah. I'm sorry you lost your mother. You're just a little kid and you need her. It's not right.

Jack continued in this vein, with encouragement and suggestions from the therapist.

THERAPIST: Jack, that little boy lives inside of you. He's been quiet for a while, but now that you are 12 and can do a lot of things, I think he has been trying to get your attention. I think he's been stuck at that age because he never expressed (or even knew) his feelings. He needs you now. When you are scared, when your father goes away, it's really him thinking something will happen to his dad. It's really him keeping you from sleeping. But now he has you and, of course, you will never leave him since he's part of you. He needs you now. So every night this week when you go to bed, I want you to talk to him and tell him you will never leave him and that he's a very good kid. And maybe you can tell him a story while you're lying in bed.

JACK: My mother used to tell me stories.

THERAPIST: Now you can do it. You're good at this kind of thing, so try it. This is your homework for the week!

Jack declined to practice this exercise in the therapist's office and agreed he would do it at home.

Session 5

At the fifth session, Jack reported that he was sleeping better but not really well yet. The therapist asked Jack to close his eyes and imagine he was in bed at night, and to report the feelings he experienced. Jack said there was still some fear but that he was not sure what it was about. The therapist asked Jack to draw the fear using colors, lines, curves, and shapes.

JACK: This is how I feel. Lots of weird lines and circles, mostly black. I think I'm afraid my father will die, like you said last week.

THERAPIST: Jack, no one knows really what will happen in the future about anyone. But when a boy loses someone close, especially his mom, he can get pretty worried and anxious and naturally begins to think that it will happen to someone else close, especially his dad. You need to let the little boy in you know that it's OK to be afraid—that you understand it. Here he is (*drawing a quick stick figure*)—tell him.

JACK: Yes, it's OK to be afraid.

THERAPIST: Do you believe that?

JACK: Well, it's OK for him to be afraid. I don't think I should.

THERAPIST: That's why I'm asking you to talk to him. I think if you give him permission to be afraid, maybe it will help you not to be so afraid. Though really, Jack, it's OK if you are too.

JACK: OK, you can be afraid. It's natural. You're a little kid.

THERAPIST: Remind him that you are with him and will never leave him, and that you know how to do a lot of things he couldn't do.

Jack practiced this for a while.

Session 6

At the sixth session Jack reported that he fell asleep before he finished talking to his 7-year-old self and forgot to worry about his dad. He was too busy. The therapist reminded Jack that every now and then he would feel lonely for his mom and to remember that he needed to let himself do that, and maybe do something nice for his 7-year-old self.

Session 7

At this last session Jack and his parents participated. Everyone talked a bit about what Jack had learned. Jack was anxious to enlighten them, particularly about stages. Jack reported that he felt happy that he was not so tired now. A follow-up session was held 1 month later—all was well.

This work was accomplished in a total of seven sessions, including the last one. The first session involved the family, while the next two were for relationship building, as well as providing a base for focusing on the death of Jack's mother. The therapist made the assumption that this was the cause of his present symptoms, particularly because of his attachment disorder. The issues that emerged spontaneously were fear of abandonment, anger, and sadness. Learning to nurture the self and gaining skills to take care of the self are important and effective.

Case 2: Susan

Ten-year-old Susan lost her father to suicide. Her parents had been divorced since Susan, the youngest of three children, was a baby. Despite the divorce, Susan's dad was very involved in Susan's life and she was very close to him. They made an agreement that she would live with him for a year, but just prior to her move he killed himself. Susan's mother brought her into therapy 6 months later, when Susan's behavior appeared to deteriorate into angry, aggressive outbursts and the teacher complained that she was not doing her work and had become quite belligerent. It is common for parents to bring a child into therapy after a traumatic loss such as this after a few months have gone by and symptoms emerge and accelerate.

Session 1

The first session took place with mother and daughter. The mother stated that ever since het father died, Susan has been having difficulties at school and their own relationship has deteriorated. "Things are getting worse," she said, "and not better as I thought they would with time." At this session, Susan was quite withdrawn and would not participate. The therapist asked the mother to go into the waiting room, and then asked Susan to draw a house and tree and person on a single sheet of paper. Susan, relieved that she did not have to talk, worked diligently.

THERAPIST: Susan, this is really a test, but I'm not using it that way—I'm using it to get to know you better. It tells me some things about you and I would like to check them out with you to see if it's right.

SUSAN: What does it tell you?

THERAPIST: Well, for one thing, it tells me you keep a lot of things to yourself.

SUSAN: It's true. How do you know that?

THERAPIST: Your house has very small windows and dark shades and sometimes when someone draws windows like that, it could mean that.

SUSAN: (*showing interest*) What else does it tell you?

THERAPIST: It also might show that you keep in a lot of anger because maybe you don't know how to get it out. Does that fit for you? The person looks kind of angry.

SUSAN: Yes!

THERAPIST: See how the house is tilting? Maybe you don't feel very sure about anything right now. And the girl is at this corner, far away from the house. Maybe you don't know where you belong.

SUSAN: (*very low voice*) That's right.

The therapist noticed tears in Susan's eyes and gently told her that they would try to work these things out together in the sessions. She wrote her findings on the back of Susan's paper and read them back to her. Susan listened intently. The therapist then suggested that they spend the final few minutes of the session playing a game. Susan selected "Connect Four"; the relationship appeared to be taking hold.

Session 2

At the second session, the therapist asked Susan to make her family out of clay. Susan fashioned her two sisters and her mother. When asked to include her father, she refused. "He's not here anymore." The therapist quickly fashioned a rough figure. "This is your father," she said. "He'll be over here." The therapist placed the figure at the far corner of the clay board.

THERAPIST: I would like you to say something to each person.

SUSAN: (*to her oldest sister*) You don't care anything about me. You're always off with your friends. (*to her middle sister*) I wish you wouldn't tease me so much. (*to her mother*) I wish you didn't have to work so much and could be home more.

THERAPIST: Now say something to your father.

SUSAN: I don't want to.

THERAPIST: OK. You don't have to. Susan, sometimes when a parent commits suicide, kids blame themselves and are ashamed to tell anyone. I wonder if that's true for you.

SUSAN: Other kids feel those things too?

THERAPIST: Yes, they are very common feelings!

SUSAN: I don't know what I did, but I was supposed to move in with him and then he went and killed himself. I thought he was glad I was coming. And I don't want anyone to know. They'll know it was because of me.

THERAPIST: It's hard for you to feel those things. I'm sorry.

Susan nodded and closed down. This was obvious by her lack of contact, her body posture, and her decreased energy. The therapist suggested they stop talking and play "Connect Four" again. Susan visibly brightened and took down the game with renewed energy. The therapist told Susan that her mother would be joining them at the next session.

Session 3

At the third session, with the mother present, the therapist asked Susan and her mother each to draw something that made them angry. Susan watched her mother draw and then finally began to work on her own picture. The mother drew an incident that happened at work and talked a little about it.

SUSAN: I didn't do what you asked me to. I just drew my family.

THERAPIST: OK. I notice that you didn't draw your father. Just make a little circle up here in the corner for him. Susan, tell each person in your family something that makes you angry or you don't like that they do.

Susan complied, but again refused to talk to the father figure.

THERAPIST: (*to Susan's mother*) I wonder if you would be willing to say something to your ex-husband over here. It is hard for Susan to do it. Anything you would like to tell him.

Susan's mother immediately began to express intense anger at him for killing himself, causing so much hurt and pain to his children, especially to Susan, and leaving her solely responsible for the three children.

Susan began to cry and said she was angry too, and that she was sure it was all her fault. The therapist directed Susan to tell this to the father figure. Susan's mother voiced astonishment and emphatically assured Susan that this was not the case, that her Dad had financial problems and that she thought that was why he probably did it, and that he loved Susan very much. But it just got to be too much for him. Susan continued to cry as her mother embraced her.

Session 4

At the fourth session, the therapist suggested that Susan draw a picture of something she had enjoyed doing with her father. She drew a picture of a swimming pool and talked about how much fun they used to have swimming together. She then asked if she could do a sand tray and proceeded to make a graveyard scene, announcing that one of the graves belonged to her father.

THERAPIST: Susan, I would like you to talk to your father's grave.
SUSAN: Dad, I hope you are happy where you are. I miss you a lot. I'm sorry things were rough for you.
THERAPIST: Could you tell him you love him?
SUSAN: Yes! Dad, I love you. (*long pause*) Goodbye. (*to the therapist*) Do we have time to play a game?

Session 5

Susan and the therapist had one more session together. Her mother was unable to attend and sent a note saying that Susan was behaving appropriately. The therapist asked Susan what she would like to do at this goodbye session, and Susan opted for clay. She made a birthday cake, with toothpicks for candles, stating with much gaiety that her dad's birthday was coming up and she wanted to have a cake ready for him.

This work took five sessions. Here again, as with Jack, the relationship was established quickly and Susan was quite responsive in spite of her initial resistance. The issue of responsibility for her father's death appeared to be dispensed with quickly. Anger and sadness were expressed. The therapist called Susan's mother to tell her that Susan had worked on the loss of her father at her particular developmental level but that deeper feelings might emerge at later developmental levels, involving issues that Susan did not have the self-support to deal with now. How she functioned in her life was the best measurement for whether or not Susan needed further therapeutic work.

Case 3: Jimmy

Six-year-old Jimmy was brought in by his dad. Jimmy's sister, 2 years younger, had been killed in an automobile accident, and Jimmy and his parents had sustained minor injuries. The father said that Jimmy seemed to be functioning well, but he felt that Jimmy needed help to deal with his sister's death, since he never spoke of her. Jimmy's mother, extremely grieved and barely functioning, was under a psychiatrist's care. Jimmy remained stoic. The therapist assumed that Jimmy was afraid to show his grief for fear of losing his mom—he needed to be strong for her. Jimmy's dad told the therapist that the children had related quite well, played together all the time, but that Jimmy loved to tease his sister, sometimes hit her, and seemed to enjoy making her cry. Jimmy, still at an egocentric developmental level, probably blamed himself for her death, particularly in light of his behavior toward her. The therapist felt that this latter issue, plus Jimmy's fear of losing his mother's love and attention, seemed to be priorities for their work together.

Session 1

At the first session, while the father talked to the therapist, Jimmy refused to talk and sat at the sandtray, running his hands through the sand. The therapist could see by Jimmy's body posture that he was listening intently. The therapist asked Jimmy if it was OK with him if his father waited in the waiting room. Jimmy nodded, his back still to the therapist. The therapist drew Jimmy's attention to the shelves of miniatures, inviting him to set them in the sand to make a scene. Jimmy proceeded to put all the trees he could find in the sand, and under one of them he placed a very small rabbit. "I'm done," he said on his own.

THERAPIST: Jimmy, could you tell me about your scene?

JIMMY: It's a forest with lots of trees.

THERAPIST: What about that little rabbit?

JIMMY: He's hiding under that tree.

THERAPIST: I'd like to talk to him. Would you be his voice, you know, as if he were a puppet? Rabbit, what are you doing?

JIMMY: I'm hiding.

THERAPIST: What are you hiding from?

JIMMY: Sometimes big animals eat rabbits. I'm hiding from them.

THERAPIST: You have a good hiding place. Do you feel safe?

JIMMY: No, I'm still scared.

THERAPIST: Is there anyone around to help you?

JIMMY: (*very low voice—body scrunched*) No.

THERAPIST: Oh, that must be hard for you.

JIMMY: Yeah.

The therapist at that point told Jimmy that they could play a game for the 5 minutes until the session ended. She asked him if it was OK if she took a picture of his scene and postponed putting the objects away so she could look at it. He readily agreed.

Session 2

Jimmy came in, asking if he could make another sand scene, and proceeded to make the exact scene he had made the previous week, except for another rabbit that he placed near the first one. "Now the rabbit has someone to help him," he said. It was the therapist's guess that Jimmy was acknowledging the help he might receive from the therapist.

THERAPIST: Jimmy, I am so sorry that you lost your sister. I would like it very much if you would draw a picture of her so I could have an idea of what she looked like.

Jimmy drew her picture willingly, explaining as he drew about the color of her hair, her eyes, the clothes she was wearing, and other details.

THERAPIST: Jimmy, I am going to make a list of some of the things you and your sister did together. Tell me one thing.

JIMMY: Well, we colored pictures from a book she had. We played Captain

Hook and Peter Pan—I was Captain Hook. We built stuff with blocks. She was only 4 and I had to show her how to do things.

THERAPIST: I know you were a good big brother. Big brothers sometimes tease their sisters too. Did you do that? I know my son used to tease his little sister and she would run crying to me. Now they are grown up and good friends. I bet you and Julie would have been very good friends as you got older.

JIMMY: Your son teased his sister? Yeah! I teased Julie a lot! I could make her cry easy. She bugged me sometimes too, and I would hit her. Then she would cry and run to my mom, who would get mad at me. I liked her really.

THERAPIST: I bet you miss her a lot.

JIMMY: (*nodding with tears in his eyes*)

The therapist offered to do a puppet show for Jimmy. In the first scene, two animal puppets—a dog and a cat—were playing and the dog began to call the cat silly names. The cat began to cry. In the second scene, a larger animal, an eagle, told the dog that there had been an accident and the cat had died. The dog began to cry, saying he did not mean to tease her. The eagle assured him that the cat did not die because of his teasing. In the third scene, the dog told the eagle how sad he was to lose his sister. The eagle hugged him.

Jimmy watched this simple show intently and immediately asked if he could do it himself. His show was actually more involved, with the dog telling the eagle about hitting the cat and being mean sometimes, and the eagle continuing to assure him that these actions did not cause her death. Jimmy's last statement on leaving this session was "I loved this puppet show!"

Session 3

The therapist asked Jimmy if he thought his mother was very mad at him, since she was so upset. Jimmy began to cry. Because of his developmental level, it was logical that Jimmy would feel that his mother's intense grief was his fault.

THERAPIST: Jimmy, I think your mom is just so sad about losing Julie that she is sick from it. I don't think she's mad at you at all. Is it OK if we ask your dad into the session so we can talk about this?

Jimmy nodded. The therapist asked Jimmy to tell his dad about thinking his mom was mad at him. Jimmy looked at the therapist, who then asked if she could tell him. He nodded vigorously. Jimmy's father was horrified at this idea, and with much emotion told Jimmy how much he and his mother loved him. Jimmy climbed on his dad's lap and sobbed.

Session 4

Jimmy told the therapist that his mother seemed a little better. She had smiled and hugged him that morning, he reported. The therapist guessed to herself that Jimmy's dad spoke to his mom about their last session. The therapist told Jimmy to make his sister out of clay and to talk to her. Jimmy told the clay figure that he missed her very much, was sorry she died, and that he would think about her a lot. He then spontaneously picked up the figure, kissed it, and said goodbye. "I want to play that game ['Blockhead'] before I leave today."

This was actually the last session. Jimmy's dad called to say that he felt Jimmy did not need any more sessions. The therapist advised him to watch for any new symptoms that might emerge, since there were many issues that had not been addressed that might affect Jimmy. He was also advised that developmentally, perhaps, Jimmy had expressed as much as he could handle at this time, and that as he became emotionally stronger, some of the other issues might need to be addressed.

Case 4: Sally

Another situation involved Sally, a 9-year-old girl whose mother had been physically abused by her father; finally, the mother had managed to escape to a new city where there was no contact at all with the father. At their new location, however, Sally had become sullen, abusive, and aggressive toward her younger sister and mother. The mother advised the therapist that they could only come in for five or six sessions. Based on previous experiences with similar situations, the therapist felt that the child might have conflicted feelings involving the loss of her father, and anger at her mother for taking her away from him as well as her friends, her school, and her previous home.

Session 1

At the first session, Sally appeared quite anxious as her mother spoke, sitting with hunched shoulders and pursed lips. The therapist directed her "intake" questions to Sally, writing the answers on the pad on her clipboard. "Do you sleep OK? Do you have bad dreams sometimes? What's school like here?" and so forth. The therapist had found that many anxious and resistant children responded to a form or paper clipped to a board as she wrote the answers. This seemed to place some distance between the therapist and child, helping to reduce any apprehension the child might have. Furthermore, asking the child pertinent questions directly, in a casual, conversational manner, rather than asking the parent, involved the child immediately. Sally responded readily, visibly relaxed, and then asked why all the toys and "stuff" were in the room. The therapist explained that they were used, along with drawings and clay and the sandtrays, to help kids express what was going on inside of them instead of just having to talk. The mother was very nervous at this session and seemed anxious to leave. The therapist invited her to wait in the waiting room while she and Sally got acquainted.

The therapist encouraged Sally to go around the room and look at everything. After a thorough examination, Sally was drawn to the dollhouse and began arranging and rearranging furniture. After some time the therapist suggested that she choose a family that would live in the dollhouse. Sally selected a mother, father, small boy, and medium-sized girl, and placed them in various parts of the house. The therapist remarked that the family appeared to be a pleasant, happy one. Sally agreed, and suddenly, clearly, lost her energy and enthusiasm with the dollhouse. The therapist suggested that they play a game and Sally, with renewed contact, selected "Uno."

When a child suddenly loses interest in a task, breaks contact when there had been good energy toward the task, it is generally a fairly reliable clue that something has occurred that has caused the child to close down. It seemed evident that the "happy family" in the dollhouse touched a painful spot in Sally. This type of closing down is actually a positive event in the therapeutic process since it indicates that just behind this resistance, feelings are coming closer to the surface.

Since the mother had been emphatic regarding the limited number of sessions, the therapist mapped out a program for the therapy, always cognizant of the fact that expectations would be anathema. Her plan for Sally consisted of the following:

At the next session she would present a nonthreatening mode of expression such as the scribble technique, which is fun and easy, and can lead to important projections. At the third session, the therapist thought she might ask Sally to make figures of her family, including her father, out of clay, and request that Sally dialogue with each of them. The therapist might help her to focus on anger, self-blame, and sadness at the loss of her father, as well as her familiar home. At the fourth session, the therapist thought she might incorporate all of these feelings, including, perhaps, any confusion Sally might feel, through drawing or painting. In this way, the varied feelings became more explicit, making it easier to work through them. Furthermore, in time, the percussion instruments could be used to "play" with feelings, providing a nurturing, enjoyable atmosphere around these emotions. At the fifth session, the therapist would suggest that Sally make a sand scene about her life. Finally, at the last session, the therapist would meet with Sally and her mother and spend some time giving the mother suggestions for helping Sally to express her feelings appropriately, as well as refining their communication skills.

The following is a summary of what actually took place.

Session 2

The therapist introduced the scribble technique, asking Sally to make a scribble and find a picture to color within this scribble. Sally appeared to enjoy this task and found a picture of a large cat surrounded by trees. She told this story about the cat:

> "Once upon a time, there was this cat who lost her way. She was walking home from a visit to a friend and somehow got lost. She had taken a shortcut through the forest and now she was lost. She didn't know where she was or which way to go to get home. It got dark and she heard all kinds of noises and got very scared."

THERAPIST: Then what happened?

SALLY: She got very tired and curled up under a tree and went to sleep.

THERAPIST: What happened when she woke up?

SALLY: When it was morning, the cat knew where she was and ran home. The family was very happy to see her and pet her and fed her. The end.

THERAPIST: That was a good story! Sally, is there anything about your story that fits for you and your life?

SALLY: I don't know. (*long pause*) Well, maybe I don't know where the home I used to have is.

THERAPIST: Tell me about the home you used to have.

Sally began to describe the house she lived in, her neighborhood, her school, and her friends. She was very animated while doing this, watching the therapist carefully (for her reaction?). The therapist realized that it was not possible for Sally to talk about these topics when she was with her mother since any mention of her previous home was probably very upsetting to her mother. In the last 10 minutes of the session the therapist decided to introduce instruments, and she and Sally played, with much gaiety, music that was happy, sad, crazy, lonely, and especially mad.

Session 3

At the next session, the therapist had put out the pottery clay, boards, and tools. They sat at the table playing with the clay. After a while, the therapist asked Sally to make her family out of clay. Sally ignored this direction and proceeded to make various kinds of food. The therapist dropped her plan and joined Sally in pretending to eat the food. Sally giggled at the therapist's dramatic enjoyment of the food. In between bites, the therapist fashioned rough figures of Sally's family: mother, sister, as well as father, whom she placed some distance from the rest of the family.

THERAPIST: Sally, I want you to say something to each person here; maybe something you like about them, something you don't like, or just anything you want to say.

SALLY: (*to her sister*) I like to play with you sometimes. I don't like it when you take my stuff. (*to her mother*) (*long pause*) I like it when you play with me. (*to the therapist*) She's always working and tired.

THERAPIST: Maybe that could be the thing you could tell her you don't like.

SALLY: Yeah. I don't like it that you are always working and tired and don't have time to play with me very much anymore.

THERAPIST: Now say something to your father over here in the corner.

SALLY: I don't want to talk to him now.

With this statement, Sally picked up the rubber mallet and began to hit a nearby mound of clay.

THERAPIST: Sally, show me how hard you can hit the clay. Stand up if you have to.

Sally began to pound the clay with all her might, holding the mallet with both hands.

THERAPIST: What are you thinking about, Sally, when you do that?

SALLY: Nothing.

THERAPIST: I bet there are a lot of things in your life that make you mad. Just hit the clay—you don't have to tell me what they are.

Sally continued to hit the clay as the therapist cheered her on. When the time was up, they cleaned up.

Session 4

At the fourth session, Sally's mother told the therapist that there could only be one more session since she had changed jobs and could not bring her daughter in after that session. The therapist urged her to accompany Sally for the last session and she reluctantly agreed.

Feeling desperate because of the lack of time, the therapist decided to offer Sally a puppet show. The show consisted of three scenes, which the therapist hoped would address some of the issues relating to Sally's situation. In the first scene, a mother puppet was singing to herself, "I'm cooking dinner, I'm cooking dinner." The father puppet came in yelling, "What's for dinner? I'm hungry! I hope it's ready." The mother puppet replied, "It will be ready very soon, dear. It will just be a few more minutes." The father yelled, "I want it now!" and hit the mother squarely on the head. Sally murmured from her place in the audience, "That's just like my life." The therapist did not respond to this remark and changed scenes. Then, two furry animal puppets, a monkey and a dog, were conferring. The monkey (the smaller of the two puppets) said, "Did you see Daddy hit Mommy again? I wish he didn't do that. It scares me." The dog replied, "Yeah. It scares me too. I'm mad that he does that. Why does he have to hurt Mommy like that!" The monkey replied, "You need to tell him to stop. After all, you are the older one. You can tell him. Maybe he'll listen if he knows how we feel." The dog agreed he would try. In the next scene, the dog called Dad, who said, "Yes, son, what is it?" With a great deal of difficulty and emotion the dog said, "Daddy, you have to stop hitting Mommy. It scares me very much and it scares my little brother. And Dad, it makes me mad that you do that!!!" The father puppet acted very upset but finally said, "I guess I do lose control. I'll try to stop. I don't want you and your brother to be scared of me." "Thanks, Dad," the dog said, and they hugged.

This was the end of the show and Sally immediately asked if she could do it herself. Sally repeated the show, adding her own words. The therapist offered to do another show in the remaining time of the session. This time, the dog called his mother and said, "Mommy, I have to tell you something. Don't get mad." She replied, "Honey, you can tell me anything." "OK," the dog said, "I miss Daddy." The mother puppet became very flustered. "You know we can't see him!!" The dog quickly said, "I know we can't see him. I just wanted to tell you I wish I could and that I miss him. And sometimes it makes me mad at you that you took us so far away from everything." The mother, quiet for a few seconds, then said, "I know you miss him. After all he was an OK father to you. Maybe after a while you'll be able to see him. I know I can make you mad sometimes. That's OK. I get mad at things too." The dog said, "Thanks, Mommy. I just wanted to tell you." And they embraced.

Sally was equally thrilled with this little show and soon made it her own. The therapist was aware that Sally had been too afraid to tell her father about her anger and other feelings she had, but she wanted to at least help Sally know that her feelings were normal and acceptable.

Session 5

At the last session, Sally wanted to put on both shows for her mom. The therapist warned the mother that she might not like the content but that it was important to understand that Sally had hidden feelings that might be the cause of her behavior, and that expressing them through fantasy at least was very relieving and healing for Sally. Sally did the shows with great gusto and her mother applauded generously as she dabbed at the tears in her eyes. The therapist talked a little about the need for Sally to express her feelings while her mother listened without judgment.

A month later the therapist called Sally's mother, who reported that Sally was much calmer and easier to live with, was no longer unusually belligerent, and in general was doing quite well. The mother, who seemed calmer herself, thanked the therapist profusely. The therapist advised the mother to be alert for new symptoms as Sally reached new developmental stages.

I have often used puppet shows, such as those described for Sally and Jimmy, particularly in situations where the child has much difficulty expressing feelings. Children are fascinated by such shows, and are very forgiving if they are not "perfect." Significant issues can be presented dramatically in simple scenes and the metaphorical messages are quite powerful. They seem to reach the child at a very deep level.

SUMMARY AND CONCLUSIONS

In this chapter, I have attempted to offer some effective methods for working with children around the issues of loss and grief on a short-term basis. These methods have at their base the theory, philosophy, and practice of Gestalt therapy. These projective techniques (drawings, clay, and fantasy; storytelling, sandtray scenes, music, and puppetry) make it possible for children to express their deeper feelings in a nonthreatening, often fun, way. The therapist must have an understanding of the myriad issues involved in traumatic loss, and determine which ones are most essential for immediate focus in the service of brief therapy. The therapist must do this gradually, even when the time is short, to allow the child to feel safe and disclose the deeper parts of him- or herself slowly. The therapist must take care not to intrude or push the child into doing or expressing anything he or she resists. This resistance is usually an indication that the child does not have enough self-support to deal with the material presented; it must be honored regardless of the short-term requirements. Though the therapist may have goals and plans, expectations can be toxic. The therapist must be infinitely sensitive to the child.

Prerequisite to any work is establishing some thread of a relationship. This relationship will build with each session. Contact, as described in this chapter, must be present each time in order for any significant work to take place, and the therapist must carefully observe the breaking of contact in order to deflect the work into something less intimidating for the child. With practice, the therapist can anticipate the loss of contact through the child's body responses: lack of energy, deflation, glazed eyes. It is futile for the therapist to attempt to ignore this evidence that the child is not fully present in the encounter. The child must be allowed time to withdraw from contact as needed. It is the therapist's responsibility to be fully contactful with the child, regardless of the child's inability to do so. However the child presents the self, the therapist meets him or her with respect, with no anticipation for a particular response. He or she must be gentle, authentic, and respectful, without becoming enmeshed or confluent with the child.

In short-term work, many other issues that cry out for attention may emerge or become obvious to the therapist. If the mandate is for brief therapy, priorities need to be followed. If good results are achieved, that is, if the child appears to make some closure regarding the loss incurred, the work must be deemed successful. Often, what the child experiences in these few sessions will carry over into other areas of his or her life.

Children do not know how to grieve and often are confused about the various feelings within them. The metaphors that emerge from projective techniques offer a safe distance to children, allowing the therapist to gently help them own the feelings that are fitting. It is through this ownership that children can move through the grief process. Therapists who work with children are privileged to have the opportunity to help them ease through difficult passages in their lives.

ACKNOWLEDGMENTS

This chapter is adapted from the book *Hidden Treasure: A Map to the Child's Inner Self,* by Violet Oaklander. Copyright 2006 by Violet Oaklander. Adapted with permission from Karnac Books.

REFERENCES

Bowlby, J. (1973–1983). *Attachment, separation, and loss.* New York: Basic Books.
Buber, M. (1958). *I and thou.* New York: Scribner.

Kübler-Ross, E. (1973). *On death and dying.* New York: Macmillan.

Worden, W. J. (2001). *Children and grief.* New York: Springer.

Worden, W. J. (2008). *Grief counseling and grief therapy.* New York: Guilford Press.

Latner, J. (1986). *The Gestalt therapy book.* New York: Gestalt Journal Press.

Oaklander, V. (1982). The relationship of Gestalt therapy to children. *Gestalt Journal,* *1,* 64–74.

Oaklander, V. (1988). *Windows to our children.* New York: Gestalt Journal Press.

Perls, F. S. (1969). *Ego, hunger and aggression.* New York: Vintage Books.

Perls, F. S., Hefferline, R., & Goodman, P. (1951). *Gestalt therapy.* New York: Julian.

Polster, E., & Polster, M. (1973). *Gestalt therapy integrated.* New York: Brunner/ Mazel.

Terr, L. (1990). *Too scared to cry.* New York: Basic Books.

Chapter 7

Solution–Focused Sandtray Therapy for Children

Elizabeth R. Taylor

*S*olution-focused (SF) therapy, a constructivist, systems-oriented, strength-based approach to therapy, relies primarily on clients' verbal skills. However, by integrating SF therapy and sandtray therapies, clients are provided with a dynamic communication device through which they can express their concerns in a kinesthetic, three-dimensional field; see and play with possibilities; note their personal and contextual resources; and project themselves into the future to a place and time where they have reached their goals.

SF SANDTRAY THERAPY

Jack, a 13-year-old middle school boy, was referred for counseling because his grades indicated a steady decline over the semester. His parents had divorced, and Jack and his two younger brothers spent their week divided between the mother's and the father's residences. Frequently, Jack took care of his younger brothers when either parent was not home. Jack's sole pleasure was playing soccer with his team that his father also coached. When he first came to therapy, the therapist asked Jack to create his world in the sand. He completed the task in 10 minutes. In the middle of the sandtray was a toilet. On each side, some distance from the toilet, were two army men, crouched and aiming their bazookas at one another. Pointing to each soldier, Jack said, "This is my mom, and this is my dad." Pointing to the toilet, he said, "This is me. My life is in the toilet." Aside from these three miniatures, nothing else was in the tray. Words were hardly needed to gain an understanding of Jack's feelings, his lack of resources, and his view of life at that moment.

The therapist sat quietly with Jack for a few minutes and then stated, "You are really having a tough time right now. How do you do it? How do you get up and go to school every day?" Jack described how he took care of himself and his brothers when they were at his mother's house, got them dressed for school, and made sure they had their backpacks. He also talked about how hard his father worked to take care of the family because his mother was an alcoholic who was always trying to quit drinking but had not been successful. Jack spoke of how much he liked soccer, how he spent afternoons practicing his skills against the side of the house, and how much he enjoyed playing soccer with his dad as coach. The therapist noted aloud that she was amazed at his independence and sense of responsibility and also by his determination to be a good soccer player. She asked Jack to expand on the relationship he had with his father, who was obviously a strong support for Jack.

This session could have gone down a different path. The therapist could have asked about the toilet he placed in the sandtray or about his mother's drinking, how he felt when she drank, or what it was like to live in an alcoholic family, to go through a divorce, or be responsible for his two younger brothers. However, none of these paths would change the situation in which Jack found himself, or help him solve his problems at school. Going down this different path would not have been the wrong thing to do, but Jack might have left feeling like he still had no resources and his problems were more difficult than he thought. Instead, the therapist, using SF therapy, took note of the capable young man and his sense of responsibility. Through sandtray and SF therapy, the client was able to communicate his physical and emotional burdens for the therapist, yet leave with a sense of pride in his accomplishments and a little hope that things might get better.

THEORETICAL APPROACHES

SF Therapy

SF therapy, a poststructural, constructivist approach, focuses on clients' strengths and resources to help them set their own goals, open possibilities, and build hope. Influenced by the communication approaches of Don Jackson and Milton Erickson, as well as by the interactional and systemic approach of The Mental Research Institute in Palo Alto, California (De Jong & Berg, 2008; de Shazer & Dolan, 2007), Insoo Kim Berg and Steve de Shazer recognized the value of how questions were worded, the focus of conversations, and the slightest innuendos in content and tone that might influence positive changes and empower individuals, families, and organizations. Rather than basing their approach on past theories and philosophies, Berg and de Shazer based SF therapy on what clients said was helpful (de Shazer & Molnar, 1984; De Jong & Berg, 2008).

The SF therapy approach relies on the therapist's view of the client as one of competence, resources, strengths, and resiliencies. Resiliency, defined as "the process of, capacity for, or outcomes of successful adaptation despite challenging or threatening circumstances" (Masten, Best, & Garmezy, 1990, p. 426), describes individuals who have been able to overcome difficult circumstances using individual and environmental resiliency mechanisms and processes, and who will continue to do so in the future (Masten & Coatsworth, 1998). The SF therapist aims to assist clients in uncovering these resiliencies, these "buried treasures," and to embrace them.

Overall, SF therapists rely on three basic principles: (1) "If it is not broken, don't fix it"; (2) "If it is not working, do something different"; and (3) "If it is working, do more of it" (de Shazer & Dolan, 2007, pp. 1–2). These principles guide the therapist to listen for what is working or has worked in the past, while at the same time taking notice of the client's strengths and resources that might be useful in addressing current challenges.

SF therapists focus on building nonjudgmental, sensitive, and genuine relationships with clients. As much as possible, the therapeutic relationship is one of equality rather than one in which the therapist is the "expert." The client is the real expert on his or her own life and the solution to the problem, though it may not always be evident (De Jong & Berg, 2008). The therapist intervenes by asking carefully worded questions that help the client see new perspectives, change behaviors, and reach goals.

The focus of therapy is on present and future challenges and solutions rather than the past, except to the extent that the client has solved similar problems but was able to cope with them or find solutions. The therapist attends to what the client is currently doing that is working, what is occurring when the problem is not present, and how the client is coping. It is assumed that the more the therapist focuses on the problem, the more the client focuses on the problem, but when the therapist focuses on exceptions to the problem and solutions, the client begins to see new possibilities (Berg & de Shazer, 1993).

Traditional assessment often involves diagnosing a client's problems and assigning a diagnostic label. Contrary to this approach, the SF therapist assesses strengths, resiliencies, and resources that the client has used in the past or is currently using to solve problems. Then, through carefully crafted questions, comments, and affirmations, the therapist asks questions and makes comments to shed light on these assets and strengths that have existed but may not have always been evident to the client. As this light brightens, the landscape of possibilities comes into focus, so that the client feels more empowered and open to possibilities for handling current and future challenges.

Limitations

Reliance on words in talk therapy, specifically SF therapy, limits the range of its effectiveness with various populations. For example, some clients may not have the maturity to understand or express themselves verbally, have language and learning differences, struggle with speech impediments, or have experienced traumatic or shameful histories that preclude the ability to use words. For those who have suffered neglect and abuse, accessing the cognitive skills needed for verbal expression may not be possible until lower levels of brain functioning are first addressed, including those areas responsible for self-regulation, impulsivity, and attention (Perry, 2009). To work with the SF model, the therapist needs to be flexible and open to other modalities and approaches that make therapy more understandable and developmentally appropriate (Selekman, 1997).

   Challenges with developmentally appropriate language have been particularly problematic in family therapy with young children; however, when the therapist employed family art and play interventions, such as creating a family picture together or having family members draw individual pictures of the family, children were more likely to engage (Selekman, 1997). Berg and Steiner (2003) recognized the developmental needs of children and introduced concrete materials into the SF therapy process, such as "power hands," cartoons, the "Scribble Game," making up stories, and "The Most Wanted Person." Similarly, Nims (2007) described the application of SF therapy to play therapy using developmentally appropriate techniques, such as puppets, art, and sandtray. Recently, sandtray has been offered as a tangible approach to SF therapy (Homeyer & Sweeney, 2011; Nims, 2007; Taylor, 2009).

Sandtray

The therapeutic use of sand and miniatures dates back to the early 1900s, when Margaret Lowenfeld used sandtray as a nonverbal alternative to assist clients in communicating and resolving internal and external conflicts and experiences. She called her approach the "world technique" (Turner, 2005). Dora Maria Kalff, a student of Lowenfeld's and a Jungian therapist, applied Jungian concepts to the world technique and developed "sandplay." Although Lowenfeld and Kalff equally valued the use of sandtray as a nonverbal approach to therapy, their views of process and outcomes differed. For Kalff, the important aspect of sandplay was healing at the unconscious level. Her approach was to sit quietly and observe as the client created the sandtray and then to interpret the symbols provided by the child's sandtray creation. On the other hand, Lowenfeld saw sandtray work as a type of dialogue for children who had difficulty expressing themselves; therefore, she actively engaged with clients, asked questions, and refrained from interpreting symbolism. Instead, she let the child identify the sandtray's meaning (Hutton, 2004).

The use of sand and miniatures in therapy have been viewed through the eyes of different therapeutic approaches—Gestalt therapy (Oaklander, 2003), Adlerian therapy (Bainum, Schneider, & Stone, 2006), Jungian therapy (sandplay) (Peery, 2003), and constructivist therapies (Freeman, Espston, & Lebovits, 1997; Spooner & Lyddon, 2007), particularly SF therapy (Homeyer & Sweeney, 2011; Nims, 2007; Sweeney, 2011; Taylor, 2009). Just as the philosophy behind each of these theories differs, so does their application to sandtray, including the therapy goals, therapist roles, client directives, and whether or not to use interpretation.

Sandtray offers a number of advantages over talk therapy alone. First, sandtray appeals to most all developmental levels. This reality can be seen at any beach, often crowded with toddlers, children, teens, and adults playing in sand and water, creating structures, digging holes, and burying and unburying themselves and objects. Lowenfeld (1935/2008) stated that of all the equipment used in a play room, the most important is that of the "world cabinet" which includes the sandtray and miniatures in a space that is easily accessible by the client. Supporting this opinion, Ray and colleagues (2013) recently found that of over 100 play materials in the playroom, 72% of the children in client-centered play therapy chose to play with the sandbox and its tools.

The use of a sandtray facilitates a positive relationship with the client by quickly putting the client at ease. Since the materials are familiar to children, they are less likely to be intimidated by the therapy process and more likely to associate these familiar objects with the therapist, thus providing a catalyst for the rapport- and relationship-building processes (Gil, 2006). Because using sandtray does not require artistic talent, working with the sandtray creates less self-judgment regarding "right" and "wrong" ways of creating (Gil, 2006). This freedom facilitates the client's sense of acceptance by the therapist but also acceptance of the process through which therapy is initiated.

Due to the playful nature of sandtray, clients freely express what may have been difficult to express verbally due to shame, guilt, or fear. Instead, they creatively merge fantasy and reality and expand on possibilities, often surprising even themselves (Mook, 2003). Yet the sandtray provides structure and safety due to the sandtray's concrete boundaries, which can be particularly helpful with those who have aggressive and impulsive tendencies (Sweeney & Homeyer, 2009).

One of the most important benefits of sandtray work is the client's control over the sandtray process and materials. This control is important for children and adolescents who lack influence over the circumstances that affect their lives, particularly those who have been sexually, physically, or emotionally hurt or who are experiencing grief and loss due to parental divorce or the death of a close family member. The client's control over the sandtray often allows this reconstruction of meaning and purpose in the safety of the therapeutic relationship.

Although children begin to prefer more verbal modes of expression as they mature (Gil, 2006), some still gravitate toward the sandtray and miniatures even in middle and high school, perhaps feeling that they won't really give anything away if working through a nonverbal modality. When adolescents hesitate to participate in the sandtray process, the therapist can initiate play by sifting the sand between his or her fingers. This often results in the client mirroring this activity, playing with the sand while talking, eventually selecting miniatures and placing them in the sandtray. Even just running the hands through the sand can be relaxing enough that the adolescent begins to verbally engage with the therapist or the sandtray materials.

For some, the use of words can be emotionally difficult, causing shame and embarrassment (Kestley, 2005), but in sandtray the client communicates through the materials, distancing the self from the emotional content yet communicating the essence of the experience. By gaining emotional distance, the client may be able to rely more on cognitive processes to focus on what meaning this experience may have, what may be learned from it, and possible solutions and alternative paths toward change.

Through sandtray, experiences can be accessed through all the senses, three-dimensionally, so that what the client expresses through sandtray more closely resembles reality than verbal descriptions alone (Kestley, 2005). In sandtray, the miniatures and the sand, as well as the process and placement of the miniatures, constitute the language through which clients (and sometimes therapists) communicate their stories, problems, and solutions.

The integration of SF therapy and sandtray offers other advantages as well. SF therapy, based on systemic practices, emphasizes the contextual and relational influences of the client(s). Through sandtray, these influences become tangible, visible, and dynamic, as clients select miniatures and place them in the sandtray to illustrate past, current, and future challenges and solutions. Using this miniature world, the client can safely practice new behaviors before trying them outside of the therapy room. They can also see the influence these behaviors may have on significant others and address how others' reactions might impact them. Finally, clients might consider other resources yet to be uncovered until seen in a visual, tangible field. Many other advantages exist in the use of SF therapy with sandtray, since the client is able to see and control the miniatures and create a world of possibilities.

STAGES OF SF SANDTRAY

The SF sandtray process encompasses six stages that are based on solution-focused (De Jong & Berg, 2008) and sandtray therapies (Homeyer & Sweeney, 2011). When applying these stages, the therapist should remain flexible and attentive to clients' personal frames of reference, strengths, and contexts. How the therapist moves through the stages and what techniques are used should be in response to individual clients, since clients are the experts on their own problems and solutions. Although these stages are presented in linear fashion, clients may move in and out of different stages. For example, it is not unusual for the therapist to refocus on the client–therapist relationship (see Stage 2) when clients deal with difficult and traumatic events in order to reinforce the therapist's support of the client.

Stage 1: Preparing for the Client

The first stage, preparing for the client, involves not only reviewing notes from past sessions and making a plan for the current session, but also "setting up the room" (Homeyer & Sweeney, 2011, p. 34) with a thoughtful selection of sandtrays and miniatures. Standard sandtrays, approximately 30″ × 20″ × 3″ and painted blue on the bottom to represent water, should be large enough for the client to express what is meaningful, but not so big that they become overwhelming to the client. Two sandtrays are recommended, one with wet sand and another with dry sand. However, if only using one sandtray, it is important to have a container with water to be used with the sandtray (Homeyer & Sweeney, 2011).

An advantage of using two sandtrays is their use in making contrasts and comparisons, such as making sandtrays illustrating the difference between problems and solutions, the problem and its exception, or the problem and hypothetical outcomes. If only using one tray, a rectangular tray is more beneficial than a round tray, because it can be divided easily (Homeyer & Sweeney, 2011) to compare scenes. For example, Lynn, a seventh-grade boy wrestling with acceptance by his peers, spontaneously created a sandtray to describe his dilemma. On one side of the sandtray, the standard rectangular-size container, was a young man standing with three or four other young men with scattered beer bottles and a grave. On the other side of the sandtray, he placed a young man, woman, and several biblical miniatures. He stated, "This is me. I can go ahead and hang out with my friends and go to parties and drink and do drugs, or I can go to church and quit doing drugs." The therapist asked the client, "Which of these do you think would help you reach your goals?" The discussion then focused on the client's goals, other choices, and the influence of his choices on himself, others, and what he wants.

Miniatures

Miniatures should be carefully selected and organized. Categories of miniatures include people (variety of ages, ethnic groups, and family types), animals (prehistoric, zoo, farm/domestic, birds, insects, sea life), buildings, vehicles, vegetation, fences, signs, bridges, nature items, fantasy figures, landscaping items, household items, and other miscellaneous items, such as medical pieces, alcohol containers, brushes, and spatulas. Homeyer and Sweeney (2011) provide a comprehensive list of items and categories but state that the therapist need not have all items to do sandtray. Rather, it is best to select several items from each category to begin, being sure that items are placed in categories for selection and are relevant to the client's world. For example, Jack, whose mother struggled with alcohol, needed to have those items that would help him express his thoughts about his mother, including beer and wine bottles to use with the sandtray. Jack often illustrated his current situation by placing many or a few of the alcohol miniatures around the figure that he used to represent his mother, indicating how bad the drinking had been the week before the session.

When using SF therapy, numerous miniatures should be included that reflect strengths, resources, miracles, and goals, including treasure boxes, a lighthouse, a wishing well, gems and crystals, an Aladdin's lamp, different types of sports goals (e.g., soccer, basketball, football), magicians (male and female), and superheroes or animals that reflect strength and power. Materials can be collected from dollar stores, craft stores, play therapy resources, and even grocery stores among cake decorating items. These items are helpful in describing client strengths and resources, what will be better when the client reaches his or her goal, or what will be different when the problem is no longer present. One neglected middle schooler depicted his counselor as Superman. The school counselor had become a major source of support at school and the counselor's office a place he could go for a respite when he became overwhelmed by social and academic demands.

Stage 2: Introducing the Sandtray Process and the Presession Change Question

First and foremost, the beginning of the first session should focus on building the client–therapist relationship. "Sandtray therapy should involve a dynamic interpersonal relationship. Regardless of the specific therapeutic and theoretical approach one takes to the sandtray process, the evolution and development of a dynamic interpersonal relationship is crucial" (Homeyer & Sweeney, 1998, p. 4). Lambert and Cattani-Thompson (1996), reviewing the research regarding the effectiveness of counseling overall, suggest that aside from client variables, the counselor–client relationship is the best predictor of client outcomes. The relationship is indeed the "major mediator of therapeutic experiences" (Perry, 2009, p. 252).

Clients differ in terms of their approach to therapy. Some are eager to begin, whereas others tend to resist engaging in the sandtray process or the therapeutic relationship overall. This may depend on the attachment style of the client, what the client has been told about therapy, the client's temperament, and how the client experiences the problem that brought him or her to therapy. If a younger client appears reluctant, the therapist might spend the first 5 or 10 minutes reading a book, coloring or drawing together, or talking about the child's interests before introducing the sandtray. However, younger children are often less hesitant than older children since they tend to use these materials in their personal play time in kindergarten, at home, or in day care.

For older children who are somewhat hesitant, it is helpful if the therapist casually plays with the sand while talking with the client. This gives the client permission to do the same. With some clients, playing with sand allows the client to relax enough to verbally communicate with the therapist. Later, the client may be more open to suggestions to use the miniatures.

To introduce the sandtray process, the therapist might state, "Here is the sandtray and here are the miniatures. You can use any of the miniatures you want and place them in the sand." Many SF therapy techniques can be utilized in sandtray work (see Table 7.1). For example, the first SF suggestion given to the client may be the "presession change question," a technique that immediately creates a positive, goal-focused direction to therapy. The question "What changes have you noticed that have happened or started to happen since you called to make an appointment for this session" (de Shazer & Dolan, 2007) focuses clients on the exceptions to the problem rather than the problem itself. Using the sandtray, the suggestion might be, "In this tray, make a sandtray that shows how things were when you found out you were coming to see me. In the second tray, make a sandtray that shows how things are better." Ron, an 8-year-old boy, illustrated how things were better by placing only one parent in the second tray rather than the two parents that were in the first tray. He stated, "The police came and took my dad to jail last night." When asked what made this better, Ron discussed the domestic abuse his mother had endured for several months.

Although the presession change question can be helpful, it can also be confusing to children who do not know how much time has elapsed between the time of the referral and the first session. Sometimes, children do not realize they are going to therapy until they arrive. In one first session, when the child and parent entered the room, the child looked up at his mother and stated, "I thought we were going to the dentist."

Stage 3: Listening to the Client's Story

If the client completes the presession change sandtray or the therapist determines not to use the technique, one of the most common starting suggestions is "Create your world in the sand." This was the suggestion given to Jack, who discussed his life in the toilet, and it was all that was needed to gain an understanding of his world, the problem, his resources, the dynamics of the family, and the possible direction for therapy.

The Therapist's Role

The SF therapist listens carefully while clients tell their stories. Bliss (2010) described this technique as "extreme listening" (p. 219). To be an extreme listener, the therapist enters the therapy session without any preconceived notions, believes in the client's knowledge about the goals of therapy, asks questions for understanding, and listens "like a person possessed" (p. 111). Listening does not necessarily involve words; it may be sitting quietly but intensely focused on being with the client as he or she constructs the sandtray, asking questions to clarify meaning in order to understand exactly what the client intends when using such words as "bad," "sad," or "angry." As the therapist asks these questions, the client is empowered as a teacher (Bliss, 2010) and an expert on his or her own problem.

A SF therapist is more active in the sandtray process than a client-centered or Jungian therapist. Similar to other approaches to sandtray, the therapist listens and validates the story through nonverbal behaviors, such as nodding or leaning in, but SF therapists may also express validation by asking clients to give more information or letting clients know the therapist is listening. For example, the therapist might say "Tell me more about this [miniature]" or "I can tell you are really thinking about this" or "Who else might be in the scene who could be helpful?" Although SF therapy focuses on strengths and resources, SF therapists hear the client's concerns, pain, and challenges.

WHO AND WHAT ARE IMPORTANT

Since SF therapy places importance on the systemic and interactional world of the client, SF sandtray focuses on who and what are important in the client's world, who the client sees as resources, and how these relationships and the client reciprocally influence one another.

One approach to gaining information is by having the client create a sandtray of his or her family and important others (Taylor, 2013). The therapist might begin by stating, "I want to know more about you, so I want you to create a sandtray of your family. You can choose any of the miniatures you wish to represent the different family members. You can also include your pets or other people who are important to you." The therapist takes notice of what miniatures are selected to represent significant others and how they are placed in relation to one another.

Kate, a 15-year-old middle school girl, placed the people in her family using the entire sandtray. As she placed the figures, she told the story of the evolution of her family. Her mother and father divorced while living in Florida and she now lived with her mother and her mother's partner in New Mexico, as well as Kate's biological older brother and the partner's younger son. She placed these figures in close proximity to one another and her father on the other side of the tray since he still lived in Florida. She also placed another young man in the tray between herself and her mother's partner. She talked about this young man, a 20-year old quadriplegic and the partner's son, who had died a year earlier while Kate was caring for him. Because Kate, then 13 years old, complained about having to stay home and supervise the young man, she had suffered a great deal of guilt when he died the next day. Through sandtray, she was able to externalize her pain and express what she had not told anyone over the past year. Using SF therapy, the therapist validated Kate's pain, her love and concern for this young man, and her ability to cope with the situation in spite of her guilt. Within several sessions, Kate's countenance considerably improved as did her grades, as the burden of her guilt was lifted and she finally could grieve his loss.

COMPLIMENTS

As the therapist gains more information about the client and validates his or her struggles, the SF therapist gradually shifts the focus of the session from the problem, to times when the problem does not exist, to the client's strengths and resiliencies, and to the helpful behaviors the client uses to cope with problems (DeJong & Berg, 2008). The therapist listens carefully and appropriately compliments the client on exceptions to the problem, strengths, resources, and resiliencies. These might be internal resiliencies, such as courage, problem-solving skills, the ability to form good relationships, academic achievement, and perseverance, or external resources, such as social supports, involvement with community or church groups, or participation in extracurricular activities (Werner & Smith, 1992).

As appropriate, the SF therapist uses three different types of compliments—direct, indirect, and self—to help the client recognize and use his or her strengths. For example, a middle school boy, Ben, was locked in his house basement with his three younger brothers for almost 5 years. Ben described how he took care of himself and his siblings and would sneak into the kitchen to steal food for them when the parents were out. The therapist responded with amazement and an indirect compliment, "Wow! How did you manage to be so responsible?" Ben stated that he just knew it was the right thing to do, so he listened for times when his parents had gone to their second story bedroom to sneak around in the kitchen for things they needed. The therapist stated, "I can tell you really care about your brothers," another indirect compliment. The third type of compliment, the self-compliment, might happen spontaneously or the therapist might ask the client directly about his or her strengths. The self-compliment, often quite difficult for clients until they feel accepted and comfortable with the therapist, involves making direct statements about personal strengths and talents, such as, "I am good at playing soccer" or "I am really good at building Legos."

Stage 4: Goal Setting

The next stage of SF sandtray, goal setting, might be accomplished in a number of ways; however, SF therapy uses specific techniques to address general and specific goals, including future-focused questions, the miracle question, scaling questions, relationship questions, and exception questions. Several SF questions are particularly useful in this process and can be easily applied to sandtray (see Table 7.1 for examples).

Future Focused Questions

Future-focused questions might involve directly asking about the future, for example, "Make a sandtray that shows what you want to be better in your life" (de Shazer & Dolan, 2007). Another approach would be to come at the solved problem looking from the future to the present, such as, "I want you to make a sandtray of what will be better when you no longer have to come to see me"; or "Make a sandtray of what it might look like if next week I came into your classroom, and the problem was solved";

or "Make a sandtray of how things will be better when this problem is solved."

The Miracle Question

One of the most interesting SF questions used to set goals is the miracle question, which allows clients to suspend limitations and doubts about the future by opening up possibilities in a type of "what if?" scenario. Answers to the miracle question often lead to the client's goal for therapy. When asking the miracle question, the therapist should employ a bit of flair and excitement, speaking slowly (De Jong & Berg, 2008):

> "Suppose that today you go home [pause], do what you normally do when you get home [pause], perhaps have something to eat, do some homework, go out and play [pause]. Then, you go to bed. While you are asleep a miracle happens [pause], only you don't know this miracle has happened [pause]. The miracle is that the problem that brought you here is solved [pause]. When you wake up in the morning, what will be first thing that you will notice that's different, that lets you know the problem is solved?"

The client can then construct the sandtray illustrating the miracle. It is important to state "the problem that brought you here is solved," not "all of your problems are solved." To ask that all problems would be solved would be unrealistic and would not point the client in the direction of a goal. However, focusing on just one problem increases the possibilities of a goal that can be solved or at least get better.

The miracle question should be asked objectively and for the purpose of gaining the client's perspective on the goal rather than that of the therapist or the person who referred the client. If the therapist rephrased the miracle question, for example, stating "The miracle is that you are no longer getting into trouble," then the therapist determined the goal and not the client, and the client may describe behaviors in the classroom or with peers, when in actuality the client's miracle might be something that is occurring at home. This distinction illustrates how the client, not the therapist, is the expert on the problem. For example, a teacher once referred a 5-year-old student for disrupting the classroom. When the therapist asked the miracle question, the student stated, "My dad would come home." The night before, without saying goodbye, his father had left his mother, and when the little boy woke up the next morning his mother told him his father was gone. The child was extremely tearful when arriving at school, but by lunch time, he was kicking his peers, throwing his things off his desk, and creating problems for the teacher and the class. Similarly, Jack, who felt his life was in the toilet, was originally referred for failing grades but when the therapist asked Jack about the problem, the real issue surfaced and could be addressed.

Scaling Questions

Scaling questions provide another way to set goals, assess the client's current status, and scale progress. The purpose of scaling is to facilitate therapeutic growth, provide motivation and encouragement, and illuminate the client's perceptions of progress and potential (Berg & de Shazer, 1993). For example, when asking a child how he was getting along with his brother, the therapist might state, "On a scale of 1 to 10 with 1 being you and your brother fight all the time and never have a moment of peace, and 10 being you and your brother never fight and love to play together all the time, what number would you give yourself?" (see Table 7.1).

Almost anything can be scaled including goals, motivation, progress, closeness with others, likelihood of success, and effort. Generally speaking, lower numbers on a scale should represent what is not wanted or the negative aspects of a goal, and the higher numbers should represent achieving the goal or success. When asking scaling questions, it is important to clearly define the upper and lower anchors.

One of the most visual approaches in using scaling questions to create goals is the use of a basketball or soccer goal at one end of the tray and having the client place himself in the tray where he is in relation to the goal. The therapist can then ask the client what it would take to move up just a little to reach the goal. The sandtray and miniatures become a vivid picture of progress.

Another useful approach, particularly with middle and high school children, is to have them place miniatures that represent themselves reaching their ultimate goals when they are older. Many place on one end of the tray a house, car, and spouse as the ultimate goal. Some may not reach so far into the future but include graduation or a car. At the other end of the tray, they use miniatures to represent where they are right now. In between, miniatures are placed to represent what next steps might be taken to reach their goals. As these young people place their miniatures, they vicariously bring to life their dreams and ambitions but also come to realize what may be keeping them from realizing their goals. Even the impediments can be placed in the sandtray using miniatures representing the obstacles, so that the client considers what might be needed to overcome them.

Another approach to scaling is to ask the child the scaling question and have the child illustrate the scaled number using the sand and miniatures.

This provides a picture of where the child is currently but also a way to set goals for the future by asking the child about how the scene would be different if the child was one number higher on the scale. For example, Ellen, a 7-year-old girl, stated her number was a "2" and as an example she placed two girls in the sandtray, one who was kneeling and praying and the other standing with her back to the first girl. Ellen tearfully stated that she was the praying girl, and the second girl represented her friend, who was ignoring her and acting like she wasn't going to be her friend anymore. This vivid picture clearly stated how Ellen saw herself in the relationship, so the therapist asked Ellen to make a sandtray that would show what it would like if the problem was solved. Ellen chose two other girls to join the miniature representing her friend and stated that they would all be playing together and she wouldn't be left out. This clear illustration led the therapist to ask, "What is one thing that would be different if you were playing together?" Ellen stated, "I would be laughing and having fun." The therapist pursued this further by asking about when she had had fun in the past, what she was doing, and what might be one step she could take to have fun again. This shifted the conversation and the goal from focusing on Ellen and her friend, whom she could not control, to helping Ellen find things to do with others that she could control.

Relationship Questions

Relationship questions provide a different way to access client goals, strengths, and resources (De Jong & Berg, 2008). To assist in generating goals, the therapist might ask the client to select miniatures and put them in the sandtray that represents those with whom the child feels close. The therapist can then ask a direct relationship question: "Who will notice when you are able to reach this goal?" The second type of relationship question asks about the goal from the viewpoint of another person(s)—for example, "Make a sandtray that shows what your teacher [significant other person] might say you are doing when you reach your goal." A third type of relationship question would ask about the goal as if another person made it—for example, "What would your teacher say you need to do to go back to class?" (see Table 7.1). Asking these questions, using the miniatures that the client has placed in the sandtray, creates and expands on goals and the reciprocal relationship between goals and significant others.

To reach goals, clients most often need resources. Illustrating the family in the sandtray is an excellent method for providing a visual display of who is available. Rather than focusing on what might be negative about relationships, the therapist could ask, "Show me someone you feel safe to talk to"; "Show me the people you like to spend time with"; and "Who could you ask to help you with your homework?" (see Table 7.1).

TABLE 7.1. Solution-Focused Therapy Techniques Utilized in Sandtray Therapy

Solution-focused questions	Solution-focused sandtray therapy suggestions
Future-focused questions	• Make a sandtray of what you want to be different when you leave my office. • Show me one thing that will be better when you no longer have to come to see me. • I want you to make a sandtray of what it might look like if next week I came into your classroom and the problem was solved. • Pretend I see you in line at the movies, and you are no longer having this problem. Make a sandtray to show me what would be different.
The Miracle question	Suppose that today you go home [pause], do what you normally do when you get home [pause], perhaps have something to eat, do some homework, go out and play [pause]. Then, you go to bed. While you are asleep a miracle happens [pause], only you don't know this miracle has happened [pause]. The miracle is that the problem that brought you here is solved [pause]. When you wake up in the morning, what will be first thing that you will notice that lets you know the problem is solved? [The client can then construct the sandtray illustrating the miracle. The miracle can be modified to make it easier to understand—for example, "the wizard raises his magic wand and the problem is gone" or "the fairy sprinkles magic dust over you while you are sleeping and when you wake up the problem is gone."]
Exception questions	• Make a sandtray of what it would look like if you didn't have this problem right now. • Make a sandtray of your day when you don't have this problem.

Relationship questions	• Make a sandtray of . . .
	  □ What your [important other] will notice when you are no longer having this problem.
	  □ What you will have to do to convince [important other] that you no longer have this problem.
	  □ Show me who would notice if things were better. Is there someone missing who might also notice? Find a miniature to represent that person and place him or her in the tray.
	  □ Who could you go to for help if you needed it? Who is someone you feel safe with? Who do you like to play with?

Scaling questions	Place a sport's goal (e.g., goal post, basketball hoop, soccer goal) on one end of the sandtray. Tell the client: • This is the _____ field. Put the miniature that represents you in the sandtray that shows how close you are to getting to your goal, followed by. . . . *(continued)*

TABLE 7.1. (*continued*)

- What could you do next to move closer to your goal?
  On a scale of 1 to 10, where are you right now, with 1 being you have not reached your goal and 10 you have reached your goal? Create a sandtray that shows what that looks like.
- On one end of the sandtray make a scene showing where you are right now. On the other end of the sandtray make a scene that shows where you want to be when you are grown up or no longer in school. Choose some miniatures that represent what you will be doing between now and in the future to get to your goal and place them in the middle.

Use different miniatures to represent the scaling question. Tell the client:
- Choose which miniature represents where you are right now.
- We are going to make a scale from 1 to 5, with 1 being the worst and 5 being the best. I want you to choose a miniature that would represent each of the numbers on the scale from 1 to 5 and place them in the tray. [The client can then use these to answer scaling questions about goals, motivation, confidence, or other notions of current status.]

Sometimes, these questions lead the client to add miniatures to the sandtray to represent other resources. For example, when asking a child who was a survivor of sexual abuse "Who could you talk to about your experience," the child added a nurse to the sandtray.

Exception Questions

One of the best ways to set goals is to focus on the exceptions to the problem rather than the problem itself. Exception questions ask about times and places when the problem might have happened but did not (de Shazer & Dolan, 2007). For example, a child is referred to the counselor for not doing his work and causing problems with other students. Rather than focus on these problems, the therapist might state, "Make a sandtray that shows me what it is like when you are having a good day in class." Using the miniatures, the student is able to create a successful day. The therapist then more fully expands on differences during these exception times rather than focusing on the lack of success.

Stage 5: End-of-Session Feedback—Compliment, Bridge, and Suggestion

About 10 minutes before it is time for the child to leave, the therapist takes a "thinking break" (De Jong & Berg, 2008, p. 121). The therapist states, "I want to look again at your sandtray and take some notes and maybe some pictures, so I won't forget our session. Is that OK with you?" The therapist uses the time, not more than 3 or 4 minutes with younger children, not only to record the information but also to think about feedback for the client. The silence in this brief interlude often sets a tone of anticipation for what is to come.

Compliments

Feedback should begin with compliments, direct or indirect (De Jong & Berg, 2008). The most natural compliment is to state something about the client's work in the session such as "Thank you for putting so much thought into what you created." This might be followed by more specific descriptions of the creation, specifically those areas that demonstrate strengths and resources. Pointing these out in the sandtray helps the client to see him- or herself in a positive, and perhaps a more capable light, affirming but also encouraging. For example, the therapist might choose a superhero, such as Superman, that represents a strength of the client, and then place it in the sandtray, explaining how the client demonstrated great courage in continuing to face specific challenges.

Bridge

The bridge provides a link between the compliment and the suggestion and gives a rationale for the suggestion. Often, it begins with "I agree . . . " followed by a statement about the challenges the client is facing or something the client is already doing that is working (De Jong & Berg, 2008).

Suggestion

The therapist then makes a suggestion based on how the client sees him- or herself in relation to therapy. If the client does not want to come to therapy or demonstrates that he or she might not return, it is best to just end with a compliment and thank the client for participating in the process. If the client does not mind coming to therapy but does not think he or she has a problem, then the suggestion might be an observation, such as, "I want you to watch for things you like about school, and then come back and tell me about them." However, if the client seems to be a willing participant, sees the need for change, and seems motivated, then the suggestion might be discussed as a type of experiment (De Jong & Berg, 2008).

One of the easiest methods in considering which suggestion to make is to lean on the three basic rules of SF therapy:

1. "If it's working, do more of it" (de Shazer & Dolan, 2007, p. 1); that is, when the client speaks of successes, encourage the client to continue doing what works. After all, why would the client do anything else if he or she is already solving the problem?

2. "If it's not working, do something different" (de Shazer & Dolan, 2007, p. 2); that is, work with the client to identify what the client thinks might work and then phrase the task as an "experiment." The therapist might suggest something but would do so only tentatively beginning with, "I wonder what would happen if. . . . "

3. "If it's not broken, don't fix it" (de Shazer & Dolan, 2007, p. 2); so the therapist might ask the client to observe the things the client would like to continue to happen and then come back and talk about those things that are already working. This is often assigned as a presession task for the client to do before ever attending therapy or can be a way of beginning termination of therapy and reinforcing changes that have already been made.

The following is an example of the compliment–bridge–suggestion sequence. Ben, who had been locked in a basement for much of his early life, had struggled academically and socially. After making a sandtray of his world with only four miniatures representing his teacher, his counselor, and two cousins, the therapist gave the following compliment, bridge, and suggestion:

> "I am so impressed with how far you have come since you started school. You have learned to count money, read, and write short stories. I know it has been difficult to come to a new place, and I admire you for your hard work and how you don't give up. I agree it is difficult to come to a new place and meet new people, so I was wondering if you might try an experiment. Between now and the next time we meet, I want you to say 'Hello' to three people at school and see what happens. When you come back, we can talk about it and see what worked."

Suggestions can even be rehearsed in the sand as a type of role play before the client leaves the session. So in some sense, the client has already been successful and may be more confident to try the new behaviors.

AFTER THE FIRST SESSION

SF therapy is a brief therapy, five being the average number of sessions (de Shazer, 1985). The client may make just a small amount of progress, but it can quickly cascade into other areas, so that sometimes only one or two sessions are needed. Studies have yet to be conducted regarding the length of SF sandtray, but it would be reasonable to assume that it too is a briefer form of therapy. Considering this, it would be appropriate to adopt Oaklander's (2000) recommendations for brief therapy and apply them to SF sandtray. She suggests that the therapist (1) plan each session but remain flexible; (2) set priorities for what will be covered according to the developmental stage of the child and what the child determines to be most important; (3) let the child know that you only have a brief time together; (4) keep boundaries, remaining careful about becoming enmeshed in the child's life; and (5) include parents in the therapy whenever possible. Since the SF therapist quickly leads clients to reveal goals and priorities and their strengths and resources, as well as gaining an understanding of the child's developmental level, planning and setting priorities for future sessions may be much clearer once the client and therapist have met one or two times.

Next Sessions: EARS—Eliciting, Amplifying, Reinforcing, Starting Over

EARS—Eliciting, Amplifying, Reinforcing, Starting Over—is a simple acronym for remembering the process of second and subsequent sessions. Eliciting exceptions to the problem often begins with "What's better since the last time you were here?" In SF therapy sandtray, this might be stated as "I want you to make a sandtray to show what's better since you were here last time." Clients are not specifically asked about suggestions from the prior session for three reasons: (1) the client is still the expert, and it is up to the client to decide to follow the suggestion; (2) the client might have done something different that was even more effective than the suggestion; or (3) events might have occurred that made the suggestion irrelevant (De Jong & Berg, 2008). A fourth reason, particularly with children, is that by checking up on whether the client followed the suggestion, the relationship can quickly be perceived as a student–teacher relationship rather than a client–therapist relationship, implying an imbalance of authority, knowledge, and power that can harm the therapeutic relationship.

The most useful approach for checking progress is scaling. Using the sandtray for scaling provides a vivid picture of progress and may be used to scale home, school, or other significant contexts. For example, Jack, the young man who felt his life was in the toilet, scaled his progress using 10 of the miniatures and placing them in a line in the sandtray. Each time he did this he represented himself in different ways. Usually, he would place wild animals and dragons to represent the lower numbers and superheroes to represent the upper numbers. He often used city workers to represent himself, yet, over time, how he scaled himself changed. In his first scale, he chose a street cleaner to represent himself at a "4" on a scale of "1 to 10."

After the first session, he generally scaled himself at a "5" or "6," continuing to use street workers. By the end of therapy, he used regular people to represent himself and scaled his progress at an "8." This transformation became evident in his overall disposition, as he seemed happier and more capable to address academic concerns.

To check progress, the therapist might ask the client to create a sandtray using the same suggestion given in an earlier session. For example, the therapist might ask the client to re-create a sandtray of the client's family or use another intervention, such as the future-focused question or even the miracle question. This way the client and therapist can take note that change occurs, as well as what changes the client might like to see continue.

Amplifying the exception involves asking about how this is different from the problem and then expanding on the exception. For example, if Jack demonstrated he was higher on the scaling question, the therapist might ask him how he was able to do this, for example, "Show me in the sandtray how this is different from last time you were here." The therapist then focuses on reinforcing the successes and exceptions by asking relationship questions, such as "Who noticed?" or "What did your [mom, dad, sister, brother, dog] say or do when that happened?" Each of the miniatures can be placed in the tray or even outside the tray if they are not already included in the original setup, so that the client can see how the exception might have positively affected others. Hypothetical questions can also be posed, such as "What if your sister had been there, what would she have seen you doing?" It is also good to ask the child's perspective on his or her behavior, for example, "What does that say about you that you were able to do this?" Asking these questions creates new perspectives on the client's view of the problem, the solution, and even him- or herself.

The last step, "starting over," means the therapist returns to the first question and asks "What else is better?" and restarts the same sequence. As the client and therapist continue to discuss and amplify the exceptions, these exceptions become rehearsals for future exceptions, and by using the sandtray the client can see or rehearse other possibilities and anticipate positive changes. Interestingly, over time, children begin to enter the counselor's office, quickly stating what's better or answering the scaling question. They learn to focus on these indicators of progress more than their failures.

RECORDING

The child's sandtray work should be respected as a progress note, as the miniatures and their placement in the sand are the client's words in therapy. Once the client has completed the tray, the therapist takes a picture of the sandtray, particularly from the client's perspective. The use of smartphones and various small cameras make it easy to digitally record the sandtray from different perspectives, load the photos onto a computer, and insert them into the progress note. It is important that the therapist notes whether it is the client's or the therapist's perspective that is being photographed and the suggestion that was used to complete the tray. Over time, the pictures become a valuable resource for monitoring progress and noting what is different or better since earlier sessions. For example, after the client has made the tray in the third session, the therapist might show the client the picture of the first tray and ask about what is different, what has gotten better, and what else the client would like to see changed. The photographic note then becomes part of the session, not just a filed progress note. Of course, when working with children, the therapist remains cognizant that photographs and their accompanying progress notes may be accessed by adults in the child's life, particularly parents. For this reason, the therapist may elect to not take pictures or only sketch the location of miniatures.

The therapist will also want to note the various responses to the SF therapy suggestions and interventions, including the miracle question, relationship questions, and scaling questions. These responses remind the therapist and client just how much progress has been made. Similarly, it is important to note strengths and resiliencies that may have been complimented or could be complimented in the future. This list tends to grow, as the client and therapist open new treasures in the field of possibilities and solutions.

CAVEATS

Several caveats to the SF therapy approach should be noted. First, not all children enjoy playing with the sandtray or at least not in every session. If the therapist insists on its use, power struggles may ensue and impair the client–therapist relationship. Second, the SF therapist carefully leads the client from one step behind, meaning that it is the client who determines the pace and content of therapy, and the therapist follows closely, leading through questions that demonstrate genuineness, curiosity, and respect for the client's perspectives on the problem but also its solution (Cantwell & Holmes, 1994; De Jong & Berg, 2008).

Two mistakes often occur when first learning SF therapy. The first is forgetting to view the client as a person of strength and resilience. After all, the client did something that allowed him or her to cope with the current problem to get to this point and time. A second common mistake is for the SF therapist to use *questioning techniques* without any regard for the client's responses. Instead, the questions become more important than the client's answers, as the process takes on an air of interrogation rather than therapy. The therapist would do better to slow down, listen to and paraphrase what the client says, and ask questions based on the client's responses, all the while taking stock of the client's strengths and frame of reference.

A final consideration in using SF therapy sandtray is the pace of the session. Clients require time to create their sandtrays, so that care needs to be taken in making any comments or asking questions until there appears to be a pause in the client's work. Since the client is communicating through the sandtray and its miniatures, the therapist should respect this communication as a two-way dialogue, showing the same respect as if the client was communicating verbally. This means that the therapist should be careful to not interrupt the client or ask questions at inappropriate times or too frequently.

SUMMARY AND CONCLUSIONS

SF sandtray, a strength-based brief therapy approach for working with all ages, holds particular advantages for those who may not have the language or developmental skills for verbal expression. It provides a dynamic visual, tactual, and three-dimensional frame for viewing problems and creating solutions within the context of relationships. Using sandtray and miniatures, the therapist can bridge the gap between perceptions and oral language, fantasy and reality, the impossible and the possible, allowing for a sensory expression of the client's view of challenges and their solutions.

REFERENCES

Bainum, C. R., Schneider, M. F., & Stone, M. H. (2006). An Adlerian model for sandtray therapy. *The Journal of Individual Psychology, 62*(1), 36–46.
Berg, I. K., & de Shazer, S. (1993). Making numbers talk: Language in therapy. In S. Friedman (Ed.), *The new language of change: Constructive collaboration in psychotherapy* (pp. 5–24). New York: Guilford Press.
Berg, I. K., & Steiner, T. (2003). *Children's solution work.* New York: Norton.
Bliss, V. (2010). Extreme listening. In T. S. Nelson (Ed.), *Do something different* (pp. 109–116). New York: Routledge.
Cantwell, P., & Holmes, S. (1994). Social construction: A paradigm shift. *Australian and New Zealand Journal of Family Therapy, 15*, 17–26.
De Jong, P., & Berg, I. K. (2008). *Interviewing for solutions* (3rd ed.). Belmont, CA: Thomas Higher Education.
de Shazer, S. (1985). *Keys to solution in brief therapy.* New York: Norton.
de Shazer, S., & Dolan, Y. (2007). *More than miracles.* Binghamton, NY: Harworth Press.

de Shazer, S., & Molnar, A. (1984). Four useful interventions in brief family therapy. *Journal of Marital and Family Therapy, 10*(3), 297–304.

Freeman, J., Epston, D., & Lobovits, D. (1997). *Playful approaches to serious problems*. New York: Norton.

Gil, E. (2006). *Helping abused and traumatized children*. New York: Guilford Press.

Homeyer, L. E., & Sweeney, D. S. (1998). *Sandtray: A practical manual*. Royal Oak, MI: Self-Esteem Shop.

Homeyer, L. E., & Sweeney, D. S. (2011). *Sandtray: A practical manual* (2nd ed.). New York: Taylor & Francis.

Hutton, D. (2004). Margaret Lowenfeld's "world technique." *Clinical Child Psychology and Psychiatry, 9*(4), 605–612.

Kestley, T. (2005). Adolescent sand tray therapy. In L. Gallo-Lopez & C. E. Schaefer (Eds.), *Play therapy with adolescents* (pp. 18–29). New York: Jason Aronson.

Lambert, M. J., & Cattani-Thompson, K. (1996). Current findings regarding the effectiveness of counseling: Implications for practice. *Journal of Counseling and Development, 74*, 601–608.

Lowenfeld, M. (2008). *Play in childhood*. Portland, OR: Sussex Academic Press. (Original work published 1935)

Masten, A. S., Best, K. M., & Garmezy, N. (1990). Resilience and development: Contributions from the study of children who overcome adversity. *Development and Psychopathology, 2*, 425–444.

Masten, A. S., & Coatsworth, J. D. (1998). The development of competence in favorable and unfavorable environments: Lessons learned from successful children. *American Psychologist, 53*, 205–220.

Mook, B. (2003). Phenomenological play therapy. In C. E. Schaefer (Ed.), *Foundations of play therapy* (pp. 260–280). Hoboken, NJ: Wiley.

Nims, D. R. (2007). Integrating play therapy techniques into solution-focused brief therapy. *International Journal of Play Therapy, 16*(1), 54–68.

Oaklander, V. (2000). Gestalt play therapy. In H. G. Kaduson & C. E. Schaefer (Eds.), *Short-term play therapy for children* (pp. 28–52). New York: Guilford Press.

Peery, J. C. (2003). Jungian analytical play therapy. In C. E. Schaefer (Ed.), *Foundations of play therapy* (pp. 14–54). Hoboken, NJ: Wiley.

Perry, B. D. (2009). Examining child maltreatment through a neurodevelopmental lens: Clinical applications of the neurosequential model of therapeutics. *Journal of Loss and Trauma, 14*, 240–255.

Ray, D. C., Lee, K. R., Meany-Walen, K. K., Carlson, S. E., Carnes-Holt, K. L., & Ware, J. N. (2013). Use of toys in child-centered play therapy. *International Journal of Play Therapy, 22*, 43–57.

Selekman, M. D. (1997). *Solution-focused therapy with children*. New York: Guilford Press.

Spooner, L. C., & Lyddon, W. J. (2007). Sandtray therapy for inpatient sexual addiction treatment: An application of constructivist change principles. *Journal of Constructivist Psychology, 20*(1), 53–85.

Sweeney, D. S. (2011). Integration of sandtray therapy and solution-focused techniques for treating noncompliant youth. In A. A. Drewes, S. C. Bratton, & C. E. Schaefer (Eds.), *Integrative play therapy* (pp. 61–73). Hoboken, NJ: Wiley.

Sweeney, D. S., & Homeyer, L. E. (2009). Sandtray therapy. In A. A. Drewes, *Blending play therapy with cognitive behavioral therapy* (pp. 297–318). Hoboken, NJ: Wiley.

Taylor, E. R. (2009). Sandtray and solution-focused therapy. *International Journal of Play Therapy, 18*, 56–68.

Taylor, E. R. (2013). Postmodern and alternative approaches to genogram use with children and adolescents. *Journal of Creativity in Mental Health, 8,* 278–292.

Turner, B. A. (2005). *The handbook of sandplay therapy.* Cloverdale, CA: Temenos Press.

Werner, E. E., & Smith, R. S. (1992). *Overcoming the odds.* Ithaca, NY: Cornell University Press.

Chapter 8

৵

Short-Term Animal-Assisted
Play Therapy for Children

Risë VanFleet
Tracie Faa-Thompson

*A*nimal-Assisted Play Therapy (AAPT) has grown in practice during the past decade. AAPT represents the true integration of play therapy and animal-assisted therapy, where appropriately selected and trained animals join play therapists to deliver treatment. It can be conducted with individual child clients, families, and groups, and it can take the form of nondirective or directive play therapy. It is far more complex than many initially think. This chapter is designed to outline the competencies required, the basic principles and goals, and the methods used to implement it. Although many species can be involved in different ways, this chapter focuses on the involvement of dogs and horses in the practice of AAPT.

Animal-assisted interventions have become more popular and accepted in recent years, perhaps because of their frequent use with veterans of the wars in Afghanistan and Iraq. With that popularity has come risk, however, and practitioners who are not fully trained in the modality might find themselves in untenable situations. The involvement of animals can provide huge contributions to play therapy with children experiencing a wide range of social, emotional, and behavioral difficulties, but the practice of AAPT involves an understanding of guiding principles, methodologies, and the animals themselves. Practitioners who wish to add AAPT to their cache of treatment methods are likely to experience the profound benefits of this approach when they are fully prepared to use it.

RATIONALE AND DESCRIPTION
OF THE TREATMENT APPROACH

Jalongo (2004) has written, "Companion animals should matter to educators, if for no other reason than that they matter so much to children" (p. 17). This could just as readily apply to play therapists. Melson (2001; Melson & Fine, 2010) has clearly shown the developmental importance of animals to children. Children are attracted to animals, and animals figure prominently in their artwork, stories, and even their dreams. Furthermore, studies of companion animals in families have demonstrated increased self-regulation, lowered blood pressure, increased levels of responsibility, enhanced empathy and care giving, more frequent initiation of positive or prosocial behaviors, and improved social functioning through the social lubricant effects of animals (Beck & Katcher, 1996; Chandler, 2012; Esteves & Stokes, 2008; Fine, 2010; Podberscek, Paul, & Serpell, 2000; VanFleet & Colţea, 2012). Play interactions with animals afford opportunities for the use of touch in the play therapy process; moreover, it is possible that the production of oxytocin that occurs when humans touch familiar animals (Olmert, 2009) can contribute to feelings of relaxation and safety in the therapeutic process. Many practitioners of AAPT have commented that the presence of an animal facilitates the development of rapport with the therapist.

AAPT represents the full integration of two empirically supported approaches: play therapy and animal-assisted therapy (AAT). Although initially defined in VanFleet (2008), the definition has been slightly revised as follows:

> Animal Assisted Play Therapy is the integrated involvement of animals in the context of play therapy, in which appropriately-trained therapists and animals engage with child, family, and adult clients primarily in play interventions aimed at improving the client's psychosocial health, while simultaneously ensuring the animal's well-being and voluntary engagement in the process. Play and playfulness are essential ingredients of the interactions and the relationship. (VanFleet, 2013, p. 15)

AAPT can be used with clients of all ages, although this chapter is limited to its use with children and adolescents. It can be delivered in individual, group, or family sessions. The therapist creates a climate of playfulness to ensure the emotional safety necessary for child clients to express and master their difficult emotions and problems during therapy. As with other forms of play therapy, a light, playful atmosphere readily engages clients and enhances the therapeutic process. AAPT can be used in child-centered play therapy, and it can be used to teach skills or address specific problem areas through more directive forms of play therapy. Families are often involved at least some of the time as well. Because AAPT is essentially a play therapy approach, it has the same versatility as other play-based interventions do. AAPT can be helpful in addressing clinical problems (VanFleet, 2008; VanFleet & Faa-Thompson, 2010) and in humane education programs (Jalongo, 2014; VanFleet & Faa-Thompson, 2014).

AAPT has become more formalized in the past decade, but there have been play therapists who have involved animals in their work for much longer (e.g., Marie-José Dhaese, personal communication, 2012). Other play therapists have independently discovered the value of including animals in their play therapy sessions and have written about their experiences (Parish-Plass, 2008, 2013; Thompson, 2009; Trotter, Chandler, Goodwin-Bond, & Casey, 2008; VanFleet, 2008; VanFleet & Colţea, 2012; VanFleet & Faa-Thompson, 2010, 2012, 2014; Weiss, 2009).

PRINCIPLES OF AAPT

To ensure that the best interests of the child are met, along with the welfare needs of the animals involved, adherence to AAPT's guiding principles is necessary for play therapists to become certified animal-assisted play therapists. Whenever nonhuman animals are asked to perform tasks under human direction, their welfare needs to be considered. Too many therapy animals are exposed to debilitating levels of emotional stress or exhaustion without any recognition by their owners, a state of affairs that disregards the animal's welfare and presents a very poor model of caring to children. Similarly, when therapists bring dogs into the playroom or take children out to work with horses, they must think about additional factors that impact the child and the therapeutic process. To ensure the physical and emotional well-being of children and animals as well as the therapy itself, the following principles have been developed (VanFleet, 2014; VanFleet & Faa-Thompson, 2010).

Respect

To the greatest degree possible, AAPT ensures the equal and reciprocal respect of children and animals. The needs of humans and nonhuman animals are considered equally important.

Safety

AAPT activities must be physically and emotionally safe for all involved. The therapist places a limit upon, or stops immediately, any activity that is not safe. The therapist is responsible for maintaining the safety of all participants in the session.

Enjoyment

AAPT sessions must be enjoyable and pleasant for the animal therapy partner as well as for the child client. Children or therapy animals have the option of nonparticipation; they may opt out of any activities they wish. Tired or bored dogs can lie down. Children can choose to play without the dog. Child and animal decisions are respected within the boundaries of safety. The therapist facilitates the session to ensure its therapeutic value regardless of these choices.

Acceptance

In AAPT, the therapist accepts the child and the animal for who they are. The therapist accepts and works with children's needs, feelings, and process without pushing them in a different direction or at a faster pace. Similarly, the therapist does not expect the animal to become something he or she is not. For example, AAPT dogs are not expected to become so docile or controlled that their individual personalities and interests are denied. While therapists need to train their dogs for good behavior and ability to tolerate children and the many activities of the playroom, they do not overtrain them to relinquish their essential canine and individual natures. Some dogs are more suited to nondirective play therapy while others are better candidates for directive play therapy approaches, and therapists consider this difference and act accordingly. The same principle of acceptance also applies to other species involved in play therapy.

Training

Therapists train their therapy animals using positive reward-, play-, and relationship-based methods. Aversive equipment or procedures, such as the use of whips; choke, prong, and shock collars; or physical corrections of the animal, have no place in the training, the therapy sessions, or the lives of these animals. This principle serves the welfare of both animal and child.

Relationship

The AAPT process focuses on relationship, not control. Just as the animals are taught to behave politely and respectfully with children, children learn to treat the animals with tolerance and respect. The therapist helps children learn to recognize and respond to the animal's feelings while developing a healthy relationship with the animal. All interactions with the animal therapy partner follow the same principles for the development of humane, empathic, healthy human relationships. The essential playful nature of interactions during AAPT permit this to happen readily.

Process

AAPT is a process-oriented form of therapy. While sessions might focus on specific tasks or goals, such as teaching something new to the dog or horse or other animal, the process of getting there is considered of much greater importance than achieving any single outcome. The therapist knows how to facilitate and use the process to help children overcome their difficulties or develop new skills. Unexpected events are woven into the texture of the session so that child and animal needs are met.

Foundations

AAPT is grounded in well-established theories and practices in terms of child development, child clinical intervention, play therapy, and humane animal treatment. Adherence to these foundations and the other AAPT principles is designed to ensure a positive, relationship-oriented, best-practices approach for each child and each animal involved in the therapeutic process.

GOALS OF AAPT

Five major goals can be addressed through the use of AAPT (VanFleet & Faa-Thompson, 2010). In many cases, two or more areas can be addressed simultaneously.

Self-Efficacy

Children learn many skills that can build their competence and confidence and their sense that they can act and make a difference. These include learning how to keep themselves safe as they approach and interact with animals, how to teach animals using positive approaches, and how to accomplish a new task in partnership with an animal. It is quite common to hear children involved in AAPT say, "I'm a really good dog trainer!" or "I know a lot about horses now!" or "I'm not afraid anymore because I know what to do!" They stand a little straighter and taller, and are happy to share what they've learned with their families.

Attachment/Relationship

Relationships with animals mirror relationships between humans in many ways. Children who have disrupted attachment relationships due to neglect and maltreatment can trust animals when they are not yet ready to trust human adults. The presence of a dog was found to help children in the foster care system drop their defenses readily and engage more with other people, the so-called social lubricant effects of animals (Gonski, 1985). As children learn to build healthy, mutually respectful, and fun relationships with the play therapy animals, they are learning how to do the same with their peers and families. Georgie, a 12-year-old girl with serious auditory processing problems and posttraumatic stress disorder, giggled whenever Kirrie, a therapy dog, licked her face. She told the therapist, "No one ever liked me as much as Kirrie before!" Before children can express empathy for others, they need to feel it themselves. Hide-and-seek with the dog searching for the child is a favorite play therapy activity that is played repeatedly by some children needing to know that someone will always come looking for them.

Empathy

AAPT has the potential to build children's capacity for empathy. During sessions, it is common for therapists to draw children's attention to the animals' feelings, as well as to how the children's behavior affects the animal. Over time, children show more caring for the animals, and more recognition of their feelings. Quieter activities such as petting a dog, grooming a horse, or using massage or other forms of therapeutic touch can show children the value of physical contact and caring, perhaps through the release of oxytocin (Olmert, 2009). There is evidence that children who develop humane attitudes toward animals can transfer them to humans (Ascione, 1992; Ascione & Weber, 1996).

Self-Regulation

Emotional and behavioral self-regulation can be influenced by AAPT work. Play therapy animals often exhibit some unpredictable behaviors or do not perform tasks perfectly, requiring patience and flexibility on the part of the children. For example, when a child teaches a dog a new trick, such as jumping through a hoop, the dog might walk around the hoop or go under the hoop. This is a challenge for children without sufficient self-regulation. The therapist can assist them in helping the dog try the trick again, adjusting their expectations, or understanding that learning new things takes time for everyone. Children learn to use shaping, giving treats for small steps in the right direction, which in turn might be a skill they can use themselves to tackle complex tasks one step at a time. There are also some impulse control games one can play with dogs, such as ones where the child and dog play in a lively manner, and then the child and dog move into a sit-stay position as quickly as possible, alternating energetic expression with calmer periods. Horses can be excellent partners in self-regulatory activities. It takes calmness and patience to get a horse to walk through an obstacle course, but the animal's presence seems to make it easier for children to accomplish such things.

Problem Resolution

In addition to the more process-oriented goals described above, AAPT can be used to resolve specific problems. Nearly any emotional, social, or behavioral problem can be addressed more directly through AAPT. For example, a 6-year-old girl who was selectively mute learned to give a dog verbal cues when teaching a new trick, and later generalized that to her classroom.

AAPT can be very effective in tackling some of the specific problems associated with trauma and attachment disruption (Parish-Plass, 2008; VanFleet, 2008), anxiety, anger and aggression, attention-deficit/hyperactivity disorder (ADHD), social fears, depression, divorce, domestic violence, disasters, and so on, and in building specific skills such as frustration tolerance, social interaction skills, paying attention, and the like. There are also some problems involving animals themselves that can be addressed through AAPT: overcoming fear of dogs or horses, recovering from facial bites from a dog, grieving the loss of a family pet or therapy dog, and eliminating behaviors associated with the abuse cycle, such as animal cruelty.

DESCRIPTION OF AAPT

AAPT can take different forms, depending on the therapist, the animal(s) involved, the client(s), and the therapeutic goals. Typically, it involves the play therapist bringing an appropriately selected and trained dog into the playroom for part or all of a play session, or it may involve a play therapist taking the client(s) to a setting where appropriately selected horses are available. In the case of equines, the therapist might work in tandem with a professional with expertise in horse behavior, training, and safety.

There are many ways that a therapist can put the play into AAPT; these are described below. Some are more common in nondirective play therapy, while others reflect a more directive play therapy approach.

- Through words, tone of voice, body language, and design of the play space, the therapist creates a light, playful, emotionally safe climate that permits children to express themselves freely.
- The therapist shows empathic acceptance of naturally occurring play

that child clients and animals develop on their own. This refers to spontaneous expressions of play and playfulness, initiated by either the child or the animal but engaged in by both of them.

- The therapist encourages the child to interact playfully with the animal, perhaps showing the child how to do so if needed.
- The therapist suggests playful tasks and activities to be conducted.
- The therapist facilitates the session using a playful tone of voice and demeanor.
- The therapist models playful behaviors with the animal.
- The therapist responds to child–animal interactions and/or processes them with the client in a light-hearted manner.

As can be seen from this list, the play therapist uses the many skills acquired in the process of becoming a play therapist to include the animals and to set up and process the therapeutic interventions toward the accomplishment of therapeutic goals.

AAPT can be used in a nondirective or child-centered manner, or it can be applied as a more directive intervention. As with play therapy without the involvement of animals, the nondirective portion of the therapy is conducted separately from the directive portion because the underlying assumptions and "rules" are different, but the two can be incorporated within the same session as long as the therapist informs the child when the it is the "child's choice" or the "therapist's choice" for the activity. This is often best accomplished in separate rooms, but a temporal separation is also possible, where half of the session is conducted as a nondirective session and the other half as more directive. The key is that the principles of both major types of play therapy are not compromised by blending the two in the same moment. In addition, many of the therapeutic skills used by therapists in nondirective play therapy can be incorporated into directive interventions, such as empathic listening, imaginary play, structuring, and limit setting (see, e.g., VanFleet, Sywulak, & Sniscak, 2010).

NONDIRECTIVE AAPT

In nondirective AAPT, the child selects the activities and toys to be used, and the animal is involved only if the child requests it. If the child is playing alone, the therapist provides empathic listening responses through the dog some of the time, such as, "Kirrie, Lori is a princess, and she's very pleased with her beautiful shiny gown. . . . She has a magic wand now." Other empathic responses are delivered directly to the child as usual. If the child requests that the dog participate in an imaginary play role, and if that request is appropriate (i.e., the dog is comfortable and capable of playing that role), the therapist does whatever possible to follow the child's lead. For example, if a child asks the dog to become a police dog and search for survivors of a disaster, the therapist uses verbal or gestural cues to tell the dog to "Search!" or "Go find it!" Any time that a child attempts to do something inappropriate with the dog, the therapist sets a limit, "Billy, one of the things you may not do is grab Kirrie's tail, but you can do almost anything else." There are times when the child asks the dog to perform a behavior the dog does not know or cannot realistically perform. In that case, the therapist continues to follow the child's lead as much as possible, while pretending that the dog is doing as asked. For example, when Nancy asked Kirrie to fly through the air on an imaginary horse with her, the therapist simply helped the dog to follow Nancy around the room. In most cases, children simply see this as part of their imaginary play and don't expect the dog to act out the actual impossible feat. Despite these minor variations, the play therapist using nondirective AAPT tries to remain true to the principles and practices of nondirective play therapy.

DIRECTIVE AAPT

The directive forms of AAPT are many and varied. Here, the therapist has more leeway in deciding the activities and interactions that will help the child meet specific therapeutic goals. Within the many forms of directive AAPT, there is a "continuum of directedness," where the therapist might provide relative structure in setting up the activity and processing it, or there might be a great deal of structure provided for specific skill acquisition, for example. In directive AAPT, the therapist matches the specific technique to the child's therapeutic goals as well as to the personality and abilities of the animals. Dogs are often suitable for both nondirective and directive AAPT, but some seem more suited to one than the other. For example, a dog who initiates activities and invites interactions with the child might be better suited to directive AAPT work.

Because of their large size and the need for at least a little more structure for safety purposes, equines tend to be included in more directive AAPT. As noted before, there can be different levels of directedness, and all of them can involve horses. Horses are often included in group or family AAPT, and this process typically requires a little more structure provided by the therapist.

In directive forms of AAPT, the therapist usually suggests a specific task or activity, provides some instruction if needed, and verbally reflects the client's reactions during the activity. Sometimes there is a short debriefing period at the end, where the focus is on the participant's experience and feelings during and after the activity. Some activities are rather vague, allowing children to solve the problem in their own way; others require some instruction for skill building or safety purposes.

Some forms of directive AAPT are described briefly below for each of the goal areas. It should be noted that all goal areas can also be addressed through the use of nondirective AAPT.

Directive AAPT for Self-Efficacy

Anything that develops new skills for the child, or allows the child to help the animal build new skills, can assist with this goal area. Some AAPT activities might include teaching children about animal body language, helping them learn to greet a dog safely, showing them how to use clicker training or other positive reinforcement methods to teach the animal a new behavior, or allowing them to select a new trick for a dog and then helping them teach it over the course of a few sessions.

Directive AAPT for Attachment/Relationship

Here, the therapist can suggest ways for the child to (1) interact in mutually beneficial ways with the animal, (2) play safely and respectfully as in a game of fetch, (3) play hide-and-seek activities with the child hiding and the dog seeking, (4) touch the animal appropriately (such as avoiding the front of a horse's face or stroking instead of patting), (5) notice the animal's reactions to the child's behavior, and (6) use cues creatively, such as a hand target (animal touches child's hand) with the cue "Kiss me!" Imaginary roles where the dog becomes a "search and rescue dog" or a "guard dog" can help children feel more cared for during the process, often a first step toward the enhancement of empathy. Throughout the process, the therapist can respond with the metaphors in the child's play with the animal.

Directive AAPT for Empathy

Children in AAPT often spontaneously show empathy toward the animals, especially after they have developed a relationship with them. In nondirective AAPT, the therapist reflects their actions and feelings when they arise. In directive AAPT, the therapist can ask the child to engage in caregiving activities, such as feeding, watering, exercising, or grooming the animal. The therapist not only provides some basic information about animal body language, but facilitates the child's ability to read it in real time, often asking the question, "How do you think (animal's name) is feeling right now?" They can also prompt children to notice animal reactions, "When you just shouted loudly, what did Sparky do?" or "I noticed when you shouted right by Sparky's ear, he moved away from you—what's up with that do you think?" To foster empathy, the therapist might also prompt the child for empathic action, such as: "Sparky seems rather nervous around that toy. Can you think of a way to help Sparky feel safer and happier?" Another example of an empathy-building activity comes with the involvement of animals who might have some physical limitations, such as blindness or deafness, and helping the child work with the animal while accommodating the limitation.

Directive AAPT for Self-Regulation

In directive AAPT, the therapist can ask the child to work with an animal who needs a little extra patience, invite the child to play some self-control games with the animal (requiring self-control of both animal and child), or encourage games that involve alternating arousal and calmness, such as "Red Light/Green Light" with the animal.

Directive AAPT for Problem Resolution

These interventions depend on the nature of the specific problems that the child might have. These can include slow-motion games for children with ADHD, "On Light/Off Light" (dog turns a tap light on and off at the child's bidding) to help with fear of the dark, "Slobber Ball" (child plays fetch with the dog) for tactile defensiveness, eye contact games for social skills, and a whole host of initiative games and activities designed to bring out metaphors related to the child's problem. VanFleet and Faa-Thompson are currently working on a manual with a wide range of activities to be included. Ideas are also available in Trotter (2012).

RISKS OF AAPT

While there are many benefits to children from AAPT, there are also risks (VanFleet, 2008). Taking one's nice pet dog to work or exposing children to horses that are sociable is not enough, and can be fraught with ethical concerns. It is vitally important that therapists obtain full training for themselves and their animals to ensure the safe and ethical practice of AAPT. The next section outlines some of the competencies required for the practice of AAPT.

COMPETENCIES

It is an ethics requirement that clinicians practice within the scope of their training. As with any approaches new to a practitioner, it is vital that they become trained and receive supervised practice of that method. It is not sufficient to just read a book and begin taking one's pet dog to work or to expose clients to one's horses. The practice of AAPT is far more complex than most realize. In addition to the therapist mastering the method, the animals must be properly vetted for their suitability for the work asked of them. The competencies required of the therapist as well as the animals are listed below.

The Therapist

In order to competently practice AAPT, the therapist needs competency in the following areas. They must have working knowledge of:

- All major forms of play therapy, including nondirective, directive, family, and group. This includes competence in selecting the right play therapy methods to meet child and family needs.
- Each species involved, including the ethology, communication signals, and stress signals, and the ability to observe and comprehend these immediately as they are happening.
- Animal selection, handling, husbandry, and training. This includes knowing the temperament and personality features of animals appropriate for AAPT, how to handle them safely, the many facets of caring for them to ensure health and well-being, and how to train them using only positive, relationship-building methods.
- The therapeutic facilitation of the various AAPT interventions used, including the development of the child–animal relationships, modeling and helping the client engage in healthy interactions, and how to structure, process, and otherwise facilitate all interactions in the service of therapeutic goals. They must know how to combine core therapy skills with play therapy modalities and the various activities involving the animals, and to do this with individuals, families, and groups.
- How to split their attention effectively between the therapeutic work being done and the welfare of the humans and animals involved. This is one of the more difficult aspects of AAPT to master.
- How to recognize and deal with unique countertransference issues that arise when one works with one's own animals in therapy.

The Animals

The competencies or behaviors needed from the animals depend to some extent on the species involved as well as the type of therapy in which they will be engaged. In general, the following conditions must be met. The animal needs to be:

- Assessed by an objective source in terms of appropriateness for the work being required. This involves assessment of stress reactions and the therapist's ability to recognize and take appropriate action when the animal is uncomfortable or distressed.
- Shown to have good health and to be pain-free.
- Unafraid, unreactive, and sociable with people, and specifically with the age groups with whom the animal works.
- Assessed by an objective source for specified trained behaviors that are needed for good behavior and for tasks required during the AAPT sessions.
- Included in a therapeutic involvement plan (International Institute for AAPT Studies, 2014) that shows therapist awareness of the strengths and needs of the animal and how they will be used or accommodated during the animal's involvement in therapy sessions.

These competencies take time to develop, even for animal-savvy therapists. The process can be rewarding, especially as therapists expand their skills and ideas for involving animals in such a way that their child and family clients benefit. A certification program in AAPT was begun in 2013 after several years of development. See *www.internationalinstituteforaapt.org* and *www.playfulpooch.org* for more information.

PRACTICAL MATTERS

Depending on the therapeutic goals, the animals involved, and the specific interventions used, AAPT sessions might be as short as 20 minutes (as part of a session involving other interventions) or as long as 2 hours. Furthermore, most therapy animals are not expected to work a full week. They need downtime and often work on a part-time basis. Even when they are on-site all the time, they need a location in which they can relax or sleep without being disturbed by other staff or clients. This means that sufficient space is needed, not only within the playroom, but also in the office area for dogs to have a bed or crate. Horses need shelter, areas to graze, and places where they can retreat from the work some of the time as well. At all times, an "escape route" is necessary for any animals involved, so they can remove themselves from the work. When this happens, the therapist helps the client process any issues and feelings that arise for the child, and helps the child understand the animal's point of view.

Only humane, noncoercive training methods are sanctioned for animals involved in AAPT. Equipment that is distasteful to the animal, such as choke chains, prong collars, and shock collars for dogs, and bits, spurs, or whips for horses, is never used. Not only does this have the potential for causing stress for the animal, but it also provides a very poor role model of relationship to the client and fails to teach a humane way of interacting with animals. Therapists must always model empathy for clients and animal partners alike.

CASE ILLUSTRATIONS

Identifying information in the case illustrations that follow has been disguised completely. In some descriptions, the case represents a composite of several cases, but the depictions represent realistic examples of AAPT at work.

AAPT with a Foster Child and an AAPT Dog[1]

Background

Brandon was 8 years old and had lived as a foster child for 2 years in three different families. He had been with his current family for 9 months. He had been seen in our practice for individual play therapy and Filial Therapy prior to the time the AAPT was implemented with him. In his family of origin, his mother's boyfriends had frequently threatened him, and there were several documented cases of severe physical abuse that eventually resulted in his placement in foster care. His mother continued to live with one of the abusers, so return to her had not been possible. His current foster family had expressed interest in adopting him. His presenting behaviors had included acting out at home in the form of destructive tantrums, difficulty talking about himself or his experiences, and some recent incidents at school in which he had retaliated against a child who had bullied him. He had struck the child in the face, and the school had suspended both boys for several days and requested counseling.

In play therapy, he had done well. He engaged readily with the toys in nondirective play therapy, and he had eagerly participated in some directive interventions that his regular therapist used to help him develop better social and coping skills. The Filial Therapy sessions had largely reduced the home tantrums and helped stabilize his placement with his family. Even with all this improvement, however, he remained reluctant to talk with adults and experienced residual fear during conflict situations, including the occasional arguments that his foster parents had. There were three other foster children in the family, and Brandon got along reasonably well with them, but he mostly avoided contact. His foster parents and the school counselor described him as "painfully shy and withdrawn."

---

[1] The therapist for this case was Risë VanFleet.

Therapeutic goals that remained included continuing work on building secure attachment, developing self-efficacy, and helping him with his social relationships at home and at school. He had enjoyed interactions with the family pet dog, and his regular therapist, the foster parents, and the foster care social worker all agreed that AAPT might help him overcome some of his remaining difficulties.

Interventions

Because Brandon was already participating regularly in nondirective play sessions at home with his parents through the Filial Therapy being conducted with his regular therapist, I chose to use mostly directive AAPT interventions with him. His parents met with his regular therapist to discuss the home play sessions and other progress and obstacles, and I met with him for approximately 30–40 minutes per session.

During my first session with Brandon, he said very little. He was cooperative and did as I asked, but he answered any lightly stated questions with single-word answers, with his eyes cast downward. Seeing his discomfort, I moved quickly into the AAPT process. During our first session, I taught Brandon how to greet a dog safely, how to deliver treats with an open hand, and how to give the cues for some behaviors that my AAPT dog, Kirrie, already knew. He watched my brief demonstrations and then did what I asked, smiling shyly as Kirrie took the treats from him and paid close attention to him. I also taught him how to use the clicker in marker training—to click when the dog did the requested behavior and then provide a treat. He brightened up considerably during the clicker training. I showed him some options of new behaviors to teach Kirrie, and he selected one where we would teach her to jump into a large box and lie down. We planned to begin the following week.

During the second session, we reviewed the things that he had learned the prior week, mostly with Brandon showing me what he remembered. He had remembered everything in great detail and was eager to start with the new behavior. In this case, I had provided him with enough details about what Kirrie knew that I thought he might be able to teach her the first step of getting in the box without much input from me. I suggested he ask Kirrie to sit-stay, and then for him to figure out what cue she already knew that would get her into the large box that I provided. He immediately realized the "over" cue (jump over a barrier) would work, and he quickly taught her to jump into the box and sit for a treat. During this second session, he began talking much more to me, excitedly pointing out how Kirrie was responding to him and how he wanted to be a dog trainer. I empathically responded to most of the things he was saying. Near the end of the session, we worked on helping Kirrie lie down, a behavior she had learned but not

thoroughly at that point in her life. For this, we used lure–reward training, where he positioned the treat in a manner that led to her lying down,
and then released it when her belly was touching the floor. We did this on
the rug to solidify her understanding of what we wanted when we said
"down." To close out the session, we played a game of fetch with Kirrie,
and Brandon laughed aloud every time she brought back the ball and spit
it into his open hands.

In the third session, we completed Kirrie's training of getting into the
box and lying down, and Brandon was delighted. We then put up a chair
barrier and taught Kirrie to jump over that as well. When Kirrie began
walking around the chairs instead of jumping over them, I let Brandon
handle it (giving no treats), but I also realized that the dog was probably
getting tired. I asked Brandon why he thought Kirrie might not be jumping
over the chairs anymore, and he replied, "Because she is tired?" I agreed,
and without my asking Brandon got up to put the chairs away. Because this
was a directive session, I was able to reinforce him for considering Kirrie's
feelings and moving on to something else.

Brandon continued to talk excitedly about the things we were doing in
the fourth session. He stood taller, looked at me when talking, and immediately got the treats and other items ready for our activities without being
told. He was showing initiative, enthusiasm, and pleasant social interaction. Brandon learned a few other, more complex, tricks that Kirrie could
do, such as opening and closing the door on cue. Most of the activities were
geared toward self-efficacy goals, but they also required that he be sensitive
to the dog's needs (empathy) and self-regulation so that he could manage
the levels of arousal for the dog. He did well with all of these, particularly because his attention was focused so much on the dog and she was so
responsive to him. We added one activity during this session. His mother
had told me that he occasionally had taken money from her purse, and the
regular therapist had helped her deal with that. Even so, I had an opportunity to work on this as Kirrie had taken a loaf of bread from the counter the
night before. We engaged in an activity called "Help Kirrie," where I lightly
explained that Kirrie had seen and taken something she wanted without
asking, and that I wanted to help Kirrie remember to ask so she wouldn't
ever get in trouble. Brandon and I were seated, and Kirrie was in a down-
stay on the floor. After telling Brandon Kirrie's story, without referring to
his own behavior in any way, I asked Brandon what advice he could give
Kirrie the next time she saw something she really wanted. With just a little
prompting, Brandon was able to give several suggestions, all of which had
been part of the things his foster mother had worked with him on. I was
able to reinforce his advice, often saying things like, "I hope you're listening
Kirrie, because Brandon has some really good ideas for you. We don't want
you to get into trouble!" When Brandon's foster mother came into the room

to take him home, he proudly told her how much he had helped Kirrie with her problem. This represented a playful intervention designed to help him internalize some of the things that they had discussed previously. There was no need to draw verbal parallels back to his own behavior. It was clear that he understood the metaphor, and it was emotionally safer for him to do it with the focus on the dog.

During the fifth session, Brandon and I invited his foster mother to come in with us for a demonstration. He stood tall and proudly explained each activity or trick to her, and stated clearly that he had taught Kirrie several of them, which he had. There was no sign of shyness or fear. At the end, he proclaimed, "I'm a good dog trainer!" His foster mother was pleased that he seemed so proud of himself.

When Brandon and his foster parents arrived for his sixth AAPT session, his foster father told me that Brandon had told him all about the demonstration that he had given his foster mother. We took a few minutes for Brandon to provide a brief demonstration for his father as well. Again, there was no sign of his typical shyness or withdrawn behaviors. At this point, his parents were reporting that they had no further meltdowns at home and that the school had reported that he had opened up more at school. His teacher said that he had done a little report about dogs and read it to the class without hesitation, which had surprised her. She wondered if the family had gotten a new dog, as it was such a departure from his usual behavior.

Outcomes

The following week, I was out of town for a speaking engagement, but his regular therapist who had recently acquired and trained her own dog (and who had been through the AAPT training program) asked Brandon if he could teach a targeting cue and an eye contact game to her dog, who did not yet know these particular behaviors. She reported that Brandon remembered every step and showed her just how to teach those two things. Again, his pride and ability to look after the dog's welfare while interacting were notable. The therapist, too, said that he seemed like a different child with the new confidence he was displaying.

Because most of the goals we had set for AAPT had been accomplished, I met with Brandon just one more time, and we took photos and a video for him to have of his work with Kirrie. Not long after this, his foster parents adopted him. Kirrie and Henry, the dogs he had worked with, "gave" him a present of a tote bag with a photo of him and Kirrie on it (carefully selected to provide no hint of a therapeutic setting), and a message of congratulations. He was very pleased. He was discharged from therapy entirely after it was clear that the adoption was working out well.

In this case, AAPT was used to augment his other play therapy work and to achieve some elusive goals. In just eight sessions, he was transformed from a shy, withdrawn child with poor self-regulation under stressful conditions to a much more confident, openly happy, and socially interactive child. These changes transferred to his home and school environments readily. There had been few changes in his life at that time, other than the AAPT work, so his parents, his regular therapist, and even his foster/adoption social workers attributed these particular changes to his experience with AAPT.

AAPT with a Family of Three and an AAPT Horse[2]

Background

The family was comprised of a mother, father, and their adopted teenage son. The family had experienced behavior and relationship problems with the son for quite some time. They had not been physically or emotionally close for as many years as they could remember, and the adoption was on the verge of breakdown. A large part of their family disharmony was a breakdown of communication, and although they thought they were communicating with each other, no one was actually hearing the others clearly. They had received a wide range of therapeutic services over several years, but they reported that "nothing has helped." They reluctantly agreed to try equine-assisted play therapy (EAPT).

Horses were incorporated into their sessions, which were held in a farm environment and conducted by an adoption social worker and qualified play therapist with experience in equine-assisted interventions, including EAPT (Faa-Thompson). I had met with them for two sessions where they engaged in interventions designed to achieve more effective communication, teamwork, partnership, and physical and emotional closeness. Their sessions lasted 1½ hours each. There had been some improvements over these first sessions, and they seemed at least slightly more motivated to participate.

AAPT Intervention during the Third Session

To continue work on the goals noted above, I selected an activity called "Extended Appendages," adapted slightly from the intervention by the same name developed by the Equine Assisted Growth and Learning Association (EAGALA; see *www.eagala.org*). Adaptations included the infusion of a playful tone into the overall climate and the methods of reflecting the family's experiences as they went along, both of which were drawn from

---

[2]The therapist for this case was Tracie Faa-Thompson.

my background in nondirective play therapy. Extended Appendages is a directive play therapy activity in which the therapist initially provides the structure and tells the family what they are to do, and then stands back, observes, and reflects on how it is going.

To start the activity, I asked the family to link their arms together and to choose someone to be "the brain." The brain stands in the middle and is the only one who has the ability to speak. The other two serve as "the appendages," the arms and legs of the trio, and they move only when the brain tells them to. I explained that their task was to catch a horse, put a halter on it, brush it, and then to put a saddle on it. While this might sound simple, it is not when you are linked together in this manner, with only one person permitted to talk, and the other two limited to the use of one arm and one leg each (except for very general movement). To dissuade the appendages from "cheating," I placed brightly colored oven mitts on the hands they were not supposed to use (the ones on the side linked to the brain).

The family chose the mother to be the brain. She was only 4 feet 11 inches tall, whereas the father and son serving as appendages were both over 6 feet tall. Off they went, struggling to walk together in some type of harmony and to "listen" to the brain only. At first they went around in circles, and it was difficult for them to listen to the brain and to avoid making their own comments. I remarked on these difficulties with humor and wondered aloud whether the appendages might need gags too. Soon everyone was laughing. They eventually got around to deciding which of several horses they would catch. The horses had been watching this strange, uncoordinated six-legged, three-headed creature with interest. The family approached their chosen horse slowly, as they were still having some difficulty coordinating their walking together as a unit and under command of the brain. As they finally reached the horse, they realized that they had not brought any of the equipment to catch and halter the horse with them. They struggled to turn around and then walked all the way back across the arena.

They then went back and approached the horse they had selected and tried to catch him. What seemed easy for one person to do now seemed impossible with three. The brain (mother) was getting frustrated, and the arms (father and son) were waving around like jellyfish tentacles. Laughter was also impeding the process. At the same time, a small pony had quietly come up behind them and was pulling hard at the loose parts of their clothing with his teeth.

After much gesticulating, they nearly had the halter in place, and the horse shook his head and the halter dropped onto the ground. This happened several times with the horse shaking his head or moving away at the last minute. The teenaged boy tried to "cheat" with the halter by using both of his hands, but the pony intervened by leaning against him and alerting me to what was going on so I could gently, and with humor, remind them of the "rules."

All three sighed together loudly when the headcollar was finally secured in place. They then worried about the next task, brushing the horse. They had learned from past mistakes, however, and collected the brushes first and brought them to the horse. The brain provided clearer direction as they brushed the horse, with the pony still standing by to seemingly adjudicate further efforts to cheat. Now it was time for the saddle. The family had never saddled a horse before. Over the course of the session, however, they had been working better together, and they put the saddle in place and secured it more efficiently and effectively than they had done with the headcollar and brushing.

Outcomes

At the end of the session, the family remained physically linked together as I briefly discussed the activity with them. (All were able to speak now.) They described how difficult it had been to really listen at first and how frustrating it had been for them. They stated how they now felt much more connected, as well as much closer. The boy described how he had wanted to cheat, but how he had found it funny that the pony had caught him out each time.

There had been much laughter within this session, something that had been missing from this family's life for a very long time. At their next meeting with coordinated services (treatment team meeting), they explained that they had gone from a 3 to a 10 in closeness during and after this third EAPT session (on a scale where 1 is "not close" and 10 is "very close"). The family took part in four more EAPT sessions, during which these gains were maintained. They also reported, not only to me, but to other members of their services team, that the breakthrough in their relationship made during their third EAPT session and cemented during the subsequent sessions had completely changed their relationships with each other for the better. Listening, laughter, and appreciation for each other had continued as their relationships with each other deepened. The problems with which they had struggled for so long had virtually disappeared as their relationships became healthier and stronger.

EMPIRICAL SUPPORT FOR AAPT

Although there is empirical support for play therapy (see, e.g., Bratton, Ray, Rhine, & Jones, 2005; Reddy, Files-Hall, & Schaefer, 2005) and for AAT (see, e.g., Fine, 2010; Nimer & Lundahl, 2007; Parish-Plass, 2013), AAPT is relatively new as a treatment modality. There have been some promising preliminary studies (Thompson, 2009; VanFleet, 2008), and clinical measures of improvement have been notable. In fact, in an unpublished, informal survey of 18 foster parents of children who had hurt animals in their homes, all of them reported that the animal maltreatment had stopped after involvement in AAPT. There is much anecdotal evidence of effectiveness, but more controlled research is needed. Before controlled research can be conducted, however, practitioners must be fully trained in the method. This has been happening in both the United States and the United Kingdom, and a certification program that is based on demonstrated competence is in place (International Institute for AAPT Studies, 2014; *www.internationalinstituteforaapt.org*). A study of the effectiveness of the training program is currently underway by a doctoral student. It is hoped that in the next several years more rigorous, controlled research can be completed on this promising integration of approaches known as AAPT.

SUMMARY AND CONCLUSIONS

AAPT involves the full integration of play therapy with animal-assisted therapy. Animals, most frequently dogs and horses, are involved in play therapy sessions with children, teens, adults, and families, individually and in groups. The sessions involve playful interactions designed to meet therapeutic goals, and they can be facilitated by therapists using nondirective, directive, and family play therapy modalities.

Therapist and client response to the use of AAPT has been universally enthusiastic. A wide range of presenting problems has been shown to be clinically responsive to this approach, using both behavioral and self-report indices. Anecdotal evidence and preliminary studies have been very promising. The field has been moving forward with extensive professional training, supervision, and competence-based certification. More rigorous research is needed, and there will soon be sufficient numbers of certified animal-assisted play therapists available to participate in such studies. The International Institute for AAPT Studies has been established to help the field develop further as a professional endeavor. More information can be found at *www.playfulpooch.org* as well as at *www.internationalinstituteforaapt.org*.

REFERENCES

Ascione, F. R. (1992). Enhancing children's attitudes about the humane treatment of animals: Human-directed empathy. *Anthrozoös, 5*, 176–191.

Ascione, F. R., & Weber, C. V. (1996). Children's attitudes about the humane treatment of animals and empathy: One year follow-up of a school-based intervention. *Anthrozoös, 9*, 188–195.

Beck, A. M., & Katcher, A. H. (1996). *Between pets and people: The importance of animal companionship* (rev. ed.). West Lafayette, IN: Purdue University Press.

Bratton, S. C., Ray, D., Rhine, T., & Jones, L. (2005). The efficacy of play therapy with children: A meta-analytic review of treatment outcomes. *Professional Psychology Research and Practice, 36*(4), 376–390.

Chandler, C. K. (2012). *Animal assisted therapy in counseling* (2nd ed.). New York: Routledge.

Esteves, S. W., & Stokes, T. (2008). Social effects of a dog's presence on children with disabilities. *Anthrozoös, 21*(1), 5–15.

Fine, A. H. (Ed.). (2010). *Handbook on animal-assisted therapy: Theoretical foundations and guidelines for practice* (3rd ed.). New York: Elsevier.

Gonski, Y. A. (1985). The therapeutic utilization of canines in a child welfare setting. *Child and Adolescent Social Work Journal, 2,* 93–105.

International Institute for AAPT Studies. (2014). *Certification in animal assisted play therapy.* Boiling Springs, PA: Play Therapy Press.

Jalongo, M. R. (Ed.). (2004). *The world's children and their companion animals: Developmental and educational significance of the child/pet bond.* Olney, MD: Association for Childhood Education International.

Jalongo, M. R. (Ed.). (2014). *Teaching compassion: Humane education in early childhood.* New York: Springer.

Melson, G. F. (2001). *Why the wild things are: Animals in the lives of children.* Cambridge, MA: Harvard University Press.

Melson, G. F., & Fine, A. H. (2010). Animals in the lives of children. In A. H. Fine (Ed.), *Handbook on animal-assisted therapy: Theoretical foundations and guidelines for practice* (pp. 223–245). New York: Elsevier.

Nimer, J., & Lundahl, B. (2007). Animal-assisted therapy: A meta-analysis. *Anthrozoös, 20*(3), 225–238.

Olmert, M. D. (2009). *Made for each other: The biology of the human–animal bond.* Cambridge, MA: Da Capo Press.

Parish-Plass, N. (2008). Animal-assisted therapy with children suffering from insecure attachment due to abuse and neglect: A method to lower the risk of intergenerational transmission of abuse? *Clinical Child Psychology and Psychiatry, 13*(1), 7–30.

Parish-Plass, N. (Ed.). (2013). *Animal-assisted psychotherapy: Theory, issues, and practice.* West Lafayette, IN: Purdue University Press.

Podberscek, A. L., Paul, E. S., & Serpell, J. (Eds.). (2000). *Companion animals and us: Exploring the relationships between people and pets.* Cambridge, UK: Cambridge University Press.

Reddy, L., Files-Hall, T., & Schaefer, C. E. (Eds.). (2005). *Empirically-based play interventions for children.* Washington, DC: American Psychological Association.

Thompson, M. J. (2009). Animal-assisted play therapy: Canines as co-therapists. In G. R. Walz, J. C. Bleuer, & R. K. Yep (Eds.), *Compelling counseling interventions: VISTAS 2009* (pp. 199–209). Alexandria, VA: American Counseling Association.

Trotter, K. S. (Ed.). (2012). *Harnessing the power of equine assisted counseling.* New York: Routledge.

Trotter, K. S., Chandler, C. K., Goodwin-Bond, D., & Casey, J. (2008). A comparative study of group equine assisted counseling with at-risk children and adolescents. *Journal of Creativity in Mental Health, 3*(3), 254–284.

VanFleet, R. (2008). *Play therapy with kids and canines: Benefits for children's developmental and psychosocial health.* Sarasota, FL: Professional Resource Press.

VanFleet, R. (2013). *Animal-Assisted Play Therapy: Theory, research, and practice training manual.* Boiling Springs, PA: International Institute for Animal Assisted Play Therapy Studies.

VanFleet, R. (2014). *Animal Assisted Play Therapy philosophy and guiding principles.* Boiling Springs, PA: Play Therapy Press.

VanFleet, R., & Colţea, C. G. (2012). Helping children with ASD through canine-assisted play therapy. In L. Gallo-Lopez & L. C. Rubin (Eds.), *Play-based interventions for children and adolescents with autism spectrum disorders* (pp. 39–72). New York: Routledge.

VanFleet, R., & Faa-Thompson, T. (2010). The case for using animal assisted play therapy. *British Journal of Play Therapy, 6,* 4–18.

VanFleet, R., & Faa-Thompson, T. (2012). The power of play, multiplied. *Play Therapy Magazine of the British Association of Play Therapists, 70,* 7–10.

VanFleet, R., & Faa-Thompson, T. (2014). Including animals in play therapy with young children and families. In M. R. Jalongo (Ed.), *Teaching compassion: Humane education in early childhood* (pp. 89–107). New York: Springer.

VanFleet, R., Sywulak, A. E., & Sniscak, C. C. (2010). *Child-centered play therapy.* New York: Guilford Press.

Weiss, D. (2009). Equine assisted therapy and Theraplay. In E. Munns (Ed.), *Applications of family and group Theraplay* (pp. 225–233). Lanham, MD: Jason Aronson.

Chapter 9

☙

Short-Term Play Therapy
for Children with
Sexual Behavior Problems

Paris Goodyear-Brown
Amy Frew

*T*he task of assessing and addressing sexual behavior problems (SBP) in children produces complex challenges for the therapist. Stereotypes and generalizations can create an impression that children with SBP are loaded guns. These misperceptions can discourage families from seeking the kinds of services that would provide adequate guidance and support, leaving them feeling isolated. However, growing evidence supports the position that children with SBP can be successfully treated, particularly when a combination of behavior parent training, SBP-focused, and trauma-focused therapy (Silovsky, Swisher, Widdifield, & Burris, 2012) is utilized. This chapter lays out the necessary components of SBP treatment as well as an argument for delivering these components through the developmentally sensitive mediums of play and expressive therapies.

The Association for the Treatment of Sexual Abusers (ATSA) Task Force on Children with Sexual Behavior Problems defines SBP as sexual behaviors by children age 12 and younger that are developmentally inappropriate and potentially harmful to themselves or others (Chaffin et al., 2008). These behaviors may or may not be due to sexual gratification. They can relate to imitation, self-calming, curiosity, anxiety, and/or attention seeking and be alone or with the involvement of other children (Silovsky & Bonner, 2003).

The source and type of the behavior seen as problematic may vary for each child. It is considered harmful when it involves coercion or threats of violence or when a significant age difference exists between children. Cause for concern exists if an age difference of more than 2 years exists (Davies, 2012). When assessing the level of harm in the child's sexual behavior, physical, intellectual, and emotional development must be accounted for. Treatment for the sexual behavior may involve both the child and caregiver(s) and begins with appropriate assessment (Silovsky et al., 2012).

Sexual behaviors are relatively common in children (Kellogg, 2009). Before their 13th birthday, more than 50% of children will engage in some form of sexual behavior, with 73% occurring with another child (Larsson & Svedin, 2002; Johnson, 2007). While these behaviors are considered normal, SBP is identified when behaviors are excessive in frequency, interfere with normal social functioning, occur between children of significant developmental or chronological age differences, involve coercion or intimidation, and/or are emotionally distressing (Chaffin et al., 2008). Harmful sexual behaviors involve one or more children in sexual acts or discussions that are inappropriate for their stage of development or age. These may range from sexually explicit phrases to full penetrative sex (Rich, 2011).

Reports of SBP have risen in recent decades due to a combination of increased awareness and clearer definitions of problematic sexual behavior (Chaffin et al., 2008). Population-based figures related to incidence of problematic sexual behavior in children are not available. Reported rates of SBP are lower for children who have not experienced sexual abuse than those who have (Friedrich et al., 2001; Silovsky & Niec, 2002). Higher frequencies of behavior are consistently reported for children under age 5 than for school-age children (Friedrich, Fisher, Broughton, Houston, & Shafran, 1998). One-third of preschool students and 6% of school-age children who had been sexually abused displayed SBP (Kendall-Tackett, Williams, & Finkelhor, 1993). This higher frequency in young children may be developmental, as young children communicate more through their behavior than through their words. Moreover, preschool-age children have not been immersed for as long in the social norms that might inhibit older children from engaging in sexually inappropriate behavior. Children with SBP are quite diverse in the types of sexual behaviors displayed and in maltreatment history, mental health status, familial factors, personal demographics, and socioeconomic status (Chaffin et al., 2008). While there is no clear pattern of factors that distinguish children with SBP from other groups of children (Chaffin, Letourneau, & Silovsky, 2002), recent studies have explored family characteristics, environmental factors, and additional stressors as potential factors in increased frequency in children's sexual behavior (Friedrich et al., 2001; Silovsky & Niec, 2002). Girls and boys are equally represented in reports of children with SBP (Silovsky & Niec, 2002).

While sexual behavior is displayed with higher frequency in clinical samples of sexually abused children than their peers (Goodyear-Brown, Fath, & Myers, 2012), other risk factors impact SBP and must be accounted for (Friedrich, Lysne, Sim, & Shamos, 2004). SBP may also be part of a pattern of disruptive behavior not due to any specific abuse experience (Friedrich, Davies, Fehrer, & Wright, 2003). Sexual abuse experiences are associated with 28–48% of SBP cases (Bonner, Walker, & Berliner, 1999; Kendall-Tackett et al., 1993; Friedrich, Trane, & Gully, 2005). While there is not one specific behavior indicative of sexual abuse, on average, sexually abused children display sexual behaviors two to three times higher in frequency and variety than children who have not experienced sexual abuse (Friedrich et al., 2001).

The norms of healthy sexual behavior include a broad variety of developmentally appropriate activities. Sexual behavior must be assessed with an understanding of the context in which it occurred, as there is no single standard for what is acceptable (Johnson, 1991). Utilizing the Child Sexual Behavior Inventory (CSBI; Friedrich & Gramsch, 1992), which looks at normative and atypical sexual behaviors in children ages 2–12, during the assessment phase will help clinicians in planning treatment.

Greater frequency and variety of behaviors is witnessed in children 2–5 years of age than in older cohorts (6–9 and 10–12) (Friedrich et al., 2001); this may be due to an increasing developmental understanding and awareness of socially accepted behaviors and body boundaries. Children without evidence of sexual abuse or mental illness between the ages of 2 and 5 show interest in nude or partially dressed people, try to touch their mother's or other women's breasts, and touch their own private parts (Friedrich, 2003). Genital play is a common sexual behavior seen in children up to age 6 (Larsson & Svedin, 2002). Playing games such as "doctor" and examining and touching each other's bodies may occur between siblings or peers.

Johnson (2002) identified key characteristics of healthy childhood sexual behavior. Sexual exploration is silly, spontaneous, and lighthearted, though it may result in embarrassment; it does not lead to feelings of anger, anxiety, or shame. Participation is voluntary and common between children of similar ages and developmental stages. Behavior warrants concern when it is persistent, extensive, elicits complaints from other children, and/or occurs with individuals not within 1 year of the child's chronological or developmental age (Thanasiu, 2004). Common and age-appropriate behaviors can become problematic when the behavior is disruptive or frequent in nature (Kellogg, 2009).

Rarely are a child's sexual behavior problems about sexual pleasure. Behaviors are more likely due to curiosity, traumatic experiences, anxiety, poor impulse control, or other factors (Kellogg, 2009). Jealousy and anger may motivate abuse between siblings, as opposed to sexual arousal (Yates, Allardyce, & MacQueen, 2012). A disability may also disempower another child, allowing for sexual behaviors to occur (Rich, 2011; Yates et al., 2012).

SBP originate from a multitude of factors: sexual and/or physical abuse, life stress, impaired family relationships, posttraumatic stress disorder, general emotional and behavioral problems, and dissociative symptoms (Adelson et al., 2012). Children can become normalized to acts of sexual aggression and exploitation due to their environment and have a less developed sense of appropriate sexual behavior (Ringrose, 2012).

An assessment of factors (family nudity, child care, new sibling, violence, abuse, neglect, developmental stage of the child, and parental response) is recommended (Kellogg, 2009). The greater the number of life stressors a child experiences (e.g., domestic violence, death of a significant individual, significant illness of the child or family member, incarceration of caregiver or sibling), the greater the frequency of observed sexual behaviors in the child (Friedrich et al., 2001). Additional factors may be related to heredity (Langstrom, Grann, & Lichtenstein, 2002), child maltreatment, exposure to a highly sexualized environment and media (Friedrich et al., 2003), and heightened curiosity about sexual activity after the introduction of these behaviors by peers (Friedrich, 2002). A child's curiosity may be triggered by seeing another child or adult nude, a woman breastfeeding, or the birth of a new sibling, thereby amplifying sexual behaviors (Kellogg, 2009). Poor supervision and access to pornography introduce age-inappropriate sexual language to children. Environments in which sexual activities are openly occurring, family nudity or co-bathing occur, or less privacy is given while dressing or using the bathroom affect a child's understanding of appropriate sexual behavior (Friedrich et al., 2001).

Children who display SBP share some common traits (Rich, 2011). They have poor self-regulation and coping skills, experience social anxiety and social inadequacy, have a poor understanding of social behavior, possess a poorly developed sense of morality, and exercise limited self-control. They may act out of their emotional experiences through negative and inappropriate behavior, have little insight into the feelings and needs of others, and exhibit a poorly defined sense of personal boundaries (Rich, 2011).

Individual factors and life circumstances impact the child's ability to learn appropriate boundaries and behavior. Therefore individualized assessment and treatment is necessary. Assessment within the context of the family system helps clinicians gain insight about how all members of the family perceive and contribute to the continuation of the sexual behaviors and helps to guide later intervention choices. Since children and parents are often uncomfortable with delving into sexualized material, it can benefit the overall case conceptualization for clinicians to take their time during assessment to build rapport with family members, to understand the child's world, and to approach the sexualized content in a way that minimizes shame. Gil and Shaw (2013) have developed an extended assessment process (the Assessment of Sexual Behavior Problems in Children [ASBPC]) that involves both child-centered play therapy and specific play and expressive therapy techniques, such as the Kinetic Family Drawing, Self-Portraits, play genograms, and sandtray reconstructions. One of the strengths of this extended format (four to eight sessions) is that it allows time for relationship to be built between therapist and child and for the therapist to enter in more fully to an understanding of the dynamics within the family system that may need to be addressed during treatment.

A thorough assessment will include general behavior and psychological functioning along with specific sexual behavior problems. A number of nonsexual behavior problems have been associated with children with SBP (e.g., attention-deficit/hyperactivity disorder [ADHD], oppositional or aggressive behavior) and should be accounted for when creating a treatment plan. Assessing for problems commonly related to abuse or trauma such as posttraumatic stress disorder, anxiety disorders, and/or depression are relevant because a significant number of children with SBP have relevant histories (Chaffin et al., 2008). Silovksy et al. (2012) have created a typology for working with children with SBP. Assessment of the child will determine if treatment is focused solely on SBP, on a trauma disorder with SBP, on disruptive behavior disorder with SBP, or on a combination of trauma and disruptive behavior disorder with SBP (Silovsky et al., 2012). Psychoeducation that involves both caregivers and children and targets rules about sexual behavior and boundaries, sex education, and abuse prevention skills is recommended (St. Amand, Bard, & Silovsky, 2008). Short-term outpatient treatment focusing specifically on self-control skills is effective when SBP is the sole presenting concern. Trauma-focused cognitive-behavioral therapy may be beneficial when trauma-related symptoms are present. For children with disruptive behavior disorders, such as oppositional defiant disorder, treatment that offers behavior parent training in addition to these components is helpful. Finally, a combined approach using all forms listed is suggested when a complex presentation is encountered. Effective intervention involves working directly with the parents or caregivers of the child along with the child him- or herself.

There may be situations in which the child should be removed from the home for the safety of other residential children, particularly if the sexual behavior is aggressive in nature, caregivers are unwilling or unable to follow the safety/supervision plans, significant distress is being experienced by another child in the home due to the behavior, or potential harm to self or others has been expressed (Chaffin et al., 2008). Alternative placements may include a relative's home, a foster home, or inpatient or residential treatment (Carpentier, Silovsky, & Chaffin, 2006). If the child is removed from the home, future goals include reunification with family members when appropriate and safe for all individuals. Rules for family interaction including privacy and shared activities, along with supervision, should be discussed prior to transitioning the child back into the home environment.

PLAY THERAPY FOR SBP

Children naturally learn about themselves and relationships through play (Axline, 1947; Carmichael, 2006; Landreth, 2002). Through play therapy, children can wrestle with difficult content, express feelings, and problem-solve, as well as learn about navigating relationships with others. Developmentally appropriate expression of thoughts and feelings occurs as children work through metaphors in play, art, and sand. This use of metaphor and symbol can help children create a sense of safety by psychologically distancing themselves from their problems while working to find solutions or alternative cognitions or behaviors.

As children often do not have the verbal articulation skills necessary to adequately express their feelings and experiences in words, therapists strategically use play therapy to help children articulate their experiences in the comfortable medium of play, through the vocabulary of symbols, while developing positive skills to cope with their problems (Gil, 1991; Goodyear-Brown, 2009). When directly questioned, children may have difficulty verbalizing their feelings, either because of an inability to connect feelings with experiences or because they are guarded (Hall, Kaduson, & Schaefer, 2002). In play therapy, toys become the vocabulary of children. As relationship is built through play, the child's initial defenses are lowered (Landreth, 2002).

Children's interactions with clinicians may be guarded if their trust has been betrayed. The corrective emotional experience necessary for healing can occur through the positive relationship that develops between the child and the therapist (Moustakas, 1997; Schaefer & Drewes, 2013). The power of play may initiate, facilitate, or strengthen the therapeutic process, mitigating the approach to negative and anxiety-producing content in the counseling session (Goodyear-Brown, 2009). These play-based approaches act as mediators to influence positive and desired change for a child (Baron & Kenny, 1986). These changes may include the child's emotional regulation, attachment formation, self-esteem, self-expression, and stress management (Schaefer & Drewes, 2013).

Moreover, the whole realm of sexual behavior, sexual education, and body safety training can be overwhelming for caregivers. Some caregivers are lacking in adequate knowledge, others are simply embarrassed by the content, and still others are afraid of providing too much information or further traumatizing a hurt child. For all these reasons, even the most intentional and present parent may neglect appropriate education in this area. If parents are embarrassed by the content themselves, children can pick up on these undercurrents and choose not to ask pressing questions or share troubling sexual experiences. Playfulness in therapy can invite conversation about sexual topics in a way that reduces embarrassment and optimizes fun. When parents and children laugh and play together and build their sense of connectedness, conversations related to sexual behavior and boundaries become not so scary.

Treatment

Children who receive therapeutic treatment are less likely to commit future abuse than children who receive no support (Janes, 2011). Goals for therapeutic intervention with children displaying SBP include creating a healthy and safe personal environment for the child, encouraging identification and expression of emotions, correcting cognitive distortions, increasing the child and family's awareness of underlying causes of behavior, improving emotional communication between parent and child, and teaching healthy coping strategies and alternative behaviors (Chaffin et al., 2008).

Treatment created for adults, traditionally focused on relapse prevention, the assault cycle, and arousal reconditioning has not been successful with children (McGrath, Cumming, Burchard, Zeoli, & Ellerby, 2010). Criminal justice involvement and CBT-based treatment are traditional with adult offenders, but have not proven helpful in the treatment of children (Friedrich, 2007). Current treatment focuses on similarities in children with SBP and youth offenders rather than with adult sexual offenders (Beerhuizen & Brugman, 2012; Janes, 2011; Pullman & Seto, 2012). Treatment for sexual behavior problems has traditionally focused on individual rather than relational factors. Focusing on parents rather than children as the primary source of change has proven most effective in treatment of SBP.

For the parent specifically, successful treatment includes psychoeducation for the caregiver(s) and practice of new skills and strategies, which will result in an increased set of positive interactions with the child in question. Short-term outpatient treatment with appropriate parent involvement has had positive results with lasting changes in behavior (Bonner et al., 1999;

Chaffin et al., 2008). Treatment involving parents includes four parts: behavior parent training, sexual behavior rules, sex education, and abuse prevention skills (Silovsky et al., 2012).

Behavior training for parents includes relationship-building skills and developmentally appropriate behavior management skills (Silovsky et al., 2012). Since SBP often occur within chaotic family systems, and since a subset of children with SBP also have other behavioral concerns, parent training programs and family therapy programs aimed at clarifying boundaries, consistently enforcing boundaries, and enhancing positive relationships between family members can be helpful. One empirically supported protocol that effectively increases positive interactions between parent and child and increases positive parenting skills while decreasing behavior problems and decreasing parental stress is parent–child interaction therapy (PCIT; Eyberg, 2004; McNeil & Hembree-Kigin, 2010; Urquiza & Blacker, 2012). Consisting of two phases, child-directed interaction and parent-directed interaction, the medium of play is used to help children and parents connect through the developmental language of the child (play). Parents practice a set of skills called the PRIDE skills that give their child specific labeled praises while reflecting their speech and describing and imitating their play. More humanistic in approach, Filial Therapy and the 10-week manualized format of this approach, child–parent relationship therapy (CPRT; Landreth & Bratton, 2006), allows for the parent to enter the inner world of the child while also increasing the positive interaction in the relationship. The protocol also teaches parents how to set appropriate limits when necessary. In cases where the SBP is a response to sexually abusive experiences, it is important to engage in the dyadic work needed to shore up the parent–child relationship prior to intense exploration or reenactment of trauma-related material. Especially when a child is accompanied to treatment by a nonoffending parent, CPRT can help to strengthen the bond between parent and child while coaching the parent in how to be a container for some of the sexually thematic material that may emerge (Bratton, Ceballos, Landreth, & Costas, 2012).

Sex Education

Information about sexual development, normal sexual play and exploration, and how to talk with children about sexual matters is included in the sex education component of treatment (Chaffin et al., 2008). A child's understanding of appropriate language and names for body parts contributes to better abuse prevention (Silovsky et al., 2012). Abuse prevention skills include setting sexual behavior rules, safety planning with the child and parents, establishing the correct names for body parts, training in healthy relationships, and setting and keeping boundaries with siblings and individuals outside the family. Prevention skills begin with the parent and are taught to the child to develop an understanding of how to stay safe in potentially harmful situations (Silvosky et al., 2012). Parents learn how to ensure the safety of the child and are educated on risk and protective factors related to SBP.

Sex education, aimed at the developmental level of the child, will be a necessary part of treatment in cases involving SBP. Depending on the age of the child, initial sexual education may be simply an introduction to the difference between private parts and public parts. It is important that therapists make no assumptions regarding what level of introduction a child has had to sexuality or sex education. In some cases, a child's first introduction to the correct anatomical names for genitalia may be in your playroom. It is optimal if parents can be a part of this introduction. Children are not naturally embarrassed by their bodies and if the information is delivered playfully and matter-of-factly, children can learn quickly and without shame. In fact, it is often the caregivers who need more coaching in how to speak in a straightforward way about topics related to sexuality.

Caregivers can inadvertently instill in children a belief that private parts are bad, dirty, secret, or not to be talked about. Parents may need help understanding that a child's ability to talk openly and articulately about his or her private parts and sensual responses to situations can be protective and preventative. Caregivers often use euphemisms when talking to children about their private parts—children may use words such as "pee pee," "wee wee," "weiner," "tushy," and the like. It is fine to use the child's language as a starting point while building bridges to the appropriate words for body parts. In *Tackling Touchy Subjects*, children begin by celebrating all the wonderful things that their bodies can do. Children are given a variety of pictures depicting activities such as throwing a ball, singing a song, running, and similar images on a page opposite a picture of a fully clothed child. As the therapist points to different "public" parts of the figure's body, the child guesses which activities can be completed using that body part (e.g., the mouth can sing a song, the hands can catch a ball). The client is then shown the same male and female figures without their clothes and are again given activity icons (such a peeing, pooping, and kissing) to match to various parts of the children's bodies. All of this is done very matter-of-factly. We also offer a variety of cloth and colorful, textured papers from which to make bathing suits for the figures. The figures can be traced, cut out, and made into puppets. We then talk about the parts of the body covered by the swimsuit as private parts and go over anatomical names for these parts. Again, to leach the embarrassment out of these words, we will often take a song the child and parent know, replace some words with the anatomically correct words and sing several stanzas of the song. This sometimes ends up in lots of giggles, and everyone learns the necessary information.

Playful Interventions That Optimize Support Systems during Treatment

A strong support system is important for the family of the child displaying SBP. Adult supervision at school and home, along with therapeutic support, provides the initial sources of safety planning. The amount and type of information shared with sources outside the home should be determined by the situation; it may be better to contain the information when the behavior occurs rarely and in the home environment (Chaffin et al., 2008). Specific directions related to the child's supervision should be given to school personnel and caregivers (e.g., child should use the bathroom alone, keep the child within eyesight). Next we work on helping the child identify his "Touchy Subjects Team." We explore where the child's information about sex has come from to date—these sources may include television, magazines, the computer, older siblings, or same-age (and often misinformed) peers. Using paper dolls or cardboard cut-outs, we identify the people with whom it is safe and helpful to talk to during treatment for SBP. The activities "Crowning Community" (Goodyear-Brown, 2005), "Gathering a Team" (Goodyear-Brown, 2011), and "Design a Support Person" (Crisci, Lay, & Lowenstein, 1998) can be helpful exercises in this endeavor.

Creating Narrative of Specific Events

By the time children enter treatment for SBP they may already feel shame about the sexual behaviors in which they have engaged. Expressive therapy modalities can be very helpful in encouraging children to show what happened. Children are able to project the situation that occurred into the sandtray or into drawing, mitigating the approach to content that might potentially evoke feelings of shame (Goodyear-Brown, 2010). For children who are sexually acting out as a reactive behavior related to their own sexual abuse, the sandtray can be a uniquely fitted medium for helping them explore dynamics of their own abuse. Children may choose perpetrator symbols that can be contained or otherwise manipulated. The manipulation of these symbols often results in a sense of empowerment for the child. The client may also choose self-object symbols that can be nurtured. As children articulate their experiences through the symbols, metaphors are created and become a shared language between the therapist and the client.

Establishing Sexual Behavior Rules

Family safety rules can naturally contain appropriate sexual behavior guidelines. Rules should address not engaging in sexual behavior or touching private parts in public, boundaries on privacy within the family and in public, and defining and modeling appropriate language for body parts (Silovsky et al., 2012). Parents can monitor environments for inappropriate exposure to sexualized content and recognize when rules have been broken in the past, leading to current misunderstandings by the child. Children also learn appropriate physical boundaries and healthy ways to assert themselves.

Many children with SBP benefit from having the rules of sexual behavior more explicitly defined. When family systems are chaotic, boundaries and behavioral expectations may not have been made clear for multiple areas of behavior. We are more and more convinced that boundary violations of a sexual nature often follow uncorrected boundary violations of other kinds. For example, the 4-year-old brother grabs a toy from his 2-year-old sister. If, for whatever reason, the parent is physically present but unresponsive, nonverbal messages are clearly communicated to each child. The 4-year-old is reinforced in a belief that if he wants the toy and is strong enough to take it from the younger child, it is within his rights to do so. Meanwhile, the 2-year-old girl is reinforced in the belief that others can take things from her without asking. If the rights and boundaries of each child are not clarified by the caregiver over time, dysfunctional beliefs can develop and guide later behavior.

When the 4-year-old becomes a 14-year-old and what he wants now is sexual pleasure, he may not have the internal structure to respect the body boundaries of others. The 2-year-old becomes a 12-year-old and does not understand that she has a choice in the sharing of her body. These examples are meant to describe the potential progression from a lack of boundaries early in life to difficulties in maintaining appropriate sexual boundaries with others. Unimpeded, these core beliefs can lead to dysfunctional patterns for relating to the boundaries of others and influence children's growing ability to set boundaries for themselves. Therefore, one of the treatment goals in CSBP cases is the internalization and proper application of sexual behavior rules. It is helpful if sexual behavior rules are written and posted in a location where they can be seen by the children and parents.

Many parents who are confident in structuring and correcting typical child behaviors feel stymied when behavior takes a sexual turn. Some parents find the topic embarrassing. Perhaps their parents did not discuss sex with them and they have no model for how to structure these conversations.

Many parents have experienced inappropriate sexual encounters themselves and emotions and memories surrounding their own abuse may be activated when their children engage in sexual behavior. Sometimes these parents can be soothed by open conversation with a therapist about what is healthy, typical sexual behavior. Talking to both parents and children about healthy sexual development helps to lay the foundation for creating and practicing the sexual behavior rules.

One play-based activity that can be used to teach healthy and unhealthy sexual behavior is called "Mold or Gold." The therapist begins by introducing a variety of play foods and containers of Play-Doh. The therapist invites the child (or family) to choose several play food items that represent their favorite foods. The therapist also provides a container for storing the good food and a toy trash can to throw away food that has spoiled. Client and therapist talk about the benefits of healthy food and then talk about what happens to food when it spoils. Therapist and client spend time "spoiling" some of the foods (creating mold from Play-Doh, painting the foods to look like they are spoiled or burned). The therapist will have already generated a list of healthy and unhealthy sexual behaviors specific to the client context. As the therapist reads each behavior out loud the child chooses a healthy or spoiled food and throws it into the "keep" or "trash" container. Psychoeducation is provided as needed during this activity.

Children absorb new information better if it is delivered through all three learning portals: visual, auditory, and kinesthetic. In light of this, one useful strategy is to make "Rules Bracelets" to go with the written rules. Each rule can be written in a different color and a matching bead given to the child. Each rule can be rehearsed out loud as the bead is strung onto a bracelet or necklace. While many other rules for children are stated positively, such as "Use gentle hands" instead of "No hitting," sexual behavior rules are usually stated in terms of what is "not OK." These boundaries must be made explicit. For example, "It is not OK to touch other people's private parts." However, positively stated goals can be included as well. For example, "It is OK to touch your own private parts in private." Since parents and children will be part of the session together, bracelets can be made for all family members. The colors can also be used as signals. For example, if the blue bead in the bracelet represents the rule stating that it is not OK to touch your own private parts in public, then when the child begins to touch himself while watching television in the living room, the mother can point to the blue bead on his bracelet and whisper "code blue." This gentle reminder might be all that is needed to redirect the behavior. It can also be helpful to offer the child a "fidget" (a novelty item, stress ball, or other small toy) at that time, something that will occupy him kinesthetically while watching TV.

Rehearsing the Sexual Behavior Rules

Once the sexual behavior rules have been clearly stated, the next step is to help the client practice reciting them. This will help with memorization and internalization, and will also help with desensitization of any potential embarrassment around the terms mentioned in the behavior rules. Many novelty recording devices can bring a playful element to the rehearsal. The more novel the recording device, the more likely it is that the child will practice again and again. A talking parrot is kept in our playroom for just such a purpose. The child states the sexual behavior rule out loud to the parrot and the parrot repeats it back to the child several times in a row. Children are engaged and giggling as they practice the rules. For older kids, there are several novelty applications for cell phones that encourage a child to speak into the phone and the words are repeated by the character on the screen—usually in a silly voice. Megaphone voice changers can also be used to help clients play their way through the recitation of the rules. Another variation of this rules practice is to offer several small recording devices (we keep a collection of small, round, brightly colored plastic recording devices in the playroom for this game). Children record themselves saying "Yes!" into one device, "No!" into another device, and sometimes "Only when I'm alone" into a third device. The therapist then gives variations of each of the sexual behavior rules and the child hits the recording device with the most appropriate answer as quickly as he or she can.

Exploring and Establishing Boundaries

Children with SBP often need help establishing good physical boundaries. Additionally, they may need help accurately reading and respecting the nonverbal cues of others. Many play therapy activities are useful in this regard. The simplest way to help children measure personal space is to have them use the guideline of keeping an arm's length between themselves and the people around them. While certain children with nonverbal learning disabilities may do best with this simple, straightforward approach, many situations require a more nuanced approach to physical boundaries. For example, at times a child may be asked to stand in a single-file line where there would be less than an arm's length of space between him and the person next to him. In this case, being within a foot or so of the next person may be not only appropriate, but expected. However, if two children are sharing a bench where there is a lot of space, sitting very close to each other might be awkward. Even more important than scenarios and the role playing of responses is the honing of the child's internal warning system. Using metaphors such as "the warning bell in your brain" or "the uh-oh button in your belly" can help children learn to become aware of their internal states and to trust their instincts. The manual *Tackling Touchy Subjects* (Goodyear-Brown, 2013) offers a variety of situations that help children assess their own comfort level with certain touches or physical distances. In a section titled "It All Depends," children learn that their feelings about touch and physical proximity can change based on who is doing the touching, where the interaction is happening, and how the child is feeling (see example in Figure 9.1).

Touching
It All Depends...On where you are

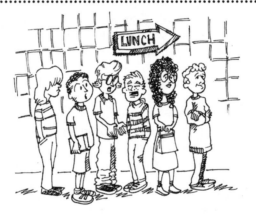

When the teacher asks you to line up for lunch, you may end up standing pretty close to others...

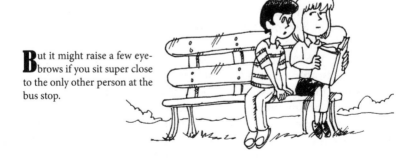

But it might raise a few eyebrows if you sit super close to the only other person at the bus stop.

FIGURE 9.1. A page from the manual *Tackling Touchy Subjects* (Goodyear-Brown, 2013). Reprinted with permission by the author.

The playroom includes a variety of playful props to assist in exploration of physical boundaries. One activity, called the "Centipede Stretch," requires a large rubbery centipede toy. Therapist and child stand facing each other, holding each end of the centipede. They back away from each other stretching the centipede to its fullest extension and then play around with what distances feel most comfortable for each participant. Another activity, one that can be fun for the whole family, is called the "Twizzler Test" (Goodyear-Brown, 2002, 2013). Individually wrapped Twizzlers are offered as units of measurement and the following questions are asked: How many Twizzler lengths would you want between yourself and a close family member? How many between yourself and a good friend? How many between yourself and someone in the grocery store line? How many between yourself and someone in a dark parking lot at night? Family members or groups of children can play around with these questions. One of the most vital pieces of learning that can emerge from this activity is an awareness that different people have different physical boundaries. Family members are likely to give a range of numbers in response to each question. The activity can be processed with a view toward how to effectively communicate with other people about your own comfort level with varying degrees of physical closeness and how to accurately assess the comfort level of others before entering their personal space.

Hula hoops are a tried-and-true prop in this kind of work. Hula hoops can be placed on the floor touching each other. The therapist stands in the middle of one and the client stands in the middle of the other. One might ask permission to step into the other's hula hoop. The person making the request must wait for a verbal cue from the other person. Once the child has become proficient at waiting for the verbal consent to enter the other person's hula hoop, nonverbal cues can be practiced. A pair of novelty gloves is also kept in the playroom. The fingertips of each glove can light up when a button is pressed. Children will wear the gloves and practice asking permission to touch the therapist with each of the light-up fingers. The client also practices accepting no as an answer when physical touch is requested.

"Blow the Whistle on 'Em" (Goodyear-Brown, 2005) is an activity that can target both verbal and physical boundaries that have been crossed with children. The child who has been sexually abused has often been involved in a grooming process in which conversation and behaviors of the perpetrator may have become slowly more and more uncomfortable for the child, but the child did not know how to express discomfort or set boundaries. In this activity, a basket of whistles and other noise-making devices (bicycle horns can be especially fun) are offered to the child. Scenarios can be role-played using puppets, and in role plays, as soon as a child begins recognizing a feeling of discomfort or associates the playful reenactment with a boundary being crossed, he or she blows the whistle. The powerful noise immediately stops the scenario. Therapist and child then work on how to translate the whistle blowing into verbiage that the child can use or safety actions the child can engage in whenever he or she feels the need to set a verbal or physical boundary.

THE ROLE OF HEALTHY TOUCH

Some children with SBP have experienced sexual abuse and neglect. For these children, sexual touch may have been the closest thing to nurturing touch that they experienced in their families of origin. In these cases, structured, therapeutically facilitated experiences of nurturing touch between child and caregiver can be invaluable. Delighting in the child and communicating this delight through nurturing touch can be reparative. Theraplay games such as "Row, Row, Row Your Boat," "Hand Stacks," "Checking for Hurts," and "Powder Prints" are games that encourage nurturing and the giving and receiving of care in nonsexualized ways. Other play therapy activities, such as the "Mood Manicure" (Goodyear-Brown, 2002) can encourage nurturing touch while enhancing emotional literacy. In this activity, a variety of nail polish colors are offered to the child. Each color is paired with a feeling word. Child, therapist, and caregiver take turns painting each other's nails while talking about a situation associated with the feeling represented by the nail polish color.

EMOTIONAL LITERACY

Some children with SBP act out in sexual ways while experiencing a specific set of emotions. As children become more aware of their own emotional states and more skilled at connecting emotional reactions to their behaviors, this new awareness can become a tool in decreasing the SBP. A multitude of interventions exist that help children expand their emotional vocabulary and explore the dynamics of their own sexualized responses. The "Color Your Heart" activity (Goodyear-Brown, 2002), "Color Your Feelings" (Gil, 2013), and "Where I Hurt" (Crisci et al., 1998) are all useful activities to promote emotional literacy.

SELF-CONTROL SKILLS

The key child-specific treatment component identified in the meta-analysis referenced above is the enhancement of self-control skills. Children with

SBP often act impulsively and can benefit from a variety of stop-and-think games. One powerful way to practice self-control skills is to utilize puppets. Any creature that can pull into itself can be useful including turtles, snails, hermit crabs, or even a kangaroo with a joey pouch. Children and parents can role-play scenarios that might tempt them to engage in inappropriate sexual behavior and practice stopping, pulling into themselves to think it over, and then completing an appropriate response. These may include relaxation skills, problem-solving skills, and routines focused on stopping and thinking before acting (Chaffin et al., 2008). Other child-friendly games, such as "Red Light/Green Light" can be played in family sessions or group therapy sessions to practice stopping quickly. Other impulse control interventions include "Freeze Bowl," "Awkward Octopus," and "Conducting Chaos" (Goodyear-Brown, 2002).

AFFECT REGULATION/SELF-SOOTHING

Anxiety management, coping skills, and social skills are included in the child-focused components of treatment (Silovsky et al., 2012). Many children use self-touch as a way to self-soothe. In many cases, as parents or other caregivers calmly set limits about when and where self-touch can happen, the issue is resolved. When children cannot stay within the set boundaries they may need to be taught other self-regulation strategies or replacement behaviors. Many play-based calming interventions exist, utilizing play materials to provide alternative sensory experiences, or as external focal points for regulation activities such as controlled diaphragmatic breathing, guided imagery, progressive tension/relaxation, or other mindfulness activities. Potential play therapy activities include "Personalized Pinwheels" (Goodyear-Brown, 2005), "Cool as a Cucumber." and the "Bubble Fall" (Goodyear-Brown, 2002).

UNDERSTANDING TRIGGERS

When children are engaging in problematic sexual behavior, there may be situations, people, bodily sensations, or visual images that trigger engagement in these behaviors. For example, if children have associated their own stimulation with visual images on a television, it may be that during the period of treatment televisions are removed from the home. If inappropriate sexual behavior has occurred with a cousin, it may be that the cousin becomes a trigger—or at least an association with—the sexual behavior. The child may have a recurring thought when he sees the cousin, such as "We play the touching game together." For a period of time, any contact between these two children would need to include a continuous visual line of supervision by a safe adult.

An example of a trigger associated with sexual behavior follows: A 4-year-old girl who had been molested by her biological mother repeatedly in front of a bathroom mirror had been moved to a foster home. Once in the new home she attempted to fondle her foster mother's breasts while the foster mom was helping her dry off after bath time. The foster parents had to cover the mirrors for the first couple of months that the child was in their care as she worked to learn new behaviors and make sense of her sexual experiences. This client chose miniature mirrors from the playroom collection and reenacted scenes of the abuse in the sandtray. Eventually a hand mirror was introduced in treatment and the foster mother would count the child's freckles while the child watched her own face in the mirror. Using the play materials, we unraveled the child's strong associations between mirrors and her own sexual reactivity. Eventually, the bathroom mirrors ceased to be triggers for this child.

Concrete materials, such as toy hooks, switches, buttons, or triggers can be hidden in the sandtray and children can be given the directive prompt to find the materials. Each time they find one they offer one object, person, situation, or whatever that "flips their switch," "presses their button," or "hooks them" into the sexual behavior pattern. The competency experience of finding the object mitigates the child's approach to this more difficult subject matter.

TAKING RESPONSIBILITY

An important part of treatment for children who have initiated inappropriate sexual contact with someone else is the taking of responsibility for their own actions, usually in the form of an apology letter. Apology letters, especially when they are a part of a potential reunification situation, need to be carefully constructed. Parts of a helpful apology letter (one that takes responsibility without assigning blame or making the other person responsible for the instigator's feelings) should be clearly laid out for children. One playful way to give structure to the letter writing is to offer a variety of inviting toy mailboxes. Inside of each of these is a sentence starter that begins a part of the letter. A larger toy mailbox can then be used to "mail" the finished letter off.

During termination, all new skill sets are celebrated. Parents and children rehearse the new boundaries in the home. There may be video monitors, alarms on doors, or new understandings that each person changes clothes and engages in toileting behaviors separately. Children are given a sample scroll of body rights (reproduced from *Tackling Touchy Subjects*).

In the office, blank scrolling paper is offered as well as an authentic feather pen set and inkwell. Children take great pride in creating their own set of body rights as we move toward termination.

CONCLUSION

Sex is an uncomfortable topic for many families. When problematic sexual behavior exists within a family system it can be associated with shame, guilt, anxiety, and other emotions that are difficult to manage. An evidence-informed, playful approach to treatment allows for the necessary components of treatment to be addressed (parent training, impulse control work, and abuse prevention skills—including body safety, sexual behavior rules, the promotion of new boundaries, emotional literacy building, and, when necessary, work related to previous abuse), while delivering the treatment through the developmentally sensitive vehicle of play. The comforting, fun, competence building nature of play therapy mitigates the approach to the sometimes difficult material covered in this work and enhances positive connections between family members while supporting deeper therapeutic change. Children who have received play-based treatment for SBP often leave treatment feeling confident in their new abilities, enjoying their family systems more, and feeling better prepared to navigate boundaries in relationships.

REFERENCES

Adelson, S., Bell, R., Graff, A., Goldenberg, D., Haase, E., Downey, J., et al. (2012). Toward a definition of "hypersexuality" in children and adolescents. *Psychodynamic Psychiatry, 40*(3), 481–504.

Axline, V. (1947). *Play therapy.* Boston: Houghton-Mifflin.

Baron, R., & Kenny, D. (1986). The moderator–mediator distinction in psychological research: Conceptual, strategic and statistical considerations. *Journal of Personality and Social Psychology, 51,* 1173–1182.

Beerthuizen, M., & Brugman, D. (2012). Sexually abusive youths' moral reasoning on sex. *Journal of Sexual Aggression, 18*(2), 123–135.

Bonner, B., Walker, C., & Berliner, L. (1999). *Children with sexual behavior problems: Assessment and treatment.* Washington, DC: Administration of Children, Youth, and Families, Department of Health and Human Services.

Bratton, S. C., Ceballos, P. L., Landreth, G. L., & Costas, M. B. (2012). Child–parent relationship therapy with non-offending parents of sexually abused children. In P. Goodyear-Brown (Ed.), *Handbook of child sexual abuse: Identification, assessment, and treatment* (pp. 321–339). Edison, NJ: Wiley

Carmichael, K. K. (2006). *Play therapy: An introduction.* Upper Saddle River, NJ: Pearson.

Carpentier, M., Silovsky, J., & Chaffin, M. (2006). Randomized trial of treatment for children with sexual behavior problems: Ten-year follow-up. *Journal of Consulting and Clinical Psychology, 74*(3), 482–488.

Chaffin, M., Berliner, L., Block, R., Johnson, T., Friedrich, W., Louis, D., et al. (2008). Report of the ATSA task force on children with sexual behavior problems. *Child Maltreatment, 13*(2), 199–218.

Chaffin, M., Letourneau, E., & Silovsky, J. (2002). Adults, adolescents and children who sexually abuse children: A developmental perspective. In J. Myers, L. Berliner, C. Briere, T. Hendrix, C. Jenny, & T. Reid (Eds.), *The APSAC handbook on child maltreatment* (pp. 205–232). Thousand Oaks, CA: Sage.

Crisci, G., Lay, M., & Lowenstein, L. (1998). *Papre dolls and paper airplanes: Therapeutic exercises for sexually traumatized children.* Indianapolis, IN: Kidsrights.

Davies, J. (2012, March). Working with sexually harmful behaviour. *Counseling Children and Young People,* pp. 20–23.

Eyberg, S. M. (2004). The PCIT story: Part I. The conceptual foundation of PCIT. *Parent–Child Interaction Therapy Newsletter, 1*(1), 1–2.

Friedrich, W. (2002). *Psychological assessment of sexually abused children and their families.* Thousand Oaks, CA: Sage.

Friedrich, W. (2003). Studies of sexuality of nonabused children. In J. Bancroft (Ed.), *Sexual development in childhood* (pp. 107–120). Bloomington: Indiana University Press.

Friedrich, W. (2007). *Children with sexual problems: Family-based attachment-focused therapy.* New York: Norton.

Friedrich, W., Davies, W., Fehrer, E., & Wright, J. (2003). Sexual behavior problems in preteen children: Developmental, ecological, and behavioral correlates. *Annals of the New York Academy of Sciences, 989,* 95–104.

Friedrich, W., Fisher, J., Broughton, D., Houston, M., & Shafran, C. (1998). Normative sexual behavior in children: A contemporary sample. *Pediatrics, 101*(4), 693–700.

Friedrich, W., Fisher, J., Dittner, C., Acton, R., Berliner, L., Butler, J., et al. (2001). Child Sexual Behavior Inventory: Normative, psychiatric and sexual abuse comparisons. *Child Maltreatment, 6*(1), 37–39.

Friedrich, W., & Grambsch, P. (1992). Child Sexual Behavior Inventory: Normative and clinical comparisons. *Psychological Assessment, 4,* 303–311.

Friedrich, W., Lysne, M., Sim, L., & Shamos, S. (2004). Assessing sexual behavior in high-risk adolescents with the Adolescent Clinical Sexual Behavior Inventory (ACSBI). *Child Maltreatment, 9*(3), 239–250.

Friedrich, W., Trane, S., & Gully, K. (2005). Letter to the Editor: Re: It is a mistake to conclude that sexual abuse and sexualized behavior are not related: A reply to Drach, Wientzen, and Ricci (2001). *Child Abuse and Neglect, 29,* 297–302.

Gil, E. (1991). *The healing power of play: Working with abused children.* New York: Guilford Press.

Gil, E., & Shaw, J. (2013). *Working with children with sexual behavior problems.* New York: Guilford Press.

Goodyear-Brown, P. (2002). *Digging for buried treasure: 52 prop-based play therapy interventions for treating the problems of childhood.* Available at *www.parisandme.com.*

Goodyear-Brown, P. (2005). *Digging for buried treasure 2: 52 more prop-based play therapy interventions for treating the problems of childhood.* Available at *www.parisandme.com.*

Goodyear-Brown, P. (2009). Strategic play therapy techniques for anxious preschoolers. In C. Schaefer (Ed.), *Play therapy with preschool children* (pp. 107–129). Washington, DC: American Psychological Association.

Goodyear-Brown, P. (2010). *Play therapy with traumatized children: A prescriptive approach.* Hoboken, NJ: Wiley.

Goodyear-Brown, P. (2011). *The worry wars: An anxiety workbook for kids and their helpful adults.* Available at *www.nurturehouse.org*.

Goodyear-Brown, P. (2013). *Tackling touchy subjects.* Available at *www.nurture-house.org*.

Goodyear-Brown, P., Fath, A., & Myers, L. (2012). Child sexual abuse: The scope of the problem. In P. Goodyear-Brown (Ed.), *Handbook of child sexual abuse: Identification, assessment, and treatment* (pp. 3–28). Edison, NJ: Wiley.

Hall, T., Kaduson, H., & Schaefer, C. (2002). Fifteen effective play therapy techniques. *Professional Psychology: Research and Practice, 33*(6), 515–522.

Janes, L. (2011). Children convicted of sexual offenses: Do lifelong labels really help? *Howard Journal of Criminal Justice, 50*(2), 137–152.

Johnson, T. (1991). Understanding the sexual behaviors of young children. *SIECUS Report,* August/September, 8–15.

Johnson, T. (2002). Some considerations about sexual abuse and children with sexual behavior problems. *Journal of Trauma and Dissociation, 3*(4), 83–105.

Johnson, T. (2007). *Understanding children's sexual behaviors: What's natural and healthy.* San Diego, CA: Institute on Violence, Abuse, and Trauma.

Kellogg, N. (2009). Clinical report: The evaluation of sexual behaviors in children. *Pediatrics, 124,* 992–998.

Kendall-Tackett, K., Williams, L., & Finkelhor, D. (1993). Impact of sexual abuse on children: A review and synthesis of recent empirical studies. *Psychological Bulletin, 113,* 164–180.

Landreth, G. (2002). *Play therapy: The art of the relationship* (2nd ed.). New York: Brunner-Routledge.

Landreth, G., & Bratton, S. (2006). *Child parent relationship therapy: A 10-session filial therapy model.* New York: Routledge.

Langstrom, N., Grann, M., & Lichtenstein, P. (2002). Genetic and environmental influences on problematic masturbatory behavior in children: A study of same-sex twins. *Archives of Sexual Behavior, 31,* 343–350.

Larsson, I., & Svedin, C. (2002). Sexual experiences in childhood: Young adults' recollections. *Archives of Sexual Behavior, 31*(3), 263–273.

Larsson, I., & Svedin, L. (2002). Teachers' and parents' reports on 3- to 6-year-old children's sexual behavior: A comparison. *Child Abuse and Neglect, 26,* 247–266.

McGrath, R., Cumming, G., Burchard, B., Zeoli, S., & Ellerby, L., (2010). *Current practices and emerging trends in sexual abuser management: The Safer Society 2009 North American Survey.* Brandon, VT: Safer Society Press.

McNeil, C. B., & Hembree-Kigin, T. (2010). *Parent–child interaction therapy* (2nd ed.). New York: Plenum Press.

Moustakas, C. (1997). *Relationship play therapy.* Northvale, NJ: Jason Aronson.

Pullman, L., & Seto, M. (2012). Assessment and treatment of adolescent sexual offenders: Implications of recent research on generalist versus specialist explanations. *Child Abuse and Neglect, 36*(3), 203–209.

Rich, P. (2011). *Understanding, assessing and rehabilitating juvenile sexual offenders* (2nd ed.). Hoboken, NJ: Wiley.

Ringrose, J. (2012). *A qualitative study of children, young people, and "sexting": A report prepared for the NSPCC.* London: National Society for the Prevention of Cruelty to Children.

Schaefer, C., & Drewes, A. (2013). *The therapeutic powers of play: 20 core agents of change*. Hoboken, NJ: Wiley.

Silovsky, J., & Bonner, B. (2003). Sexual behavior problems. In T. H. Ollendick & C. S. Schroeder (Eds.), *Encyclopedia of clinical child and pediatric psychology* (pp. 589–591). New York: Kluwer Press.

Silovsky, J., & Niec, L. (2002). Characteristics of young children with sexual behavior problems: A pilot study. *Child Maltreatment, 7*(3), 187–197.

Silovsky, J., Swisher, L., Widdifield, J., Jr., & Burris, L. (2012). Clinical considerations when children have problematic sexual behavior. In P. Goodyear-Brown (Ed.), *Handbook of child sexual abuse: Identification, assessment, and treatment* (pp. 401–428). Hoboken, NJ: Wiley.

St. Amand, A., Bard, D., & Silovsky, J. (2008). Meta-analysis of treatment for child sexual behavior problems: Practice elements and outcomes. *Child Maltreatment, 13*(2), 145–166.

Thanasiu, P. (2004). Childhood sexuality: Discerning healthy from abnormal sexual behaviors. *Journal of Mental Health Counseling, 26*(4), 309–318.

Urquiza, A. J., & Blacker, D. (2012). Parent–child interaction therapy for sexually abused children. In P. Goodyear-Brown (Ed.), *Handbook of child sexual abuse: Identification, assessment, and treatment* (pp. 279–296). Hoboken, NJ: Wiley.

Yates, P., Allardyce, S., & MacQueen, S. (2012). Children who display harmful sexual behaviour: Assessing the risks of boys abusing at home, in the community or across both settings. *Journal of Sexual Aggression, 18*(1), 23–25.

Part II

❧

FAMILY PLAY THERAPY

Chapter 10

⋧

Child–Parent Relationship
Therapy to Reduce Problem
Behaviors in Children

Kimberly M. Jayne
Garry L. Landreth

Child–parent relationship therapy (CPRT) is a short-term intervention for children in which parents learn to be therapeutic agents to address
the emotional, mental, and behavioral challenges their children may experience (Landreth & Bratton, 2006). Based on the philosophy of child-centered play therapy (CCPT) and Bernard and Louise Guerney's filial therapy model, CPRT was originally developed by Garry L. Landreth as an
intensive, short-term approach to filial therapy in which parents learn the
principles and skills of child-centered play therapy, experience the support
and process of a group therapy format, and benefit from supervised experiences through which they are able to demonstrate and integrate new parenting skills with their child. CPRT has been researched extensively since
its origination and manualization as a parent–child intervention and has
strong empirical support for use with diverse populations and to address a
variety of emotional and behavioral issues with children.

HISTORY AND DEVELOPMENT

Filial Therapy was originally conceptualized by Bernard Guerney (1964)
as a 12-month group parent training model based on the principles and

procedures of CCPT (Guerney & Ryan, 2013). Guerney believed that utilizing the natural bond between parent and child would increase the efficacy of CCPT and promote lasting systemic change in the child's family environment. In filial therapy, parents become partners in the prevention and intervention of children's behavioral, mental, and emotional challenges. Parents learn CCPT principles and skills and engage in weekly play sessions with their child at home. Play is a child's natural means of communication, so play therapy is a developmentally responsive intervention for young children (Landreth, 2012). In Filial Therapy, play is used to facilitate interaction and build the relationship between parent and child.

Landreth (2012) developed CPRT as a 10-session, short-term model and approach to Filial Therapy for parents and children. Filial therapy is defined as

> a unique approach used by professionals trained in play therapy to train parents to be therapeutic agents with their own children through a format of didactic instruction, demonstration of play sessions, required at-home laboratory play sessions, and supervision in a supportive atmosphere. Parents are taught basic child-centered play therapy principles and skills . . . and learn how to create a nonjudgmental, understanding, and accepting environment that enhances the parent–child relationship, thus facilitating personal growth and change for child and parent. (Landreth & Bratton, 2006, p. 11)

The primary focus of CPRT is on strengthening and enhancing the parent–child relationship by equipping parents with fundamental CCPT skills that are considered essential for developing healthy and adaptive relationships and have a strong history of empirical support.

RESEARCH AND EMPIRICAL SUPPORT

Many researchers have explored the effectiveness of CPRT as an intervention for behavioral and mental health concerns with diverse child and parent populations. There is strong empirical support for the use of CPRT as an intervention for children with a variety of behavioral and emotional challenges. In a meta-analysis of 28 studies examining the effectiveness of training paraprofessionals (primarily parents) to conduct play therapy with children using CPRT, Lin and Bratton (2015) found an above-average aggregate effect size of 0.59 for CPRT. Lin (2013) reported that "CCPT interventions with full caregiver involvement, in which caregivers were trained as therapeutic agents in children's psychotherapy process, provided better treatment outcomes than child-centered play therapy interventions with partial or no caregiver involvement, in which treatment was provided by mental health professionals" (p. 104). Lin and Bratton's findings were consistent with previous meta-analyses (Bratton, Ray, Rhine, & Jones, 2005) in which CPRT has consistently shown positive outcomes for children and parents and stronger evidence of treatment effectiveness than traditional play therapy in fewer sessions. These positive research outcomes appear to be the result of (1) fully involving parents as the therapeutic agents in their children's therapy, (2) parents receiving CCPT training and direct supervision from a trained mental health professional, (3) providing supervised experiences for parents to practice and integrate their skills, and (4) manualized treatment protocol of the 10-session CPRT curriculum.

CPRT has been shown to be effective as an intervention for children with a variety of behavioral, emotional, and learning challenges, including children with conduct behavior problems (Johnson-Clark, 1996); economically disadvantaged preschool children with behavior problems (Morrison & Bratton, 2011); children experiencing adjustment difficulties (Ray, 2003); children with spectrum pervasive developmental disorders (Beckloff, 1998); and children with learning difficulties (Kale & Landreth, 1999). CPRT has also been found to improve parental acceptance and empathy and decrease parenting stress (Bratton & Landreth, 2005; Ray, 2003). In addition to its effectiveness for a variety of child and parenting concerns, the effectiveness of CPRT has also been examined with a variety of diverse parent populations. Researchers have demonstrated the efficacy of CPRT with adoptive parents (Holt, 2011); Latino parents (Ceballos & Bratton, 2010; Villarreal, 2008); low-income African American parents (Sheely-Moore & Bratton, 2010); Chinese parents (Chau & Landreth, 1997; Yuen, Landreth, & Baggerly, 2002); Korean parents (Jang, 2000; Lee & Landreth, 2003); Native American parents (Glover & Landreth, 2000); Israeli parents (Kidron & Landreth, 2010); German mothers (Grskovic & Goetze, 2008); incarcerated mothers (Harris & Landreth, 1997), incarcerated fathers (Landreth & Lobaugh, 1998); and nonoffending parents of children who have been sexually abused (Costas & Landreth, 1999).

THEORETICAL FOUNDATIONS

CPRT is a parent-training model based on the principles and skills of CCPT. Originally developed by Axline (1947) as a person-centered approach to counseling children, CCPT is based on the fundamental belief that children have the innate tendency and capacity for growth. From a person-centered perspective, all thoughts, feelings, and behaviors are understood as the individual's best attempt to meet his or her needs and to maintain and enhance his or her growth (Rogers, 1957). Even problem behaviors are understood as part of the child's attempt to get his or her needs met and to move toward growth. Within the child-centered framework, the overall objective is for the parent to create a nonthreatening environment and relate to the child in ways that promote the child's internal capacity for constructive change and growth.

In CPRT parent and child play sessions, the primary goals are for the parent to:

1. *Establish a consistent and predictable environment for the child.* Limits promote a sense of safety and security in the relationship. Parents provide security and predictability through consistent behavior and responses to the child in the play sessions.

2. *Understand and accept the child's perspective, experience, and world.* Acceptance of the child's world is conveyed through the parent's eager and genuine interest in whatever the child chooses to do during their playtime. Understanding is accomplished as the parent develops greater sensitivity to the child's experience and sees things from the child's perspective.

3. *Encourage the expression of the child's emotional world.* During the playtime, the parent encourages emotional expression by accepting the child's feelings without judgment or evaluation.

4. *Establish a sense of freedom for the child.* An important aspect of the playtime is to provide an environment where the child feels free to express his or her thoughts and feelings in ways that may not be permissible at other times. Parents learn to allow their child more freedom within secure limits. Allowing the child to make choices also promotes a feeling of permissiveness.

5. *Facilitate the child's decision making.* During the playtime, the child has the opportunity to direct his or her play and the parent refrains from teaching or being a source for answers and information. The opportunity to choose which toy to play with, how to play with it, or how the play will turn out creates decision-making opportunities that promote the child's development of personal responsibility and problem-solving skills.

6. *Provide the child with an opportunity to assume responsibility and develop a sense of control.* Children are responsible for what they do during the play sessions and parents are encouraged to allow children to gain experience doing things for themselves that are within their capabilities. Children gain a sense of control and feel empowered when they have the opportunity to accomplish tasks and take responsibility for their time and actions.

OBJECTIVES OF CPRT

The primary focus of CPRT is to strengthen and develop the parent–child relationship by teaching parents skills and attitudes utilized in CCPT (Landreth & Bratton, 2006). The relationship between the parent and child is considered the vehicle for change in CPRT. Children with problem behaviors often feel misunderstood and experience disconnection in the parent–child relationship. The objective of CPRT is to help the parent develop new ways of relating to the child that will promote the child's growth in constructive, adaptive, and healthy ways and develop constructive behaviors. Parents are taught specific attitudes and skills to enhance and strengthen the parent–child relationship and to increase parental efficacy.

Therapeutic goals for children in CPRT include a reduction of problem behaviors, development of coping skills, increased sense of self-worth and confidence, and more positive perception of parents. Therapeutic goals for parents include increased sensitivity to their children's emotional experiences, more positive perceptions of their child, increased parental efficacy, and the development of more effective parenting skills.

Goals for the Parent–Child Relationship

- Strengthen the parent–child relationship and foster a sense of trust, security, and closeness for both parent and child.
- Improve family interactions and expression of affection.
- Increase level of playfulness and enjoyment between parent and child.
- Improve coping and problem solving.

Goals for Parents

- Increase understanding, acceptance, and sensitivity to their child, particularly his or her emotional world.
- Learn CCPT principles and skills.
- Learn how to encourage their children's self-direction, self-responsibility, and self-reliance.
- Develop more realistic and tolerant perceptions and attitudes toward self and child.
- Gain insight into self in relation to the child.
- Increase parental self-acceptance and confidence in their ability to parent.
- Develop more effective parenting skills based on developmentally appropriate strategies.

Goals for Children

- Communicate thoughts, needs, and feelings to his or her parent through the medium of play.
- Experience more positive feelings of self-respect, self-worth, confidence, and competence through feeling accepted, understood, and valued.
- Change any negative perceptions of the parent's feelings, attitudes, and behavior through increased trust and sense of security.
- Reduce or eliminate problem behaviors.
- Develop an internal locus of control, become more responsible, regulate emotions and behavior, and choose more appropriate ways to express needs and get needs met.
- Develop effective problem-solving skills (Landreth & Bratton, 2006, pp. 120–121).

KEY COMPONENTS OF CPRT

The facilitation of CPRT includes two critical components: a didactic, psychoeducational component and a group process component.

Psychoeducation

For the didactic, psychoeducational component of CPRT, the facilitator provides simple teaching points, assigns homework, and seeks to empower the parent through affirmation of his or her efforts. Throughout the CPRT process, the facilitator's goal is to demonstrate and integrate the philosophy and skills of CCPT in his or her presentation of the material, facilitation of the group process, and way of being within the group. Modeling is a key teaching component and allows parents to experience the impact of the philosophy and skills they are learning to implement with their child. The leader uses a strength-based approach in supervision of the parents' recorded play sessions, frequently validating and affirming the parents' efforts, focusing on what parents are doing well and providing substantial positive feedback.

Group Process

The group process component is intended to provide a safe, supportive, and nonthreatening environment that facilitates parents' exploration of attitudes, feelings, and perceptions about themselves, their children, and their role as a parent.

Maintaining a balance between the psychoeducational component and the group process component is critical to the success of CPRT and requires great skill on the part of the CPRT facilitator. The CPRT facilitator promotes the process by encouraging parents to explore their feelings more fully; encouraging interaction between group members; and building group cohesion by linking parents, normalizing and generalizing parental concerns and fears to other group members; and engaging parents in teaching and demonstrating skills to other members of the group.

Supervised Playtimes

In addition to the psychoeducational and group process components, CPRT provides a systematic and structured learning experience for parents that includes a laboratory experience of a 30-minute parent and child playtime on a weekly basis in a selected place at home or at the training site. In the playtimes, parents utilize a specific set of play materials that facilitate a wide range of play and emotional expression in three areas: (1) real-life/nurturing toys include small baby doll, nursing bottle, doctor kit (with stethoscope and three Band-aids), two toy phones, doll family, domestic animal family, wild animals, play money, car/truck, and plastic kitchen dishes—optional toys in this category include: puppets, doll furniture, and small dress-up items; (2) acting-out/aggressive release toys include a dart gun, rubber knife, piece of rope, aggressive animal or two, small toy soldiers (12–15 of two different colors), inflatable bop bag, and a mask (Lone Ranger type)—optional toys in this category include toy handcuffs with a key; (3) creative/expressive toys include Play-Doh, crayons, plain paper, child's scissors, transparent tape, egg carton, ring toss game, deck of playing cards, soft foam ball, and two balloons—optional toys in this category include a selection of small arts-and-crafts materials in a Ziploc bag, Tinkertoys or a small assortment of building blocks, binoculars, tambourine (drum or other small musical instrument), and a magic wand (Landreth & Bratton, 2006). The *Toy Checklist for Filial Play Sessions* in the CPRT treatment manual provides a more detailed description of toys. Parents practice specific skills within the time-limited format of the play session for optimal success. Parents also receive direct supervision of their skill development throughout the duration of the group training sessions.

The Child of Focus

In families with multiple children where CPRT is an appropriate intervention, parents are asked to select one child of focus for the duration of the 10-session CPRT intervention. The child of focus is typically between the ages of 2 and 10 years of age and demonstrating problem behaviors or challenges that can be effectively addressed utilizing a parent as the primary therapeutic agent. Because the focus of CPRT is on the parent–child relationship, weekly parent–child play sessions are always conducted with one child and one parent for the duration of the 10 sessions.

Weekly Parent–Child Sessions

The weekly 30-minute parent–child play session is central to the success of CPRT. The parent's consistent application of the skills and attitudes in the weekly play sessions provides the framework for learning and growth. In order to reduce anxiety and establish a pattern of success, parents are only expected to demonstrate the skills and attitudes they have been taught during the limited time of the 30-minute weekly session. Basic principles for the play sessions include:

1. The child should be completely free within acceptable boundaries to determine how he or she will use the time. The child leads and the parent follows without making suggestions or asking questions.
2. The parent's major task is to empathize with the child, to understand the intent of his actions, and to understad his or her thoughts and feelings.
3. The parent's next task is to communicate this understanding to the child by appropriate comments, particularly, whenever possible, by verbalizing the feelings that the child is actively experiencing.
4. The parent is to be clear and firm about the few "limits" that are placed on the child. Limits to be set are time limits, not breaking specified toys or other items in the room or home, and not physically hurting the parent or child (Landreth & Bratton, 2006, p. 110).

CPRT SKILLS AND CONCEPTS

Parents are taught specific attitudes and skills to enhance and strengthen the parent–child relationship and to increase parental efficacy. Skills parents learn through CPRT include structuring, reflective listening, self-esteem building, returning responsibility, and therapeutic limit setting.

Structuring

Structuring is a skill used to help the child understand the nature of the parent and child playtimes and to establish a safe, predictable, and permissive environment for the child. Structuring involves both verbal and nonverbal communication.

Examples of Verbal Structuring

1. Parent: "During our special playtime, you can play with the toys in lots of the ways you want to."
2. Parent: "We have 5 minutes left in our playtime today."

More important than the words are the nonverbal ways the parent communicates the specialness of the playtime. The parent is encouraged to enter the playtime with eager anticipation and to sit down, preferably on the floor or at the child's level, to communicate interest and a willingness to allow the child to lead and direct the playtime. The parent should move closer to his or her child when the child is intent and focused on his or her play and to join in the play when invited to do so by the child. The parent can be an involved and active participant in the child's play without physically following the child around the room by shifting body posture or leaning forward to convey interest and involvement. When the parent's whole body turns toward the child, and the parent conveys genuine interest and full attention, the child feels the parent's presence and attunement.

Reflecting a Child's Nonverbal Play Behavior

Parents respond to a child's actions and nonverbal play by describing what the parent sees, hears, and observes the child doing. When children provide little or no verbal content or emotional expression to respond to, acknowledging their behavior helps children feel the parent is interested in their world, cares about their world, and is striving to understand their world.

Toys used during the parent and child playtime should not be identified and labeled until the child has verbalized an identifying label for the item. Labeling a toy anchors the child to reality and interferes with the child's creativity and fantasy. Parents are encouraged to balance the timing and rate of their responses in such a way that conveys interest and avoids overwhelming the child. If a parent responds infrequently or is silent during the child's play, the child may feel watched or that the parent is disengaged and uninterested. If a parent acknowledges nonverbal behavior too frequently, the child may experience the parent as intrusive and disingenuous. Parents are also encouraged to personalize their responses by beginning their reflections with "You" or "You are" and focusing on the child rather than the toy.

Examples of Reflecting a Child's Nonverbal Play Behavior

1. Child: (*pushing a car across the floor*) "Vrooom."
   Parent: "You're pushing that across there."
2. Child: (*Stands the animals up in a line on top of a block.*)
   Parent: "You're lining them up on top of there."
3. Child: (*shooting at a dinosaur with a plastic soldier*) "Phew-phew."
   Parent: "Sounds like they are really fighting."

Reflecting a Child's Verbalization

To reflect a child's verbalization, the parent repeats in slightly different words something the child has said. Reflecting a child's verbalization helps the child know that the parent hears and understands the content of his or her message. It also provides the child with the opportunity to hear the message of what he or she has said to validate his or her perspective and promote the child's self-awareness and understanding.

Examples of Reflecting a Child's Verbalization

1. Child: "It's raining and lightening."
   Parent: "Here comes a big storm."
2. Child: "Today at school we had graham crackers for snack."
   Parent: "You ate graham crackers in class today."
3. Child: (*stacking the blocks to build a tower*) "It's getting higher and higher."
   Parent: "It's taller now."
   Child: "The animals want to climb up the mountain but they're too scared."
   Parent: "They want to do it, but they are afraid to go up there."

Reflecting a Child's Feelings

Reflecting feelings communicates understanding and acceptance of a child's feelings, wants, wishes, and needs and helps him or her to understand, accept, identify, and communicate his or her own emotional experience. If a feeling, desire, or need is expressed and goes unrecognized by the parent, a child might think that the feeling or expression is not acceptable. Furthermore, the child may try to express the feeling or need through problematic behaviors.

Examples of Reflecting a Child's Feelings

1. Child: "I get to play with my friends at recess."
   Parent: "You like to play with them."

2. Child: (*shooting a dart gun across room*) "Wow! It went really far."
   Parent: "You're so excited you shot it so far!"
3. Child: (*trying to take lid off the Play Doh*) "I can't get it open."
   Parent: "You're frustrated because it seems really stuck on there."

Building Self-Esteem

Parents often use praise to reinforce behavior or communicate approval to children. Praise is evaluative, nondescriptive, and promotes a child's reliance on external evaluation to feel good about him- or herself. In CPRT, parents are taught to use encouragement and self-esteem-building responses to acknowledge the child's effort and personal characteristics, and to promote a child's intrinsic motivation. Through self-esteem-building responses, the child learns to acknowledge his or her own personal qualities, commitment, and effort.

Examples of Self-Esteem-Building Responses

1. Child: (*opening a cash register*) "I opened it!"
   Parent: "You figured it out!"
2. Child: (*drawing a picture, showing it to parent, and smiling*) "Do you like my picture?"
   Parent: "You really like your picture."
   Child: "I used all of the colors in the box and filled up the whole paper."
   Parent: "You worked really hard on it and you're proud of yourself."
3. Child: (*trying to open the handcuffs repeatedly*) "This is hard. I can't get it open."
   Parent: "You are really trying hard to get it open."
   Child: (*continuing to twist and pull handcuffs*) "Oh, I think it goes this way."
   Parent: "You are figuring out how to do it."
   Child: (*opening handcuffs*) "Yes!"
   Parent: "You did it! You got them open."

Returning Responsibility and Facilitating Decision Making

Parents are usually in the position of being "the expert." Children look to parents for direction, permission, and answers. During the parent and child playtimes, the parent is not the teacher or a person who corrects children's responses. The child leads and the parent follows. Within appropriate boundaries, the child decides what toys to play with and how to play with the toys. When children ask questions or seek assistance, the parents will make a response that returns the responsibility to the child. These responses encourage children to make their own decisions and take responsibility for their choices and present concerns.

Children can learn how to make decisions and take responsibility for their choices and actions at a young age. Responsibility is learned through experience. Children who are provided opportunities to learn decision making and personal responsibility become self-directed, intrinsically motivated, and develop a sense of control and agency in their lives.

Example Responses to Return Responsibility and Facilitate Decision Making

1. Child: "What should I play?"
   Parent: "In here, you can decide what you want to play with."
2. Child: (*picking up a stethoscope*) "What is this?"
   Parent: "That can be whatever you want it to be."
3. Child: "How do you spell *giraffe*?"
   Parent: "You can spell it any way you want."
4. Child: (*picking up a paintbrush*) "I'm going to paint a rainbow."
   Parent: "You know what you want to do."
5. Child: "What color should I paint the sky?"
   Parent: "You can decide what colors to use."
6. Child: (*After struggling to tear the tape, uses scissors to cut it.*)
   Parent: "You figured out a way to do it."

Therapeutic Limit Setting

Limit setting is an essential and often challenging skill for parents to learn and apply in parent and child playtimes. Consistent limits provide structure and security for children and are critical to a healthy parent–child relationship. During special playtimes, parents try to provide a permissive and accepting environment for their child while establishing consistent limits that provide children opportunities to learn self-control, to learn to make choices, to take responsibility for their choices and actions, and to regulate their own emotions and behaviors. The parent's belief in the child's ability to follow limits and to choose positive cooperative behavior is critical to the play and limit-setting process. Children are more likely to follow limits when they experience respect for themselves and acceptance of their feelings—both positive and negative.

Limits are only presented and established within the special playtime when they are necessary, and they should be minimal and enforceable. Although a child's behavior may not be acceptable, all feelings, desires, and wishes of the child are accepted. A child's defiant, aggressive, destructive behavior often captivates a parent's attention and energy in the moment. However, the child's desire to break the limit has greater significance than the exhibited behavior. Within the 30-minute parent and child playtimes, limits (1) provide physical and emotional security and safety for children; (2) protect the physical well-being of the parent and facilitate acceptance of the child; (3) facilitate the development of self-control, and personal responsibility of children; (4) promote consistency; and (5) protect the playtime materials and room.

Parents are taught the Landreth (2012) three-step A-C-T method of limit setting to set limits in CPRT.

A—Acknowledge the child's feelings, wishes, and wants.'
C—Communicate the limit.'
T—Target acceptable alternatives.

Verbalizing understanding of the child's feeling or want conveys acceptance of the child's motivation and often helps to defuse the intensity of the feeling. Acceptance of the feeling or desire often satisfies the child, and hence the need for the behavior no longer exists. Once the parent acknowledges the child's feeling, communicating the limit specifically and clearly allows the child to quickly understand what behavior or action is appropriate and acceptable. The parent then provides appropriate alternatives for the child to express his or her feelings.

Examples of Therapeutic Limit Setting

1. Child: (*Holds up a block and threatens to throw it at parent.*)
   Parent: (A) "I know you are really angry with me," (C) "but I'm not for throwing things at." (T) "You can throw the block on the floor or you can throw it at the bop bag."
2. Child: "I'm going to paint a big sunshine on the window."
   Parent: (A) "You really want to paint a sun on the window."
   Child: "Yes, I'm going to make it beautiful."
   Parent: (A) "You really want to make it pretty." (C) "But the window is not for painting." (T) "You can paint a sunshine on the white paper or the egg carton."

TRAINING AND SUPERVISION FOR CPRT

Before utilizing CPRT with children and parents, therapists need extensive training and supervision in CCPT. In addition to training and supervised practice in CCPT, therapists also need specific training and supervision in facilitating CPRT.

PARENT SELECTION

Although CPRT is an empirically supported and highly effective intervention for a variety of child concerns and problem behaviors and with diverse parent–child populations, some children and parents may benefit more from other interventions. Parents who are experiencing a significant amount of emotional stress or personal challenges may have difficulty focusing on the needs of their children. Many parents need to engage in personal counseling before they are able to successfully learn the skills and facilitate a therapeutic play environment for their child. Furthermore, some parents may be unwilling or unmotivated to participate in their child's therapy. In addition to parental concerns that may prohibit participation in CPRT, a child's emotional or behavioral challenges may extend beyond the capability of the parent. When a child is experiencing significant challenges or distress, a parent may not be able to provide the child with an effective therapeutic experience and direct intervention from a trained mental health professional may be necessary. CPRT may often be effectively utilized as a secondary intervention to continue and maintain therapeutic change and growth once initial parent or child concerns are addressed through individual counseling and play therapy.

STRUCTURE AND CONTENT
OF THE TRAINING SESSIONS

The basic CPRT group consists of six to eight parents in a small-group format. Parents attend 10 training sessions that last 90–120 minutes. A brief summary of the content and focus for each CPRT training session is provided below as an overview of the CPRT model.

Training Session 1: Training Objectives and Reflective Responding

The primary objective in this initial session is to create a safe environment for parents, one that encourages parents to share their parenting struggles openly with each other. Toward reaching this goal, ample time is spent with parents introducing themselves and describing their families, with particular emphasis on the child they have chosen to conduct play sessions with. The therapist provides an overview of the overall objectives of CPRT, emphasizing the goal of parents developing sensitivity to their child's emotional world and increased empathy for their child's experience. The concept of reflective responding is introduced and demonstrated with a focus on identifying and reflecting feelings.

Training Session 2: Basic Principles of Play Sessions

Parents are introduced to the basic principles, guidelines, and goals for the weekly play sessions with their child. A list of toys to be used during the special playtimes is provided, with the therapist explaining the rationale for the use and inclusion of each item in the play kit. The therapist demonstrates or shows a video recording of a typical play session, followed by parents role-playing the skills observed. Parents are asked to assemble a play kit and decide on a specific time and location for their weekly play sessions by the next training session.

Training Session 3: Parent–Child Play Session Skills and Procedures

The primary intent of this session is to prepare parents for their first play session. Parents are given a handout that outlines basic "Dos and Don'ts" for conducting play sessions. The essential play session skills of structuring, allowing the child to lead, and "being with" are demonstrated by the therapist followed by parents role-playing those skills. The therapist provides parents with a play session procedures checklist to help them prepare for their sessions. Parents are instructed to conduct their first play session at home during this week and one or two parents are selected to video-record their play sessions to bring for focused supervision during the next training session.

Training Session 4: Supervision and Limit Setting

The primary goal in this session is for parents to report on their first play sessions with their children, with the majority of this time spent watching the recorded play sessions of one or two parents. The viewing of video-recorded play sessions provides a rich opportunity for vicarious learning and group empathy. The therapist uses examples from the video and from parents' comments to reinforce CCPT skills and to encourage and support parents. The primary objective is to identify strengths and positive growth in each parent's sharing. The therapist reviews and demonstrates all play session skills. The skill of therapeutic limit setting is introduced, demonstrated, and role-played by parents. Two parents are scheduled to bring video-recorded play sessions for the next training session.

Training Session 5: Play Session Skills Review

Similar to Session 4, the focus of this session is supporting and encouraging parents as they learn and practice their new play session skills. To avoid overwhelming parents, no new skills are introduced, although limit setting is a continued focus. The majority of the session is devoted to the therapist's supervision of parents' home play sessions through parent self-report and video-recorded play sessions with a focus on parents' self-awareness in relation to their children. Play session skills are reviewed and demonstrated as needed to support parents' continued learning.

Training Sessions 6–9

Training Sessions 6–9 follow a similar format. Each session begins with parents reporting on their home play sessions followed by focused supervision on the one or two parents assigned to show their video-recorded play sessions. Each week, two additional parents are scheduled to present their video-recorded play sessions. The objective is for each parent to have two opportunities to show their video-recorded play sessions and receive focused supervision and feedback over the course of training. Although no new play session skills are introduced after Session 5, related topics are presented each week to enhance parents' learning and generalization of skills to outside the play sessions.

- Session 6: Choice giving is introduced as a method of empowering children and as the fourth step in limit setting.
- Session 7: Self-esteem-building responses are presented and demonstrated.
- Session 8: Parents are taught how to use encouragement rather than praise to promote self-esteem development.
- Session 9: The goal of this session is to help parents begin to generalize the skills they have learned and apply them to everyday interactions with their child.

Training Session 10: Evaluation and Termination

The final session is used as a review and to bring closure to the group. The primary focus is on parents recognizing the progress that they and their children have made through the course of the intervention. The therapist encourages and reinforces parents' identified areas of growth and change and provides supporting examples based on parents' progress across sessions. Parents are encouraged to continue home play sessions and asked to make a commitment to continue the play sessions for a specific time frame.

A follow-up group session is scheduled approximately 4–6 weeks following the final training session.

Follow-Up Training Sessions

Parents briefly share their experiences in their play sessions since the last training session, focusing on changes they have observed in themselves and in their children. The therapist utilizes this time to briefly review the basic CCPT principles and skills. The primary aim of the follow-up session is to encourage and support parents' growth and to generalize play session skills to parenting challenges and behavior problems outside of the play sessions. Parents are asked to provide examples of times they have used their new skills successfully. If the group communicates interest, another follow-up training session may be scheduled and held in 2–3 months.

CASE ILLUSTRATION

Mary, the mother of 6-year-old Taylor, reported that she and Taylor "were always butting heads" and that he had always been a "difficult" child. Mary felt that everything from getting dressed, going to bed, and eating a healthy meal became a battle with Taylor and often ended with him throwing a tantrum, kicking and screaming at her, and her feeling exhausted and frustrated as a parent. In addition to Taylor's aggressive behavior toward her, Mary also expressed concerns that Taylor was sometimes aggressive toward other children at school; fought with his younger 3-year-old sister; and had some difficulty following his teacher's directions in class. When Mary began CPRT, she felt discouraged and skeptical about learning new parenting skills and had already read many parenting books and tried several other parenting programs to address Taylor's behavior problems without success. Mary described her relationship with Taylor as "challenging" and "exhausting" and had a hard time identifying Taylor's positive characteristics and her own parenting strengths during the initial CPRT session.

Mary participated actively in the CPRT group and connected well with other parents in the group. She was able to reflect and identify feelings in the role plays with other parents but reported that she had a hard time not asking Taylor a lot of questions and focusing on his feelings when his behavior was so out of control.

MARY: It's really hard to think about what he's feeling when he's refusing to get in the car and we are late for school in the morning.

THERAPIST: You feel frustrated and it's hard to respond to his feelings when you're under that much pressure.

MARY: Yes! Sometimes I just want to refuse to leave the house too. But I'm the mom, so I don't get to do that.

THERAPIST: It sounds like you both feel powerless.

As Mary described her interactions with Taylor, the therapist invited other parents to brainstorm feelings that Taylor may be having and that Mary could reflect to him. Although many of her interactions with Taylor were oriented around conflict, the therapist encouraged Mary to find opportunities to reflect Taylor's positive emotions as well. The following week Mary was eager to share with the group and recount her trials-and-errors and ultimate success at reflecting Taylor's feelings.

> "At first, I kept reflecting Taylor's feelings and he seemed not to care at all. He didn't respond to me and I wondered if I was getting it wrong. But I kept saying, 'You seem angry about this' or 'You feel disappointed about that.' And finally, after several times, he finally turned and looked at me, and said, 'Yeah. I *am* angry!' Even though he was still upset, I felt excited because it was so good to be able to get through to him. After I reflected his feeling, he seemed to calm down more quickly and I felt more patient with him."

Due to the intensity of Taylor's behavior and the conflict in their relationship, Mary was eager to learn new discipline strategies and limit setting. The therapist validated Mary's concerns about Taylor's misbehavior and sense of desperation to make changes in their relationship. She encouraged her to continue to focus on building her relationship with Taylor by creating more opportunities for positive interactions between them and using her new skills in their special playtimes.

Mary was nervous about her first playtime with Taylor and anxious about showing her video-recorded session to other parents in the group. After her first playtime with Taylor, Mary felt discouraged. Other parents described their children feeling excited about their special playtimes and the toys. As Mary watched another parent's recorded session, she seemed to grow quiet and appeared deflated.

THERAPIST: Mary, I've noticed you are quieter tonight than usual and I wanted to check in with you.

MARY: Oh, yeah. It's great to see and hear about everyone else's playtimes. I'm really impressed with how well you reflected feelings and behavior. But I guess I'm struggling because my playtime was a lot different than everyone else's.

THERAPIST: Would you tell us more about it?

MARY: Um. Well, Taylor and I had already had a rough morning. So when it was time for our special playtime he didn't really want to do it. I spent a lot of time setting up the toys and trying to make it fun for him. At first he refused to come into the room and then he complained about the toys.

THERAPIST: It felt like he was rejecting you after all your effort to do something fun for him.

MARY: Yes. It's hard when your own child doesn't want to play with you.

THERAPIST: It's disappointing and painful to be in this place with Taylor. I wonder if anyone else had some surprising or disappointing experiences in their first playtime?

JOANNA [Another mother in the group]: Oh, well, Katie thought all the toys were for "babies." She eventually started playing with the craft stuff and enjoyed herself, but at first I was thinking, "Oh, no. This isn't going to go well." And after all the effort of collecting all the toys too.

THERAPIST: So, Joanna, you felt some disappointment and trepidation about your playtime too when Katie didn't like the toys at first.

JOANNA: Sure. But I just kept trying to use the skills and be accepting even though it was hard.

THERAPIST: And Mary, it sounds like even though Taylor didn't want to play at first you were still able to have your playtime together. How did you get through that first tough part?

MARY: I just kept reflecting his feelings and telling him, "This is our special playtime you can play with a lot of the toys. . . . " Eventually, he came in the room and started looking around. He seemed pretty frustrated with me for the first 15 minutes or so, but I kept responding to him and trying to pay attention to what he was doing. Finally, he started setting up the animals and the soldiers to fight and he asked me for my help. So I started working with him to line them up.

THERAPIST: You were able to follow his lead and stay present with him even when it was hard. Then it sounds like he invited you to participate.

MARY: Yes. And then, when we only had 5 minutes left we were still setting all the toys up in a line. He was upset that we were running out of time and asked me for more minutes. So leaving the playtime was a bit hard.

THERAPIST: He put up a bit of a struggle at the end too, but it sounds like he really wanted to keep playing with you.

MARY: Yeah. Once we got started he didn't really want to stop. I guess I didn't really see it that way before.

As the sessions continued, Mary reported ongoing struggles with Taylor and his misbehavior but seemed to be noticing more about what motivated his behavior. When it was Mary's turn to show her recorded play session to the other parents she was very anxious. The therapist encouraged Mary to identify one skill she utilized well with Taylor and encouraged other parents to give Mary positive feedback throughout the supervision process. After watching a segment where Taylor tried to hit Mary in the face with a sword and Mary used the A-C-T model to set a limit, the therapist stopped the video.

THERAPIST: Mary, I'm noticing you remembered all the steps for A-C-T and you seemed really calm when you were setting the limit even though the sword got close to you. How were you feeling?

MARY: I was pretty anxious. I didn't want to get hit and wasn't sure I would be able to say all the steps fast enough. But I just kept repeating the steps and giving him different choices. It was hard to think of things for him to hit at first, but I picked the dolls and the puppets.

THERAPIST: And it looks like it worked. You didn't get hit and he brought himself under control.

MARY: (laughing) Yeah, I still have both my eyes. He hit the puppets instead.

BRENT [another parent in the group]: I'm impressed you stayed that calm. I'm not sure I would have been able to.

ALLISON [another parent in the group]: Yeah! I can't remember all the A's and the C's and the T's, especially not if I had a sword coming at me.

THERAPIST: I also noticed that after the limit setting you continued to play happily together.

MARY: Yeah. That would have never happened before. Usually he would get angrier and it would end in a tantrum. But this time, he hit the puppets for a while and then he wanted to play "cooking" with me. So we made "pancakes" together which is something we do on the weekends sometimes.

THERAPIST: Sounds like you felt really connected to him. You enjoyed being with him.

MARY: Yes. We really had a good time together. And I didn't know how much our weekend breakfast routine meant to him. . . . It also felt good to be able to set a limit and see him follow it without the power struggle and tantrum that usually follow.

Mary continued to have her weekly parent and child play sessions with Taylor throughout the 10-sessions of CPRT. Their play sessions became more enjoyable, interactive, and cooperative. Mary reported that they both looked forward to their special playtimes and that although Taylor tested limits, he was able to follow them more easily when she expressed empathy and provided alternatives ways for him to express himself through the A-C-T model. Although Mary continued to practice and demonstrate the skills during their playtimes, she had some challenges generalizing them to her interactions with Taylor outside of the playtimes. The therapist encouraged Mary to identify one common source of conflict between her and Taylor and to focus on approaching the issue using her new CPRT skills. Mary described an almost nightly battle about turning off the television to get ready for bed. Many of the parents in the group could relate to Mary's nightly exchange with Taylor and they all worked together to brainstorm how to address the shared problem of transitioning their children from "screen time" to bedtime. The parents role-played limit setting and giving choices for their children when they refused to turn off the television or computer. The therapist encouraged the parents to also use structuring responses like telling their children "You have 10 minutes of screen time left before it's time to brush your teeth and put on your pajamas" to help ease the transition.

The following week, Mary seemed excited to share about her week with Taylor. After three nights of emotional outbursts and consequences before bed, she almost gave up on using limit setting to help with Taylor's nightly bedtime routine. But on the fourth night, when Mary set the limit Taylor groaned and said, "I know, I know. It's time to turn it off. I choose to turn it off myself." Taylor stomped off to the bathroom, but Mary felt elated that being consistent and using her new skills had paid off.

In the final CPRT session, Mary described her relationship with Taylor very differently.

> "For the first time in a long time, I feel excited about spending time with him. Although we still butt heads from time to time, I feel a lot more calm and patient with him. I understand him a lot better than I used to too. At least, I think I do. And he seems to understand me more too. We laugh a lot more and there's a lot less yelling, and screaming, and crying in our house. We still have a couple tantrums a week, but even those seem to be shorter. He even sets limits for himself and targets alternatives for his little sister. Everything feels a lot less out of control. . . . Last week, he got to pick a prize out of the treasure box at the end of the week for having such good behavior every day at school. We still have a lot of work to do, but I'm really amazed at how far we've come together. And now instead of refusing to go in the room for our

special playtime, Taylor counts down the days till our next playtime. We are a lot closer than we used to be and I really appreciate how thoughtful, creative, and sensitive he is, something I didn't really realize before."

FURTHER APPLICATIONS OF CPRT

CPRT is an effective intervention for children and parents with a variety of emotional and behavioral challenges. As the child-parent relationship is strengthened and parents develop new ways of relating to their children, children begin to relate to their parents and behave in more healthy and adaptive ways. In addition to its use with children ages 2 to 10, CPRT can also be modified for use with infants and with preadolescents (Landreth & Bratton, 2006). The group format of CPRT provides the opportunity for parental support and vicarious learning; however, CPRT can also be adapted to meet the needs of individual clients who may not be able to participate in a group due to limitations of time, finances, or group composition.

A more thorough discussion of CPRT and specific descriptions of all the material to be taught in each of the 10 training sessions is provided in Landreth and Bratton's (2006) book *Child Parent Relationship Therapy (CPRT): A 10-Session Filial Therapy Model* and in the accompanying treatment manual by Bratton and Landreth (2006), *Child Parent Relationship Therapy (CPRT) Treatment Manual*. The process of facilitating a CPRT training group across several sessions can be viewed in Bratton and Landreth's (2013) DVD *Child Parent Relationship Therapy (CPRT) in Action: Four Couples in a CPRT Group*.

REFERENCES

Axline, V. (1947). *Play therapy*. New York: Ballantine.

Beckloff, D. R. (1998). Filial therapy with children with spectrum pervasive development disorders. *Dissertation Abstracts International: Section B. Sciences and Engineering, 58*(11), 6224.

Bratton, S. C., & Landreth, G. L. (1995). Filial therapy with single parents: Effects on parental acceptance, empathy, and stress. *International Journal of Play Therapy, 4*(1), 61–80.

Bratton, S. C., & Landreth, G. L. (2006). *Child parent relationship therapy (CPRT): A 10-session filial therapy model*. New York: Routledge.

Bratton, S. C., & Landreth, G. L. (2013). *Child parent relationship therapy (CPRT) in action: Four couples in a CPRT group* [DVD]. Denton: University of North Texas.

Bratton, S. C., Ray, D., Rhine, T., & Jones, L. (2005). The efficacy of play therapy with children: A meta-analytic review of treatment outcomes. *Professional Psychology: Research and Practice, 36*(4), 376–390.

Ceballos, P., & Bratton, S. C. (2010). School-based child–parent relationship therapy (CPRT) with low-income first-generation immigrant Latino parents: Effects on children's behaviors and parent–child relationship stress. *Psychology in the Schools, 47*(8), 761–775.

Chau, I., & Landreth, G. (1997). Filial therapy with Chinese parents: Effects on parental empathic interactions, parental acceptance of child, and parental stress. *International Journal of Play Therapy, 6*(2), 75–92.

Costas, M., & Landreth, G. (1999). Filial therapy with nonoffending parents of children who have been sexually abused. *International Journal of Play Therapy, 8*(1), 43–66.

Glover, G., & Landreth, G. (2000). Filial therapy with Native Americans on the Flathead Reservation. *International Journal of Play Therapy, 9*(2), 57–80.

Grskovic, J., & Goetze, H. (2008). Short-term filial therapy with German mothers: Findings from a controlled study. *International Journal of Play Therapy, 17*(1), 39–51.

Guerney, B. (1964). Filial therapy: Description and rationale. *Journal of Consulting Psychology, 28*(4), 303–310.

Guerney, L., & Ryan, V. (2013). *Group filial therapy: The complete guide to teaching parents to play therapeutically with their children.* Philadelphia: Jessica Kingsley.

Harris, Z. L., & Landreth, G. (1997). Filial therapy with incarcerated mothers: A five week model. *International Journal of Play Therapy, 6*(2), 53–73.

Holt, K. (2011). Child–parent relationship therapy with adoptive children and their parents: Effects in child behavior, parent–child relationship stress, and parental empathy. *Dissertation Abstracts International: Section B. Sciences and Engineering, 71*(8), 1–96.

Jang, M. (2000). Effectiveness of filial therapy for Korean parents. *International Journal of Play Therapy, 9*(2), 39–56.

Johnson-Clark, K. A. (1996). The effect of filial therapy on child conduct behavior problems and the quality of the parent–child relationship. *Dissertation Abstracts International: Section B. Sciences and Engineering, 57*(4), 2868.

Kale, A. L., & Landreth, G. (1999). Filial therapy with parents of children experiencing learning difficulties. *International Journal of Play Therapy, 8*(2), 35–56.

Kidron, M., & Landreth, G. (2010). Intensive child parent relationship therapy with Israeli parents in Israel. *International Journal of Play Therapy, 19*(2), 64–78.

Landreth, G. L. (2012). *Play therapy: The art of the relationship.* New York: Routledge.

Landreth, G. L., & Bratton, S. C. (2006). *Child parent relationship therapy (CPRT): A 10-session filial therapy model.* New York: Routledge.

Landreth, G., & Lobaugh, A. (1998). Filial therapy with incarcerated fathers: Effects on parental acceptance of child, parental stress, and child adjustment. *Journal of Counseling and Development, 76,* 157–165.

Lee, M., & Landreth, G. (2003). Filial therapy with immigrant Korean parents in the United States. *International Journal of Play Therapy, 12*(2), 67–85.

Lin, Y. D. (2011). Contemporary research on child-centered play therapy (CCPT) modalities: A meta-analytic review of controlled outcome studies. *ProQuest Dissertations and Theses, 181.* Retrieved from *http://search.proquest.com/docview/910228005?accountid=14613.*

Lin, Y.-W., & Bratton, S. C. (2015). A meta-analytic review of child-centered play therapy approaches. *Journal of Counseling and Development, 93*(1), 45–58.

Morrison, B. M. O., & Bratton, S. C. (2011). The effects of child–teacher relationship training on the children of focus: A pilot study. *International Journal of Play Therapy, 20*(4), 193–207.

Ray, D. E. (2003). *The effect of filial therapy on parental acceptance and child adjustment.* Unpublished masters' thesis, Emporia State University, Kansas.

Rogers, C. (1957). The necessary and sufficient conditions of therapeutic personality change. *Journal of Consulting Psychology, 21*(2), 95–103.

Sheely-Moore, A., & Bratton, S. (2010). A strengths-based parenting intervention with low-income African American families. *Professional School Counseling, 13*(3), 175–183.

Villarreal, C. E. (2008). School-based child parent relationship therapy (CPRT) with Hispanic parents. *ProQuest Dissertaions and Theses, 162.* Retrieved from *http://search.proquest.com/docview/304807224?accountid=14613.*

Yuen, T., Landreth, G., & Baggerly, J. (2002). Filial therapy with immigrant Chinese families. *International Journal of Play Therapy, 11*(2), 63–90.

Chapter 11

⮧

Play Therapy for Oppositional/Defiant Children

Parent–Child Interaction Therapy

Susan G. Timmer
Anthony J. Urquiza
Sharon Rea Zone

*P*arent–Child Interaction Therapy (PCIT) is a behaviorally oriented therapy for children 2–7 years of age, with the goal of changing the child's social environment to make it more reinforcing of positive rather than negative behavior. The goals of PCIT involve increasing the numbers of parents' positive verbalizations toward their children, decreasing negative verbalizations, and systematizing the discipline environment. Using social learning theory and attachment theory, developer Sheila M. Eyberg reasoned that by changing specific ways parents spoke to their children, they would also change reward contingencies and the environment of social reinforcement, and thus decrease children's disruptive behavior (Eyberg, 2004). The reader will quickly perceive that it is difficult to imagine an intervention being less similar to nondirective play therapy. Where play therapy uses play as the medium through which children can express themselves symbolically, PCIT uses play because it is an activity that children do not mind engaging in with their parents. Where play therapy focuses on the power of this symbolic expression as a way to narrate inner conflict or trauma as the key to reducing behavioral problems, the PCIT protocol focuses on changing the child's external caregiving environment. Where play therapists are the "agents" of change, observing children's play behavior, interpreting its themes, and reflecting it back therapeutically, thus helping children to resolve and understand their inner conflicts, PCIT therapists control the play environment, using it to create opportunities for the parent to practice "relating" to their children in specific ways. So, why is there a chapter on PCIT in a book devoted to play therapy? Play is the child's medium, whether play occurs in nondirective play therapy or in PCIT. Children use play for their own purposes, whether the therapist directs it or not. Traumatized children will reenact their trauma when playing with animals or other figurines, or they will act out their anger with Mrs. Potato Head. While the structure of PCIT may not seem as though it could accommodate more therapeutic strategies, particularly for traumatized children (such as those represented by play therapy), it will be demonstrated in this chapter how PCIT can address traumatized children's mental health needs, and how understanding the underlying symbolism of children's play, along with play therapy skills, might enhance the effectiveness of PCIT. First, however, PCIT is described in more detail, followed by a case illustration, and discussion of the evidence supporting its use.

WHAT IS PCIT?

PCIT is a 14- to 20-week, manualized intervention designed for children between 2 and 7 years of age with disruptive or externalizing behavior problems (Eyberg & Robinson, 1983). The underlying model of change is similar to that of other parent training programs. These programs promote the idea that through positive parenting and behavior modification skills, the parents themselves become the agent of change in reducing the child's behavior problems. However, unlike other parenting-focused interventions, PCIT incorporates both parent and child in the treatment sessions and uses live, individualized therapist coaching for an idiographic approach to changing the dysfunctional parent–child relationship.

PCIT is conducted in two phases. The first phase focuses on enhancing the parent–child relationship (child-directed interaction; CDI), and the second on improving child compliance (parent-directed interaction; PDI). Both phases of treatment begin with an hour of didactic training, followed by sessions in which the therapist coaches the parent during play with the child. From an observation room behind a two-way mirror, via a "bug-in-the-ear" receiver worn by the parent, the therapist provides the parent with feedback on his or her use of the skills. Parents are coached to practice specific skills related to their communication with the child and behavior management. In addition to practicing these skills during clinic sessions, parents are asked to practice with the child at home for 5 minutes every day.

In CDI (typically 7–10 sessions), a parent is coached to follow the child's lead in play by attending to the child's appropriate behavior in the following three ways: (1) describe the child's activities; (2) reflect the child's appropriate speech; and (3) praise the children's good behavior. The skills parents learn during this phase of treatment are represented in the acronym PRIDE, which stands for *Praise, Reflection, Imitation, Description, and Enjoyment*. By the end of CDI, parents generally have shifted from rarely noticing the child's positive behavior to more consistently attending to or praising appropriate behavior. To move to the second phase of treatment, parents must master CDI skills by demonstrating that in 5 minutes of play they can give 10 behavior descriptions (e.g., "You are building a tall tower"), 10 reflections (i.e., repeating back or paraphrasing the child's words), 10 labeled praises (e.g., "Thank you for playing so gently with these toys"), and fewer than three questions, commands, or criticisms. The following is an example of CDI coaching:

[Parent and child are playing with Legos. The therapist is watching from an adjacent observation room and talking to the parent through a "bug-in-the-ear" system.] In all dialogues, the the therapist's words are indicated by *italics*.]

THERAPIST: *Describe what Noah is doing with his hands.*

CHILD: [Plays with blue Legos.]

PARENT: You put all of the blue Legos on the table.

THERAPIST: *That was a great behavioral description!*

CHILD: Yes, I'm going to make a big blue tower.

PARENT: Oh . . . you're going to make a big blue tower.

THERAPIST: *You got it! That was a perfect reflection of what Noah said. He knows you are paying attention to what he is doing. When you give him praise and attention for his good behavior, he will do more of that behavior.*

CHILD: And I'm going to make a red barn too!

THERAPIST: *You make a red barn too, Mom.*

PARENT: That's a great idea! I'm going to make a red barn just like you.

THERAPIST: *Great imitating! He really knows you're paying attention when you imitate his play.*

CHILD: OK, you build yours right here, and the cow will go in it.

THERAPIST: *Noah is playing very gently with the toys today. And so creative!*

PARENT: Noah, you are so creative with these Legos. That's beautiful!

CHILD: Yeah!

THERAPIST: *Nice labeled praise, Mom.*

In the example, you can see that the therapist alternated between leading (and sometimes redirecting) the parent, following the parent, and giving brief bits of information: interpreting the child's behavior and explaining both the meaning and long-term effects of using the skills. These coaching strategies gently lead the parent to try out, practice, and incorporate these skills into his or her parenting.

In PDI therapists train parents to give only essential commands and to make them clear and direct, maximizing chances for compliance. Parents participating in PCIT traditionally learn a specific method of using time-out for dealing with noncompliance. Parents also may be taught "hands-off" strategies (e.g., removal of privileges) if indicated. These strategies are designed to provide caregivers with tools for managing their children's behavior while helping them to avoid using physical power, focusing instead on using positive incentives and promoting children's emotional regulation. Mastery of behavior management skills during PDI is achieved when therapists observe that caregivers are able to use the behavior management strategies they were taught without being coached and when parents report that these strategies are effective in reducing problem behaviors. By the end of PDI, the process of giving commands and obtaining compliance are predictable and safe for parents and children. Increasing predictability and safety in families helps break the cycle of violence in abusive families (Dodge, Bates, & Pettit, 1990). The following script is an example of PDI coaching:

(Parent and child are playing with Legos; the therapist is watching from an adjacent observation room and talking to the parent through the 'bug-in-the-ear' system)

THERAPIST: *It is now time to clean up the toys. Tell Noah to put the Legos back in the box.*

PARENT: Noah, it's time to clean up. Can you put the Legos back in the box? [indirect command]

THERAPIST: *Make it a direct command.*

PARENT: Please put the Legos back in the box, Noah.

THERAPIST: *That was a perfect direct command. Now Noah knows exactly what he is supposed to do.*

CHILD: [Noah starts to put a couple of Legos in the box.]

THERAPIST: *Now Noah is putting Legos away like you told him.*

PARENT: Thank you for listening, Noah! [labeled praise]

THERAPIST: *Excellent labeled praise. That will help Noah want to listen more in the future.*

As in CDI, the PCIT therapist alternates between leading, following, and explaining to the parent. However, unlike CDI, the therapist is more corrective, never ignoring mistakes, and can be more directing, particularly in the midst of a child's time-out or time-out refusal. During these mini-crises, the therapist may give the parent the words to say or prompt the parent with the beginning of a well-practiced phrase to keep the parent on track.

Therapists coach parents to recognize and provide appropriate responses for the child's behavior (e.g., recognizing and responding to praise for compliance; recognizing and ignoring minor inappropriate behavior—such as whining). As parents acquire these PCIT skills, therapists give fewer directives and instead use the coaching time to describe and praise the positive parenting they see, making connections between this behavior and the bigger picture of parenting and child development. An additional important element of PCIT coaching involves shifting *both* parent responses and cognitions about child behavior. While coaching, therapists often provide supplemental information about the child's behavior, to correct or minimize distortions in parent cognitions (especially negative or hostile cognitions). An example of this would be as follows:

[Child is coloring with a marker and paper. In the process of coloring, he accidentally moves the marker off of the paper and draws on the table.]

THERAPIST: [noticing that the child has colored on the table and the parent is irritated about the child drawing on the table] *Oh . . . that happens all of the time. It is common for a child of his age to accidentally draw on the table. The marker washes off the table easily—so no harm done. As soon as he starts to draw on the paper, give him a labeled praise for drawing on the paper.*

CHILD: [Starts to draw on the paper again.] I am drawing a truck.

PARENT: That is an awesome truck [labeled praise]; and you are doing a great job drawing on the paper! [labeled praise]

THERAPIST: *Awesome labeled praise, Dad! He wasn't misbehaving by drawing on the table—he is just not old enough to always draw on the paper. And now you've started teaching him that it's good to draw on the paper.*

Through the process of coaching, therapists can give parents immediate and accurate feedback about the child's behavior. It can be argued that when the therapist whispers into the parent's ear a different view of the child's behavior—a different interpretation of the child's intent—the therapist "interrupts" the parent's previously held negative attribution (and associated negative affect) about the child's behavior. Over time, children's behaviors that were previously viewed through a lens of negative parental attributions are viewed more positively. Parents' expectations shift to recognition and acknowledgment, then acceptance of the more positive attribution now associated with the child's behavior.

IMPROVING CHILD RELATIONSHIP SECURITY AND STABILITY WITH THE PRIMARY CAREGIVER

Helping parents by enabling and supporting a more positive parent–child relationship is another primary objective of PCIT. One of the avenues to recovery from child trauma involves eliciting support from important caregivers. Supportive parenting is associated with positive child outcomes in many domains (DeKleyn & Greenberg, 2008; Kim et al., 2003)—especially when a child is exposed to a traumatic event (Valentino, Berkowitz, & Stover, 2010). Therefore, it is essential to sustain a positive parent–child relationship and parental support in order to optimize the child's ability to deal with any adverse or traumatic experience. The combination of parental stress associated with child trauma and problematic child symptoms can erode a parent's ability to be supportive, warm, and understanding. One benefit of PCIT is that parents who use the PRIDE skills (i.e., parenting skills promoted within the first portion of PCIT) in their interactions with their children, particularly Praise and Reflection, are also more likely to be rated as sensitive, showing warmth and positive affiliation increase (Timmer & Zebell, 2006), which should strengthen the parent–child relationship. Throughout the course of PCIT, coaching focuses on helping a parent to recognize and attend to the child's positive behavior by describing and praising it. At the same time, parents are taught to ignore minor negative and inappropriate behaviors so that they can maintain a warm and supportive relationship with the child. As stated earlier, in the development of PCIT Eyberg incorporated play therapy goals and techniques proposed by Axline's (1947) and Guerney's (1964) therapeutic approaches because they promoted warmth and acceptance (Eyberg, 2004). An intervention that promotes warm, responsive, and authoritative parenting, and that combines nurturing, clear communication, and firm limit setting, may be an effective way to address a wide range of child mental health problems— including child trauma symptoms.

PARENTS AS THERAPISTS: SUPPORTING PARENT–CHILD COMMUNICATION

Although there are many perspectives on what exactly constitutes psychotherapy, a rich literature describes the benefits of parents functioning in a supportive, therapeutic-like role with their children (Guerney, 2000; Hutton, 2004). The central aspects of this type of Filial Therapy relationship include the following: (1) a positive relationship between a child and parent; (2) a focus on development of appropriate and safe expression and communication; and (3) the use of play as a central theme (Urquiza, Zebell, & Blacker, 2009). In PCIT, parents learn how to engage their children in positive and collaborative play (especially in the first component of PCIT). As a result, typically a more warm, supportive, and affectionate relationship develops between the parent and the child. Often, this new relationship includes positive verbal statements and physical affection exhibited by both the parent and the child. Similarly, the focus on safe and effective communication is a central tenet of PCIT. Parents are directed to communicate issues of safety, concern for the child's well-being, and positive regard for all appropriate and nonaggressive interactions. Because both parents and children generally perceive play activities as positive and enjoyable, sharing positive play experiences in PCIT sessions strengthens the communication between the dyad and helps rebuild a relationship history that is overall less negative and more positive.

MANAGEMENT OF THE TRAUMATIZED CHILD'S AFFECT

Traumatized young children have difficulty managing their feelings in emotionally difficult situations (Graham-Bermann & Levendosky, 1998). These young children have underdeveloped coping skills and a limited understanding of the traumatic experience they have endured (Eigsti & Cicchetti, 2004). These developmental limitations can hinder therapeutic efforts to directly address the child's trauma and traumatic symptoms, and help a child to understand his or her responses (especially his or her feelings) to the trauma. In addition to promoting a more positive and secure parent–child relationship, PCIT provides a mechanism to directly address many of the feelings that a child experiences—especially feelings associated with safety, fear, avoidance, and security. In the "PCIT for Traumatized Children" protocol, therapists are instructed to help parents identify a child's thoughts, feelings, and behaviors should the child act out the trauma in play or refer to the trauma during the treatment session. For example, if a child acted out an event, displaying anger, aggression, or fear—which are often displayed by traumatized children—parents would be coached to respond appropriately to the child. In some cases with young children, the parent might be coached to play out a resolution to the traumatic event that involves keeping the child safe. With older children, the parent might be coached to recognize and identify the feelings the child was showing. Past research has shown that distressing events that are resolved appropriately are less distressing to children than unresolved events (McCoy, Cummings, & Davies, 2009). Additionally, cognitive-behavioral research has shown that when parents label the affect connected with their children's reactions to certain experiences, their children begin to understand the meaning of the distressing affect, which is one of the first steps to being able to discuss and manage these feelings (Widom & Russell, 2008). As children continue to understand these feelings, then parents can help them engage in strategies to manage these feelings (e.g., safety planning, deep breathing, counting, progressive relaxation). An example of coaching to assist a child who has been exposed to domestic violence through this process might be as follows:

CHILD: [Is playing with a dollhouse and simulating a father coming to the door and banging hard on the door—while yelling.] Let me in! Let me in!

THERAPIST: *It looks like she is pretending through her play that she is afraid that her father is going to come back. Tell her that you understand that she is scared and remind her that there's a plan to keep both of you safe.*

PARENT: I think you get really scared when Daddy comes over to our house and is angry. But we have a plan to stay safe. I call . . .

PARENT AND CHILD: 9 . . . 1 . . . 1.

PARENT: Right! Then the police will come and we will be safe!

Therapist: *That was great. You are helping her to understand her feelings of being scared and that you can keep her safe—even if her father comes back. Maybe Mr. Potato Head can be a policeman, and you show her how the plan will work.*

PARENT: Here comes Mr. Policeman! "Let's go, Mister. No yelling and pounding doors is allowed here." [Takes away dad doll.] If Daddy comes back and you get scared, you come and find me—I'll make sure you are safe.

In order to help parents be appropriately responsive to the traumatized child's concerns, the therapist may need to have a separate "parent only" session or talk with the parent on the phone (between sessions) to educate him or her about how trauma affects children and how to respond most effectively. As with traditional PCIT coaching processes, repetition of parental responses to symptoms of child trauma increases the parent's understanding and use of supportive resources that can alleviate trauma behaviors (i.e., symptoms and cognitions).

CASE ILLUSTRATION

Samuel was just over 2 years of age when he was taken into protective custody and placed in foster care. That day his parents had been brawling: his father punched his pregnant mother in the face and belly, resulting in the mother going into premature labor, with one of her twin infants dying, and receiving 14 stitches in her face. This had not been the first time Samuel's plight had come to the attention of County Child Protective Services (CPS) social workers. His parents were known controlled substance abusers and had fallen under the scrutiny of County CPS because of their drug abuse and domestic violence. But that day, his father was arrested and incarcerated, his mother went into the hospital, and Samuel went into foster care. Samuel was first referred to PCIT 6 months after being removed from his parents' care. At this time, Samuel was reported as having severe temper tantrums when he didn't get what he wanted, banging his head and screaming loudly; he bit and hit other children, so that he was kicked out of preschool; he cried in his sleep at night and had nightmares; and he exhibited some sexualized behaviors. Though referred initially with his grandmother, Samuel began PCIT several months later with his biological mother when she began working on her reunification plan. Samuel and his mother worked for 7 months in PCIT, but were not able to move forward to the second phase of treatment because he had limited, though unsupervised, visitation with his mother. It should be noted that PCIT is not typically provided to noncustodial parents until reunification is imminent (6–8 weeks). PCIT helps build a strong and warm relationship between parents and children. But if parents are not able to reunify because of problems with addiction, the stronger relationship becomes a source of pain and possibly anxiety for the child. Additionally, noncustodial parents with limited visitation have little time to do their homework of 5 minutes a day of "Special Play Time."

Unfortunately for Sam, his mother was unable to withstand the pressures of her addiction and tested positive for hydrocodone on one of her drug tests. Consequently, her reunification plan was rescinded, and Samuel's long-term plan for reunification was converted to adoption. His foster mother, Sherri, said she would consider adopting him although she had some concerns about this course of action. His foster family agency social worker immediately requested that Samuel begin PCIT with his foster mother.

At the time Samuel began PCIT with Sherri, she reported on the Child Behavior Checklist (CBCL; Achenbach & Rescorla, 2000) clinical levels of externalizing behavior, including emotional lability, ranging from whining to anger, and screaming temper tantrums, particularly in response to being frustrated or not quickly getting what he wanted. He also continued to display sexualized behavior. In spite of his concerning emotional dysregulation, Sherri did not report that his everyday behaviors were particularly difficult for her to manage (per the Eyberg Child Behavior Inventory [ECBI] Intensity Scale [Eyberg & Pincus, 1999], the Parenting Stress Index—Self-Report [PSI-SF] Parental Distress score [Abidin, 1995], or elevated scores on the Trauma Symptom Checklist for Young Children [TSCYC; Briere, 2005] posttraumatic stress scales). During the pretreatment observational assessment, Sherri showed considerable warmth and sensitivity to Samuel, and an ability to follow his lead in play. She "managed" him using a non-directive, nonconfronting style that was effective when his affect was positive. She had less success managing him once he began to tip over into more agitated, negative affect. She did not recognize the play themes or situations that might trigger agitation, and had no idea how to handle his behavior when it began to decompensate.

Sherri learned the PRIDE skills quickly in the first phase of PCIT and also reduced verbalizations like questions, commands, and negative talk that the PCIT therapist "discouraged," per weekly 5-minute observational coding using the Dyadic Parent–Child Interaction Coding System (DPICS 3rd Edition; Eyberg, Nelson, Duke, & Boggs, 2005). According to the therapist's report, Samuel's behavior began to improve also: temper tantrums were less frequent, shorter, and less likely to involve head banging. Often, children with a trauma history begin to play out their trauma during PCIT sessions perhaps as they begin to feel safe with their caregivers; typically this occurs once the caregivers have begun to shift the way they speak and behave toward their children. Like other children, Samuel began to act out earlier traumatic experiences when playing with zoo animals in a PCIT session with Sherri. The following is a transcript of the coaching session:

PARENT: I'm going to find the zebra's mommy.

CHILD: [Picks up the zebra's mommy.]

PARENT: Oh, Samuel has the zebra's mommy.

CHILD: My mommy. Not my mommy . . . [hitting the other animal with the zebra's mommy].

THERAPIST: *Can you find another animal to be representative of you?*

CHILD: [hitting] You gotta stop it. I'm gonna fix you!

THERAPIST: *Say, "My animal can take care of the zebra until his mommy is ready."*

PARENT: My animal is going to take care of the baby zebra . . . until his mommy is ready to take care of him.

THERAPIST: *Perfect. And what you're doing is you're letting him know through symbolism that you're going to be there to protect him . . .*

CHILD: [Stops pounding with the zebra's mommy. Holds up the zebra's mommy and places it on the sill of a two-way mirror.] Aaaah! You can't be good! [Flies the zebra's mommy toward the table.]

THERAPIST: *And he's kind of playing out what's going on with him now too. We're kind of getting into a little play therapy session.*

PARENT: It took me by surprise!

THERAPIST: *You're doing fine.*

CHILD: Don't want to go! Don't want to go! Does he want to be with his mommy?

THERAPIST: *Yeah, he wants to be with his mommy.*

PARENT: Yes, he wants to be with his mommy.

CHILD: [Says something unintelligible, looking at the baby zebra.]

THERAPIST: *His mommy is still learning how to be a mommy.*

PARENT: The zebra's mommy is still learning how to be a mommy. So the elephant is going to take care of the baby zebra.

CHILD: Baby zebra?

PARENT: Yeah.

THERAPIST: *Perfect.*

PARENT: Yep. That's the baby zebra and the elephant mommy is going to take care of him.

CHILD: She looks scary.

THERAPIST: *Oh, she's safe.*

PARENT: Oh, she's safe. She's a very nice elephant.

THERAPIST: *She's strong.*

PARENT: She's a strong elephant. She's going to watch over the baby zebra. [Rubs his back.] Keep the baby zebra safe.

THERAPIST: *And the mommy can come and visit.*

PARENT: And the mommy can come and visit!

THERAPIST: *That's perfect. You're doing great, Sherri. I know that took you by surprise. [Sherri laughs.] That does happen from time to time.*

PARENT: They're just animals!

THERAPIST: *Yeah, kids will do stuff like that. And you handled it perfectly. The nice thing is that I could be here to help you through it.*

PARENT: Great!

THERAPIST: *And notice that's all he needed to deal with it right now. That was enough. Once you reassured him he calmed down, the zebra became less violent, and he was able to move on to something else.*

The above exchange represents a brief segment of coaching—no more than 2 minutes—in a typical course of PCIT. PCIT therapists would not automatically handle a situation in this way. With a child this age (and with his somewhat dysregulated style), the PCIT therapist would likely coach the parent to either model gentle behavior with her animal or to redirect the child, possibly introducing a different more interesting activity. The main goal of any strategy would be to get the child to return to appropriate play (which allows the parent to practice good parenting skills). This brief moment of play therapy-informed PCIT coaching accomplished this goal. All in all, Sherri took 8 weeks to master the skills required to move on to the second phase of treatment, and 7 more weeks to be able to manage Samuel's difficult behavior using the PCIT strategy of employing simple, positively stated direct commands to perform tasks, time-out for noncompliance with direct commands, and other skills to manage behavior when direct commands are not appropriate for the situation.

Over the course of treatment, the therapist noted that Samuel continued to have difficulties regulating his emotions, particularly when disappointed about not getting his way. The therapist referred Samuel for a developmental evaluation, to see whether these behaviors could be explained by developmental delays. In the posttreatment assessment, Sherri reported significant improvements in Sam's externalizing behavior problems on the CBCL (pretreatment T-score = 67 [clinical range]; posttreatment T-score = 52 [normal range]) and similar and normal levels of behavior problems on the ECBI intensity scale. She reported posttraumatic symptoms in the normal range on the TSCYC, significant reductions in sexualized behavior (Pretreatment Sexual Concerns Scale T-score = 69 [borderline range]; Posttreatment Sexual Concerns Scale T-score = 58 [normal range]). However,

Sherri reported that Samuel displayed significantly more depressive symptoms (Pretreatment Depression Scale T-score = 64 [normal range]; Posttreatment Depression Scale T-score = 73 [clinical range]).

The therapist noted that Samuel was more responsive to Sherri, enjoyed their play together, and was more compliant with commands. She further noted that Sherri was able to use the PCIT parenting skills she was taught in CDI and PDI. However, when under pressure, she tended to revert back to giving indirect commands and avoiding using time-out. Possibly as a result of improving the relationship and his compliance, the therapist was able to identify Samuel's need for additional developmental services as well as make a referral for additional mental health services to further address Samuel's trauma-related depressive symptoms.

EMPIRICAL SUPPORT FOR PCIT

Numerous studies have demonstrated the efficacy of PCIT for reducing child behavior problems (Eisenstadt, Eyberg, McNeil, Newcomb, & Funderburk, 1993; Eyberg, 1988; Eyberg & Robinson, 1982). Positive effects have been maintained for up to 6 years posttreatment (Hood & Eyberg, 2003). In addition, treatment effects have been shown to generalize to the home (Boggs, Eyberg, & Reynolds, 1990), school settings (McNeil, Eyberg, Eisenstadt, Newcomb, & Funderburk, 1991), and to untreated siblings (Eyberg & Robinson, 1982). In addition, research indicates that PCIT yields positive treatment outcomes with different types of cultural and language groups, including Spanish-speaking families (McCabe, Yeh, Garland, Lau, & Chavez, 2005), Chinese-speaking families (Leung, Tsang, Heunh, & Yiu, 1999), and African American families (Fernandez, Butler, & Eyberg, 2011).

While numerous studies demonstrated the value of PCIT with oppositional and defiant children, Urquiza and McNeil (1996) argued that some (if not many) of the symptoms of child victims of physical abuse or domestic violence were consistent with the disruptive behaviors of children in the PCIT studies. They proposed using PCIT with maltreated children and those exposed to domestic violence. In the last decade, research findings have shown positive outcomes with maltreating parent–child dyads (Timmer, Urquiza, Zebell, & McGrath, 2005), children exposed to domestic violence (Timmer, Ware, Zebell, & Urquiza, 2010), and children with their foster parents (Borrego, Timmer, Urquiza, & Follette, 2004; Chaffin et al., 2004; Timmer, Borrego, & Urquiza, 2002; Timmer, Urquiza, & Zebell, 2006). In summary, while PCIT was initially developed as an intervention specifically for children with disruptive behavioral problems, there is currently ample research that identifies PCIT as an effective evidence-based parenting program for high-risk and abusive families.

Traumatized young children may also come from chaotic and dysfunctional families, experiencing poor and inconsistent parenting. They exhibit defiant, oppositional, and aggressive behavior. This family history and behavioral profile qualifies them as appropriate clients for PCIT. There are also indications that externalizing behavior problems are symptoms of a traumatic response to a frightening event (Valentino et al., 2010). For some children, their traumatic response is exhibited through defiant and disruptive behaviors. It is therefore possible that by helping parents manage the child's disruptive behavior in a positive, consistent, and firm manner—a primary objective of PCIT—that the anxiety underlying that behavior may also subside, resulting in an overall decrease in trauma symptoms. In fact, recent research supports this argument, showing that young traumatized children who complete PCIT show significant reductions in trauma symptoms (Mannarino, Lieberman, Urquiza, & Cohen, 2010).

DECREASING CHILD BEHAVIORAL PROBLEMS MAY INCREASE PARENTAL COMPETENCE

For relationship-based interventions to be effective, the caregiver must be able to participate and implement the skills learned or ideas discussed during therapy sessions. When primary caregivers have other sources of stress and are trying to cope with the effects of their own traumatic experiences, these problems can not only contribute to children's mental health problems by dampening parents' warmth and sensitivity and interfering with effective parenting (Lovejoy, Graczyk, O'Hare, & Neuman, 2000), but also can disrupt treatment effectiveness (Stevens, Ammerman, Putnam, & Van Ginkel, 2002). Symptoms of posttraumatic stress, such as depression, fatigue, dissociation, and poor concentration, can interfere with the acquisition of parenting skills (Reyno & McGrath, 2006). Furthermore, parental depression increases the likelihood of early treatment termination (Kazdin, 2000), making it impossible to help the child. However, research has shown that if traumatized parents will participate in a relationship-based treatment, their own psychological symptoms can be relieved (Timmer, Ho, Urquiza, Fernandez y Garcia, & Boys, 2010).

In PCIT for traumatized children, parents are taught how to cope with the emotions that often accompany their children's disruptive behavior by using anxiety-reduction skills such as deep breathing and counting silently. They are coached to observe, notice, and react to their children's positive behavior. They are coached to show warmth, enthusiasm, and enjoyment in their interactions with their children. When traumatized parents repeatedly perform these positive and adaptive behaviors throughout the course of PCIT, it is thought that these adaptive responses may begin to generalize, or "spill over" into other parts of their lives, replacing maladaptive responses (Timmer et al., 2010).

SUMMARY AND CONCLUSIONS

Through discussion and case illustration, this chapter has described how PCIT works and the way in which PCIT uses play therapeutically. Unlike nondirective play therapy, which uses play to provide a representation of the child's psychological and emotional self, play in PCIT provides a context in which parent and child can interact in a (more or less) "power-neutral" way. When children enter PCIT with their parents, they typically do not enjoy each other's company nor appreciate each other's positive attributes. In play, parents can begin to understand their children, observing and attending to their positive behavior, and rebuild their relationships. However, when children act out traumatic events in their play, like the way Samuel hammered on the mother zebra, the two different representations of play collide. It can be difficult to ignore the meaning children give play when it triggers a traumatic memory or emotion, just as it was difficult to ignore Samuel's aggressive play. Furthermore, this aggressive play behavior can interfere with the smooth progress of the CDI phase of PCIT, typically requiring considerable amounts of "disconnection" (e.g., ignoring) instead of promoting the work of building a warm, trusting relationship. However, briefly intervening by interpreting the play for parents and giving parents the words to say to their children may help regulate the children's emotions, as well as give parents tools for later intervention. In that moment, by helping Sherri understand the meaning of Samuel's play and showing her how to talk about his anxiety about his mother, the therapist helped Sam make a little bit of sense of his confusing and scary world. Furthermore, it is possible that when the *parent* is the person who is able to help the child (i.e., the agent of change), the positive effects of treatment can be more easily sustained because the skilled parent is part of life outside of the therapy room, and will be there to intervene when the child needs help. Through this process—though not a traditional play therapy intervention—the therapist can use play to enhance communication between a parent and child, help children express thoughts and feelings about difficult and traumatic events, aid parents in understanding the concerns of their child, and build a strong and more positive relationship between a parent and his or her child.

REFERENCES

Abidin, R. R. (1995). *Parenting Stress Index: Professional manual*. Odessa, FL: Psychological Assessment Resources.

Achenbach, T. M., & Rescorla, L. (2000). *Manual for the ASEBA Preschool Forms and Profiles*. Burlington: University of Vermont, Research Center for Children, Youth and Families.

Axline, V. (1947). *Play therapy*. London: Ballantine Books.

Boggs, S., Eyberg, S., & Reynolds, l, (1990). Concurrent validity of the Eyberg Child Behavior Inventory. *Journal of Clinical Child Psychology, 91*(1), 75–78.

Borrego, J., Timmer, S., Urquiza, A., & Follette, W. (2004). Physically abusive mothers' responses following episodes of child noncompliance and compliance. *Journal of Consulting and Clinical Psychology, 72*(5), 897–903.

Briere, J. (2005). *Trauma Symptom Checklist for Young Children (TSCYC) professional manual*. Odessa, FL: Psychological Assessment Resources.

Chaffin, M., Silovsky, J., Funderburk, B., Valle, L. A., Brestan, E., Balachova, T., et al. (2004). Parent–child interaction therapy with physically abusive parents: Efficacy for reducing future abuse reports. *Journal of Consulting and Clinical Psychology, 72*(3), 500–510.

DeKleyn, M., & Greenberg, M. T. (2008). Attachment and psychopathology in childhood. In J. Cassidy & P. R. Shaver (Eds.), *Handbook of attachment: Theory, research, and clinical applications* (pp. 637–665). New York: Guilford Press.

Dodge, K., Bates, J. E., & Pettit, G. S. (1990). Mechanisms in the cycle of violence. *Science, 250*, 1678–1683.

Eigsti, I. M., & Cicchetti, D. (2004). The impact of child maltreatment of expressive syntax at 60 months. *Developmental Science, 7*, 88–102.

Eisenstadt, T., Eyberg, S., McNeil, C., Newcomb, K., & Funderburk, B. (1993). Parent–child interaction therapy with behavior problem children: Relative effectiveness of two stages and overall treatment outcome. *Journal of Clinical Child Psychology, 22*, 42–51.

Eyberg, S. M. (1988). Parent–child interaction therapy: Integration of traditional and behavioral concerns. *Child and Family Behavior Therapy, 10*, 33–46.

Eyberg, S. M. (2004) The PCIT story: Part 1. The conceptual foundation of PCIT. *Parent–Child Interaction Therapy Newsletter, 1*(1), 1–2.

Eyberg, S., Nelson, M., Duke, M., & Boggs, S. (2005). *Manual for the Dyadic Parent–Child Interaction Coding System* (3rd ed.). Unpublished manuscript.

Eyberg, S., & Pincus, D. (1999). *ECBI & SESBI-R: Eyberg Child Behavior Inventory and Sutter–Eyberg Student Behavior Inventory—Revised, Professional Manual*. Odessa, FL: Psychological Assessment Resources.

Eyberg, S. M., & Robinson, E. A. (1982). Parent–child interaction therapy: Effects on family functioning. *Journal of Clinical Child Psychology, 11*, 130–137.

Eyberg, S., & Robinson, E. A. (1983). Conduct problem behavior: Standardization of a behavioral rating scale with adolescents. *Journal of Clinical Child Psychology, 12*, 347-354.

Fernandez, M. A., Butler, A. M., & Eyberg, S. M. (2011). Treatment outcome for low socioeconomic status African American families in parent–child interaction therapy: A pilot study. *Child and Family Behavior Therapy, 33*(1), 32–48.

Graham-Bermann, S. A., & Levendoskly, A. A. (1998). The social functioning of preschool-age children whose mothers are emotionally and physically abused. *Journal of Emotional Abuse, 1*, 59–84.

Guerney, B., Jr. (1964). Filial therapy: Description and rationale. *Journal of Consulting Psychology, 28*(4), 304–310.

Guerney, L. (2000). Filial therapy into the 21st century. *International Journal of Play Therapy, 9*(2), 1–17.

Hood, K., & Eyberg, S. (2003). Outcomes of parent–child interaction therapy: Mothers' reports of maintenance three to six years after treatment. *Journal of Clinical Child and Adolescent Psychology, 32*, 412–429.

Hutton, D. (2004). Filial therapy: Shifting the balance. *Clinical Child Psychology and Psychiatry, 9*(2), 1359–1045.

Kazdin, A. E. (2000). Perceived barriers to treatment participation and treatment acceptability among antisocial children and their families. *Journal of Child and Family Studies, 9*, 157–174.

Kim, I. J., Ge, X., Brody, G. H., Conger, R., Gibbons, F. X., & Simons, R. I. (2003). Parenting behaviors and the occurrence and co-occurrence of depressive symptoms and conduct problems among African American children. *Depression, Marriage, and Families, 17*, 571–583.

Leung, C., Tsang, S., Heung, K., & You, I. (1999). Effectiveness of parent–child interaction therapy (PCIT) in Hong Kong. *Research on Social Work Practice, 19*(3), 304–313.

Lovejoy, M. C., Graczyk, P. A., O'Hare, E., & Neuman, G. (2000). Maternal depression and parenting behavior: A meta-analytic review. *Clinical Psychology Review, 20*, 561–592.

Mannarino, A., Lieberman, A., Urquiza, A., & Cohen, J. (2010, August). *Evidence-based treatments for traumatized children.* Paper presented at the 118th annual convention of the American Psychological Association, San Diego, CA.

McCabe, K. M., Yeh, M., Garland, A. F., Lau, A. S., & Chavez, G. (2005). The GANA program: A tailoring approach to adapting parent–child interaction therapy for Mexican Americans. *Education and Treatment of Children, 28*, 111–129.

McCoy, K., Cummings, M., & Davies, P. (2009). Constructive and destructive marital conflict, emotional security and children's prosocial behavior. *Journal of Child Psychology and Psychiatry, 50*(3), 270–279.

McNeil, C. B., Eyberg, S. M., Eisenstadt, T. H., Newcomb, K., & Funderburk, B. (1991). Parent–child interaction therapy with behavior problem children: Generalization of treatment effects to the school setting. *Journal of Child Clinical Psychology, 20*, 140–151.

Reyno, S., & McGrath, P. (2006). Predictors of parent training efficacy for child externalizing behavior problems—A meta-analytic review. *Journal of Child Psychology and Psychiatry, 47*, 99–111.

Stevens, J., Ammerman, R., Putnam, F., & Van Ginkel, J. (2002). Depression and trauma history in first-time mothers receiving home visitation. *Journal of Community Psychology, 30*, 551–564.

Timmer, S. G., Borrego, J., & Urquiza, A. J. (2002). Antecedents of coercive interactions in physically abusive mother–child dyads. *Journal of Interpersonal Violence, 17*(8), 836–853.

Timmer, S. G., Ho, L., Urquiza, A., Zebell, N., Fernandez y Garcia, E., & Boys, D. (2011). The effectiveness of parent–child interaction therapy with depressive mothers: The changing relationship as the agent of individual change. *Child Psychiatry and Human Development, 42*(4), 406–423.

Timmer, S. G., Urquiza, A., Zebell, N., & McGrath, J. (2005). Parent–child interaction therapy: Application to physically abusive and high-risk dyads. *Child Abuse and Neglect, 29*, 825–842.

Timmer, S. G., Urquiza, A. J., & Zebell, N. (2006). Challenging foster caregiver-maltreated child relationships: The effectiveness of parent child interaction therapy, *Child and Youth Services Review, 28*, 1–19.

Timmer, S. G., Ware, L., Zebell, N., & Urquiza, A. (2008). The effectiveness of parent–child interaction therapy for victims of interparental violence. *Violence and Victims, 25*, 486–503.

Timmer, S. G., & Zebell, N. (2006). *Mid-treatment assessment: Assessing parent skill acquisition and generalization.* Paper presented at the annual meeting of the Parent Child Interaction Therapy Conference, Gainsville, FL.

Urquiza, A. J., & McNeil, C. (1996). Parent–child interaction therapy: An intensive dyadic treatment for physically abusive families. *Child Maltreatment, 1*(2), 134–144.

Urquiza, A. J., Zebell, N. M., & Blacker, D. (2009). Innovation and integration: Parent–child interaction therapy as play therapy. In A. D. Drewes (Ed.), *Blending play therapy with cognitive behavioral therapy: Evidence-based and other effective treatments and techniques* (pp. 199–219). New York: Wiley.

Valentino, K., Berkowitz, S., & Stover, C. S. (2010). Parenting behaviors and posttraumatic symptoms in relation to children's symptomatology following a traumatic event. *Journal of Traumatic Stress, 23*(3), 403–407.

Widom, S., & Russell, J. (2008). Children acquire emotions gradually. *Cognitive Development, 23*, 291–312.

Chapter 12

❧

The DIR®/Floortime™ Model of Parent Training for Young Children with Autism Spectrum Disorder

Esther B. Hess

Playfulness is a frequent reciprocal attitude that occurs between parent and child. It represents the moment-to-moment, fully engaged interactions involving facial expressions, eye contact, voice prosody and rhythm, gestures, postures, and touch. Within this fully present intersubjective space, both parent and child experience deep joy, pleasure, and fascination with the other and with their shared activity (Hughes & Baylin, 2012). From a developmental perspective, play evolves throughout childhood—beginning in sensorimotor engagement with the physical world and culminating in the capacity to symbolically and internally represent that world. Neurotypical play frees children from physical, temporal, and spatial constraints, providing them with limitless "as-if" possibilities. When coupled with the capacity to take another's perspective (theory of mind) and to project human attributes onto inanimate objects, these children can engage reciprocally and creatively with their parents and other children.

On the other hand, children affected by autism spectrum disorder (ASD) often have great difficulties in all of these domains (Hess, 2012), resulting in repetitive, stereotypical, unimaginative, and characteristically isolated play. For many children with ASD, the various stages of play are difficult to achieve due to challenges in motor planning, expressive and receptive communication, imitation, and fine and gross motor movements (Mastrangelo, 2009). The critical question is can these children be taught how to play with family and friends? To fully appreciate the play of children on the autism spectrum, it is important to consider the various developmental functions that play subserves. From a cognitive perspective, the manipulation, organization, and later use of objects to represent people, places, and things in the real and imaginary worlds help children develop a working model for understanding and problem solving. From a social perspective, playing with objects and ideas, first alone and then with others, helps children connect. As a vehicle for emotional development, play allows children to explore and express feelings, both positive and painful. In the context of language and literacy, play provides opportunities to develop narrative and storytelling skills, which contribute to autobiographical awareness (Habermas & Bluck, 2000), and which, in turn, contribute to social connection. It is a misconception that children with autism do not play in any real sense, are not capable of pretending (which otherwise suggest symbolic capacity), and neither engage in social play or "enjoy" playing in any observable way (Boucher & Wolery, 2003). Current research points optimistically to the potential for children with autism to learn how to play. For example, in a randomized controlled study looking at the significance of joint engagement intervention, Kasari, Gulsrud, Wong, Kwon, and Locke's (2010) results suggests significant improvements in joint engagement, joint attention, and diversity of functional play acts when intervention was focused on the development of play routines in which the adult could follow in on the child's interests and then expand upon his or her play activities. The question then becomes what kind of play-based intervention helps parents bring out the best in their children with special needs so that the potential for reciprocal relationships exists?

The Developmental, Individual Difference, Relationship-based model DIR®/Floortime™ model is an interdisciplinary framework that promotes parents' ability to recognize and respect the emotional experience and expressions of their child, as shown in their actions, ideas, and intentions, and to interact in a way that helps their child use his or her natural emotions with a greater sense of purpose, building his or her capacity to engage and communicate at increasingly complex levels of functional development. The subcomponents can be summarized by looking at the three major aspects of the DIR/Floortime approach:

D—the developmental framework.
I—the individual underlying neurological processing differences of a child.
R—relationship and subsequent affective interactions.

DIR/Floortime is derived from over 50 years of study and research about child development from the fields of psychology, medicine, and education, and includes the areas of language, attention, mental health, attachment, infant development, sensory processing, and motor development.

Floortime, the heart of the DIR/Floortime model, is the play component of a comprehensive program for infants, children, adolescents, and their families with a variety of developmental challenges including ASD. This comprehensive program includes working on all elements of the DIR/Floortime model, the functional emotional developmental levels, and the underlying individual neurological differences in processing capacities, thus creating those learning relationships that will help the child move ahead in his or her development. These relationships in turn are tailored to the child's individual neurological differences that can be supported, thus providing the opportunity to move forward developmentally, mastering each and every functional emotional developmental capacity that he or she is capable of achieving (Greenspan, 2010). The DIR/Floortime model involves often not just Floortime, but different therapies like speech and language therapy, occupational therapy, physical therapy, educational programs, counseling support for parents, and home programs as well as school programs. For the purposes of this chapter, though, I will focus on Floortime, where one component is a short-term play therapy approach that helps parents create a lifestyle with the potential for a reciprocal relationship with their children. I will be including case examples and tips for overcoming problematic behaviors that are geared to help parents both get started with their Floortime regimen and learn what to do when either you or your child are feeling "stuck" in your play. This chapter also includes a summary of current evidence-based research that lends support to this developmental/relational-based play intervention for families whose children are impacted by ASD.

THE DIR/FLOORTIME MODEL

Floortime is a particular technique in which the parent is encouraged to get down on the floor and work with his or her child to master each of his or her developmental capacities. But to represent this model fairly, you will need to think about Floortime in two ways (Interdisciplinary Council on Developmental and Learning Disorders [ICDL], 2000):

1. It is a specific technique in which a parent gets down on the floor to play with his or her child.
2. It is a general philosophy that characterizes all of the interactions with the child. All of the interactions have to incorporate the features of Floortime as well as the particular goals of that interaction,

including understanding the child's emotional, social, and intellectual differences in motor, sensory, and language functioning, and
the existing caregiver, child, and family functioning and interaction
patterns.

At the heart of the definition of Floortime are two of what could be
called emphases that sometimes work together very easily and other times
may appear to be at opposite ends of a continuum.

1. Following the child's lead.
2. Joining a child in his or her world and then pulling him or her into
   a shared world to help him or her to master each of his or her functional emotional developmental capacities (Greenspan & Wieder,
   1999).

It is critical to be aware of both of these polarities, tendencies, or
dimensions of Floortime.

Following the Child's Lead

The most widely known dimension of Floortime is *following the child's
lead*—in other words, harnessing the child's natural interests. But what
exactly does that mean? By following a child's interests, or his or her lead,
we are taking the first steps in making what I have coined as a *great date*
with a child, in other words creating a validating emotional experience.
What are the elements of a great date? For most of us, it includes being in
the company of someone who is attentive, available, and fun. And when we
are with a person who incorporates all of these emotionally affirming elements, we obviously want the date to go on forever. Conversely, if we are on
a bad date, with someone who does not make us feel good about ourselves
or our experiences, most of us would attempt to escape that encounter as
soon as possible. Following a child's lead, taking the germ of his or her idea,
and making that the basis of the experience that you are about to share
with your child actually encourages the child to allow you into his or her
emotional life. Through your child's interests, by having an understanding
of his or her natural desires, parents get a picture of what is enjoyable for
the child. A child who feels understood and affirmed is a child who stays
regulated and engaged longer, one who is able to learn within the experience and ultimately move forward developmentally (Hess, 2009).

Case Illustration

Six-year-old James appears not to be able to leave his home without holding onto a stick. This seems like something inappropriate and something

a parent might want to discourage. But yet there is something about this object that has meaning for this child. Think of the stick simply as a prop that facilitates interaction. The best "toy" within a Floortime interaction is you! You are the magic, the wonder, the main attraction that entices your child into the potential for a meaningful interaction. No one has the power to reach your child in the same way that you do. So James's father is guided to start asking himself what is it about this activity that is so meaningful to his son. It is minimizing to simply attribute what we assume to be aberrant behavior on the part of a child who has a developmental delay. Not only is this short-sighted, but it does little to help us understand the underlying causes that are potentially fueling the odd behavior. The key to understanding any child is to follow his or her lead as an entry point into his or her world, thus creating the potential for an emotional connection, a relationship that allows us to pull that child into a shared validating experience. James's dad is coached to match his son's behaviors and pick up his own stick, all the while attempting to mimic the gestures of the original item. Then Dad is guided to expand the initial gesture into something socially appropriate and mutual. He begins taking the two sticks and gently pretending to fence with them. The gesture is tolerated well. Encouraged, dad now ups the ante and helps his developmentally delayed son to enter the world of symbolism by pretending that the stick has turned from a sword into the body of an airplane. Dad now guides this play experience by making the appropriate sounds and gestures of a gliding plane.

Here the two philosophies behind DIR/Floortime are at work. We are accepting the child and his or her beloved object knowing that there is something intrinsically valuable in the relationship that that child has with the object, and we are also encouraging that same child to leave his or her preferred world of isolation in favor of an experience where his or her original idea of holding onto a stick has magically emerged into a shared play experience.

Joining the Child's World

Following the child's lead is only one-half of the equation, one-half of this dynamic that we call Floortime. There is also the other half: joining the child in his or her world and pulling him or her into a shared emotional experience in order to help him or her master each of his or her functional emotional developmental capacities. Functional emotional capacities are the developmental milestones Dr. Greenspan suggested that all children need to achieve to move forward to their fullest abilities and capacities. These developmental milestones include the ability to stay focused and engaged, the capacity to be able to be regulated, the ability to have two-way verbal and nonverbal gesturing and communication, the capacity to have complex problem-solving abilities, the developmental state of being able to use ideas and symbols creatively, and, finally, to have the ability to think analytically and logically. These are the building blocks of emotional, social, language, and intellectual development. When we talk about functional emotional capacities, we're talking about the fundamentals of relating, communicating, and thinking (Greenspan, 2010).

The larger goal is having you, the parent, join the world of your child. We want to then pull the child back into our shared world to teach him or her and help him or her learn how to focus and attend, how to relate with real warmth, how to be purposeful and take initiative, and how to have a back-and-forth set of communications with us through nonverbal gestures, and eventually through words. In this fashion, parents can teach their children how to problem-solve and sequence and get their child involved in a continuing interaction with the environment and the people in his or her environment. We want to teach these children to use ideas creatively and then we want to teach them to use ideas logically, all the while progressing up a developmental ladder until they are not only using ideas logically but actually showing high degrees of reflective thinking, high degrees of empathy, and high degrees of understanding the world around them, so that they can evaluate their own thoughts and feelings. Almost all children are capable of moving forward developmentally, mastering their own functional emotional developmental capacities in regards to optimum social, emotional, intellectual, linguistic, and academic growth (Greenspan, 2001). Some parents have expressed concern as to whether or not DIR/Floortime is applicable to children who have moderate-to-severe forms of developmental delays. The direct answer is "Yes"; even children who are severely impacted with developmental delays, with the right kind of support, can move forward and upward.

Case Illustration

Jane's chronological age is 5 years, but her current developmental age is about 6 months. She has no functional language and does not appear to have the interest or the capacity to play with toys. In addition to the diagnosis of severe autism, the child also has a comorbid diagnosis of moderate-to-severe cognitive delay. She enters the playroom mostly aimless, not able to stay engaged with anything or any person for any length of time. Characteristic of the disorder, the child flaps her arms in a self-stimulatory gesture in a continuous horizontal pattern.

The difficulty that parents often face with severely impacted children is the confusion of how to follow a child's lead when the child appears to not be able to offer any lead to follow. This is the art of Floortime. You cannot do Floortime, the play therapy portion of this intervention, unless you understand the child's DIR (the developmental capacity, the child's underlying neurological processing differences, and how to use the child's relationship in the world to "woo" that child into a shared experience). By knowing the child's DIR, the parent knows how and where to enter the child's world in such a way as to create a validating experience—in other words, to experience the great date. To move a child forward developmentally, to become a more complex thinker, despite overt cognitive delays, we need to make sure he or she possesses the basic capacity to be regulated and stay engaged.

Since Jane is only offering her hand movements as "the lead," this is where the parent must enter. Playfully, Mom has been instructed to put her own hands within the child's self-stimulatory hand and arm movements. Notice that the parent is not entering the play encounter thinking that she is with a 5-year-old child; rather this mother needs to join Jane *at her daughter's own developmental capacity*. In other words, in the parent's mind, she is now playing with a child who is 6 months old and Mom must drop her intervention and her level of expectation to that level, while she uses her relationship to support the child's underlying processing challenges. As Mom slows the child's flapping gesture down, she creates a regular opening and closing rhythm to what was a moment before a chaotic gesture. As the parent slows and regulates to the beat of the activity, she also uses her voice and her facial gestures to create a high affective encounter. Mom begins to sing a classic child's song, "Open shut them, open shut them, and give a little clap." Suddenly, Jane, who up until this time appeared not to be able to focus and attend, looks with curiosity into the face of her mother. She appears intrigued and curious. The parent has just taught this child the first fundamental game of play, pat-a-cake. The developmental age of this child, and subsequently her ability to be a more complex thinker, has improved within one play session from 6 month of age to 9 months of age.

Progressing from Following a Child's Lead to Mastery

How do parents use "following the child's lead" to actually mobilize and help the child master these critical developmental milestones? To help children master the first stage of shared attention, when they are, for example, wandering away from our interaction with them, play a game that places mom or dad in front of the child, essentially blocking their child's exit from the interaction. The blocking gesture necessitates the child creating some kind of engagement with his or her play partner, even if it's a gesture of annoyance. This will form the foundation of the first act of shared attention that he or she is providing. The parent is encouraged to continue to up the ante by creating more playful obstructions (like asking for a ticket or a token from the child to assure passage before he or she moves out of the way). These types of maneuvers create multiple opportunities for shared attention as well as sustained engagement because the child is otherwise involved with his or her parent. Interestingly, this is also the beginning of purposeful action because the child is trying to move the obstruction (in this case the parent) out of the way. As the child continues to attempt to maneuver the obstacle out of the way, the parent is instructed to "play dumb," forcing the child to solve his or her way out of the current obstacle. These strategies are called *playfully obstructive strategies* and they are for the most aimless of children or the most avoidant child (Greenspan, 2010).

Case Illustration

Five-year-old Ian, affected by a moderate degree of autism, enters the play-room and appears to absent-mindedly pick up a piece of chalk, before dropping the drawing material randomly on the floor. Previously, his mother expressed concern that her son is not showing any age-appropriate interest in drawing, coloring, or cutting, and she fears that he is progressively falling further and further behind his classmates. Keeping in mind the parent's concern, the play activity is taken out of the playroom and into an outdoor play area. Mom follows Ian's lead by attempting to incorporate the child's fleeting interest in the chalk and then attempting to expand that germ of an idea into a sustained play encounter by doing some chalk drawing on the sidewalk. Once outside, mother places Ian in her lap, both to prevent flight and also to help the child become more regulated and engaged by providing proprioceptive input (deep pressure) around which he can organize and reduce the anxiety that is potentially fueling his resistance to the play activity (Ayers, 1979). She hands the child a piece of chalk, while mimicking hand-over-hand gestures in its use. Ian completely rejects the activity and withdraws his hand from any attempt to handle the chalk.

One of the basic principles of Floortime is "Never accept *no* for an answer." In other words, parents try not to back away from their child's initial resistance when they try to move their child forward developmentally. The first step in this case was for Mom to clarify her child's actual capacities to see if he had the physical ability to hold a piece of chalk in his hand. Utilizing occupational therapy strategies, the parent explored whether or not her child had an adequate pincher grasp (the ability to pinch together the thumb and the forefinger) by seeing if he was capable of handing the family dog a dog biscuit. Mom is aware that Ian loves his dog. She is counting on her son's love of the animal to be stronger than his resistance to drawing. Ian eagerly feeds the family dog using the appropriate grasp. With clinical guidance, Mom is encouraged to further expand the interaction by suggesting to her son that he draw the letters of the dog's name in chalk and then have Ian use his pincher grasp to again dot the letters of the dog's name with muffins (left over from breakfast) while instructing the dog to "eat up her name" on command. The request to draw with the chalk is now met with absolutely no resistance as Ian delights in the use of the dog as a "living puppet" to playfully overcome his resistance to the task.

The goal of playfully obstructive strategies is to follow the child's lead, on the one hand, but then to create opportunities and challenges that help the child master each of his or her functional emotional developmental goals, on the other. That is the dialectic, the two opposite polarities of Floortime: joining the child in his or her rhythms while creating systematic challenges that offer opportunities for the child to master new developmental milestones. It is in those systematic challenges that many of the specific techniques and strategies of Floortime come into play.

GETTING STARTED WITH FLOORTIME

Start Where the Child Is

The premise of Floortime is, as mentioned, to follow the lead of the child. That means we are not concerning ourselves with the child's age-appropriate or age-inappropriate behaviors. Rather we need to fine-tune the parents' ability to see what their child is interested in, however innocuous it seems, and then join in and, if possible, expand that initial "seed" of an idea. Begin by simply watching—you will learn a lot. Use your eyes and your instincts. Where is your child going? What does your child like to do? What captures his or her interest? What comes hard for him or her?

Case Illustration

Bobby, age 3 years, is sitting on his father's lap and beginning to perseverate by stroking his father's face with a glazed look in his eye. Dad is guided to start sucking on Bobby's fingers to try and create even more intimacy and closeness, but in an interactive way. Dad opens his mouth and as his son strokes his face, gets one of the little fingers in his mouth for a game of sucking on fingers. Surprised, Bobby pulls his hand away *but* with a big smile and then puts his fingers back in his father's mouth, starting a flirtatious interactive game. Later, Bobby was sucking on his own thumb and Dad, picking up on the same theme, said, "Oh let me suck on that thumb!" This time, instead of a glazed look, Bobby *intentionally* inserted his finger in Dad's mouth and let his father suck on his thumb for a moment and then pulled it back with a big smile on his face. Encouraged, Father continued to create a lovely back-and-forth scenario and playfully added more demands by asserting, "Give it to me! Yes or no!" Now Bobby is fully engaged and responds "No, no!," but this time with a big flirtatious smile, putting his thumb up to his father's face as though he wants to play the game again. Dad is suggested to offer his son his own thumb, and as the session progresses, the child begins taking more initiative, flirting more, seeking his parent out, and using simple words and phrases, becoming decidedly less perseverative and self-stimulatory.

Become a Play Partner (Not a Movie Director)

Invite yourself in to meet your child at his or her level of specific developmental ability. Put your agenda aside and attempt to "woo" your child into the opportunity for a reciprocal relationship. Parents need to be aware that when regression starts occurring, there's a common tendency that goes along with it. Mom and Dad collectively and understandably get frustrated because their child is not doing what they want him or her to do. Then the tendency is either to get more intrusive and controlling or to give up and become angry. When this happens, it is critical to understand the parents' care-giving patterns and begin reversing them by going back to the basics, where there's shared pleasure and that once again allows the parent to challenge the child to take the initiative.

Case Illustration

Stuart's mother was trying to get him to play with some colored blocks. She was anxious that her 4-year-old son was not able identify colors and she was determined to get him "up to speed." Consequently, she was being intrusive, holding his hands, and putting the blocks in her son's hands. Stuart was being more resistant and began to kick the blocks, creating chaos around the playroom. Mom was coached to use Stuart's idea of kicking blocks and incorporate her desire to get him to learn his colors, *but* this time changing the game into something fun and flirtatious. A goal area was created at one end of the playroom and then Mom was instructed to kick the blocks into the goal but use language to identify the color of the toy "Red block scores! Blue block scores!" Intrigued, Stuart stopped his tantrum and started watching Mom play this new game of block soccer. Eventually, Mom began to ask her son for help: "I need the green block now." Stuart brought his mom the correct block. Mom continued to expand on the play suggesting that now it was time for Stuart to kick in his color block. With a big giggle and smile on his face, he began kicking blocks toward the goal and saying, with some cueing from his mother, "Red block scores!" As a result there was some lovely interaction that also incorporated Mom's now thoughtful agenda.

Pacing Is Everything

Try not to move too fast or try too hard with your child. The result is tension between you and your son or daughter that is sure to lead to resistance. Try to slow your eagerness down and simply go with what the child can tolerate at first. It will expand with time and experience. The key is to pace pursuit, "wooing," to the sensitivities of your child. If he or she is a slow mover (hyporeactive to environmental stimulation), then you want to move more aggressively in pursuit. However, if you have a child who is more acutely aware of his or her environment (hyperreactive to stimulation), then you'll need to be slower and a bit more cautious with your approach.

Case Illustration

Casey is a 4-year-old who is extremely hyperreactive to environmental stimulation, what I lovingly refer to as a "rocket ship guy," a child who becomes overly agitated in a matter of moments (Hess, 2012). How does one connect with a child like Casey? A simple game of chase can be a wonderful Floortime opportunity. As you move in close to your child, he or she may scoot away. Follow after your child, again being conscious not to move too fast or in too spirited a way, so that you don't overwhelm (that takes into consideration both the "I"-individual neurological differences and the "R"-relationship of your child to the world, of the DIR model). Use your voice to be enticing "I'm going to get you." If your child can tolerate comfortably to be touched, as you catch up, capture your child in a big sweeping hug. If that gesture feels a bit too "large" for your child, then simply give a gentle squeeze or a "high five." Then release your child, allow him or her to again take the lead and ask "Now what?"

Give your child a chance to signal to you that he or she wants more interaction, in whatever way he or she can manage. Your child's signal can be verbal, but more likely it will be something more subtle, in the realm of a nuanced gesture. It means that as parents, it is important to tune in and really focus on understanding that a sideways glance or a half-smile indicates interest, even as the child appears to be darting away from you (De Faria, 2010).

HOW TO DEAL WITH PROBLEMATIC BEHAVIORS

The Escape Artist

You may be thinking, "Yeah, following my child's lead sounds great, but my son doesn't stand still for a moment to follow any kind of a lead. He is always running away from me. At best, our games together consist of me trying to catch him before he runs out of the house and gets himself into trouble." With a young child on the move, there are often initially a lot of "escape" efforts going on. He may not want to be hemmed in, or "forced" to attend to and focus on Mommy or Daddy, let alone engage. Thinking about your child's "I," his or her individual neurological differences, can help a parent understand what could be making sustained engagement really hard. If your child is sensory-reactive, then perhaps there is too much stimulation (including verbal discussion) and your child is feeling overwhelmed and overloaded (De Faria, 2010). Children react to what initially feels good or bad to their body and then behaviors follow (Hess, 2012). Perhaps in a previous experience with other therapies your child has been "forced" into an interaction. The result is that now your child has ultimately become an expert in escaping what feels bad to his body. The message is don't take resistance as a rejection. As mentioned, part of the DIR/Floortime message is that we don't accept "No" for an answer. The "art" of being a Floortimer is to use even an attempt to escape engagement as an opportunity for reciprocal interaction.

Playful Obstruction

A lot of parents misunderstand the concept of playful obstruction. It is not "OK" to simply get into your child's face and block his or her movements in an attempt to force interaction. Rather, the idea is to gently and playfully use yourself and your body as "something your child has to deal with" as he or she navigates in what may appear as purposeless wandering. Here is where it is crucial to get on the floor adjacent to your child. As your child moves away, you move in front of him or her, capturing his or her attention and gaze even if it is only for a moment. The expectation is that your child will move away again. Parent, you need to move with him or her, playfully dodging and blocking his or her escape. Above all else, DIR/Floortime is an affective-driven treatment model, which means that you need to engage in overexaggerated gestures—BIG smiles as you catch your child's attention, for example. Remember, you are not in a power struggle. Your goal is to entice that "gleam" in your child's eye that lets you know that he or she is feeling emotionally affirmed (Greenspan, 2010). That is the beginning of the great date with your child.

The Train Engineer

One often-seen aspect of autism is repetitive behaviors characteristic of obsessive–compulsive disorder. It is, for example, quite common for a child to play with toy trains by lining them up in a straight line. The play, however, appears to never move beyond the lining up of the cars. Clearly, since this is not the typical way that most children play with their toy trains, worried parents have a hard time resisting the urge to break the repetitive pattern. In Floortime, play schemas, however innocuous they may seem, are honored as the germ of the idea that will set future play into motion. The task of the parent is taking the very small (albeit repetitive) idea and enlarging the concept into the potential for social reciprocal play.

Which Hand?

Parents need to position themselves in front of their child, with the trains between both of them. Join the child as he or she starts to line up the trains, helping to create his or her lineup by adding pieces yourself. He or she may resist your efforts or even pick up the train piece that you just placed and replace it with another. However, as your child begins to realize that you are not going to intrude and redirect his or her play, your child will get more comfortable with your participation and even begin to look for your next overture.

Now you can get a little mischievous. Make sure that your child is watching you as you playfully take some of his collection of trains and place them behind your back. It is important to see that your child is visually tracking your actions. Visual tracking is the precursor for communication both verbal and social. While you are hiding your child's trains, remember to be very expansive in your affect, act as if you have this amazing secret that he or she is about to discover. You can use your body to gently block your child if he or she begins to grab. Once you have his or her attention, take a couple of the hidden trains and place one in each hand. Present your child with two clenched fists in front of you. So there shouldn't be any confusion, for an instant, open your hands, so that the train is revealed. Close your hand quickly, so that the game can continue.

If your child tries to pry your hands open, that's OK. Let him retrieve his desired object. Our objective is not to have meltdowns, rather it is to create an emotionally validating relationship. Smile encouragingly and repeat the gestures. This time, however, when you child goes for your fingers, make the play a bit more complex by asking your child "Which hand?" Even if he only remotely brushes the hand that contains the toy, that gesture will warrant the release of a train. After a few rounds of successful back-and-forth, continue to make the play even more complex. This time, present your child with both hands, but make the hands empty. Now your child has to figure out the next step and you are helping him navigate the difficult world of sequencing. Understand that no matter how time-consuming these initial back-and-forth gestures seem to be, they are all part of a the bigger strategy to help your child not be so isolated in his or her play. The beauty of this approach is that once you are able to achieve extended reciprocal play, then you will also see language developing, as your child uses various forms of communication to signal his or her interest in your interaction (touching your hand, pointing to the correct hand, etc.). What we are aiming for is social referencing where your child is now looking at your face to figure out what is going on. As mentioned, social referencing is the precursor to verbal communication and part of the building blocks for all future communication skills.

Floortime is an "affect-driven interaction." In Floortime we use our emotional expression to entice a child's interest and attention and to make an *effective* connection with a child that leads to the possibility of wooing that child into the interaction and the possibility of even further more complex connections. This means using our facial muscles in a turned-up smile to suggest that we are happy, or turning downward that same smile into a frown or even a scowl that lets the other person know that we are serious. Use your voice in a lilting fashion to suggest silly moments or speak in whispers to suggest thoughtfulness and concentration. Think of affect as both the carrot and the glue that hold the two of you together. The art is balancing your affect with the sensitivities of the child in front of you (De Faria, 2010). For example, a highly emotional and sensitive child may back off if you come on too strong. In contrast, a child who is "low tone" or presents rather flat in his or her affective abilities, needs a lot of cheerleading from you, or he or she won't take notice of your overtures.

Keeping Track

How do you as a parent create the next steps to expand play with your child so that the activity is more developmentally appropriate? A two-word answer to this problem is *spontaneous creativity*. What this means is that once you have established a back-and-forth rhythm with your child, now you need to "think outside the box" and help your son or daughter create a story around the trains. "Where are the trains going?" You can expand your initial game of guessing which hand holds the trains to which hand now holds the train tracks. Collect them as he or she chooses correctly and then be your child's assistant as your child begins to start putting the tracks together. As you build on the idea of train tracks, consider added elements of developmentally appropriate pretend play: toy houses, animals, and people along the track. The idea is that as you join in his or her play, you are beginning to break up the familiar pattern of his or her limited activity and make the play into something larger and grander than the original idea.

The Spin Master

A lot of children with autism like nothing better than to lie on their side and perseveritively spin the wheels of a toy car. Again, you need to overcome your initial resistance and the wish that your child is doing something more purposeful. Instead, join your child at his or her developmental level, get down on the floor, and together watch the wheels spin. Once your child is tolerating your presence, interfere just a bit, perhaps with a feather that you poke into the spokes of the car wheels. The game is for your child to start the spinning activity and for you to interfere by playfully inserting the feather. See if you can develop a rhythm to the interaction, "as child spins wheels, you insert the feather, wheels spin, in goes the feather." After a short time see if you are achieving a back-and-forth pattern of engagement. Congratulations, you have just completed one circle of communication (Greenspan, 2010). Once you've achieved basic reciprocity, the next step is to enlarge the play, perhaps attaching colored ribbon into the spokes of the wheels to make a rainbow racer, or the like.

The Toss Champ

Let's say that your child seems to like nothing better than to simply pick up toys and throw them in the air. How do you turn that idea into something that is playful and meaningful? Again, we return to the original premise of DIR/Floortime: following the lead of the child. It is helpful to approach the child not where he or she is chronologically but developmentally. Start off by trying to figure out what is the exact appeal that throwing objects has for your son or daughter. Often the behavior comes out of the child's individual neurological needs, his or her "I." A sensory-craving child is looking for a reaction to help his or her fragile nervous system have a clearer idea of where he or she is in space and time. That helps reduce a general state of anxiety that often accompanies ASD (Hess, 2009).

Initially, try imitating your child's gestures, so that he or she has the experience of being emotionally validated. Once the two of you are connected, then up the ante by creating a game of target practice where you take a basket and begin to challenge the child to see who can get the most points by throwing the toy directly into the basket.

Case Illustration

Marcus is an 8-year-old boy who loves to throw balls around aimlessly. Father and son were in the garage playroom when Marcus discovered several balls in the corner. He immediately began to throw them around the room aimlessly. Utilizing clinical instruction, Dad quickly emptied a small trashcan and made that the target for him and his son to aim at. This game expanded into 10 opportunities for turn taking (circles of communication). Marcus began to tire of the structure of the game and again started to toss the balls around the garage haphazardly. The garage door (which operated vertically, rising from bottom to top) happened to be open. One of Marcus's balls landed on top of the open garage door. Quickly, Dad was instructed to take the empty small child's wading pool that was located just outside the garage and use that as the next "basket" to catch the balls. As luck would have it, after throwing a couple more balls on top of the open garage door, one of the balls dropped right into the "new basket."

Delighted, Marcus immediately began to verbalize with his dad that they had created a new game! Dad and son worked on coming up with a name for this new game (moving the child into the higher developmental level of complex thought) and that evening spent the better part of playtime teaching the new game that they had created together to the rest of the family.

WHAT TO DO
WHEN A CHILD STARTS REGRESSING

Alisa is a 3-year-old girl with no verbal language and a diagnosis of moderate-to-severe autism. After several Floortime sessions she was beginning to use her words more, becoming a problem-solving communicator. However, when she returned to preschool following a month-long winter break, she became much more perseverative, self-stimulatory, passive, and avoidant at home, although she was very compliant at school. The school program was a very controlled, discrete trial program where she complied, but was unable to generalize these skills into her greater social emotional world. In fact, outside the school, there was marked regression.

Her mother had great difficulty trying to get her daughter to interact with her at home. Alisa seemed resistant, angry, annoyed, passive, and self-stimulatory, which resulted in her mother getting frustrated, becoming more intrusive and more controlling. Mom was beginning to give up trying to interact with her daughter, leading to even further regression.

After observing the child and her mother's interactive patterns and doing a quick developmental profile of the child's functional and developmental levels, individual neurological differences, and relational/interactive patterns, it became clear to me that the combination of Alisa's difficulty with transitioning back to school after holiday and her mother's fear that the regression was indicative of a permanent setback was a lethal combination. With some additional short-term coaching, where Mom was reminded to follow her daughter's lead, Alisa started to demonstrate renewed initiative to be interactive. With this change her affect began to blossom again and a smile came to her face. She began flirting and looking at her mom and began interacting in a problem-solving way, using simple words and phrases. As a general rule, relationships that provide more warmth and support tend to create more initiative taking in the other person, usually reversing the pattern more quickly.

It was important for this parent to understand that even though there was momentary regression, Alisa still had a broad range of capacities when Mom interacted with her in a very flexible manner. Additionally, when a child shows a pattern of regression, it is very important to remember to explore all possible reasons, starting first with physical causes, such as change in diet and nutrition, health/illness issues, medication, and the like. Then it's recommended to explore broad family and environmental changes. These changes can include differences in the child's ecology, for example, a new school room, painting in the house, or exposure to anything that can be ingested or smelled that could create an allergic or toxic reaction. Then it's very important to look at what's happening in the family—any changes in work status, health/illness, visits from in-laws, or the basic routines at home, as well as the sibling and marital patterns that could be underlying contributors to a child's dysregulation.

After the situation has been diagnosed with a child, it is very important to then create interactive learning opportunities that can reverse the trend. Usually, this involves going back to the basics, working up the developmental ladder during interactive opportunities. With the child in our example, it meant focusing on Alisa's basic desires and needs, having Mom validate her daughter emotionally, so that this couple was back on board to "having a great date together." Remember, it is possible to think of DIR/ Floortime as a short-term intervention for parents, but what we are really talking about is creating a lifestyle where wonderful, natural interactive moments can happen and do happen all day long. Simply allow yourself to move with your child into a playful back-and-forth interaction whenever the opportunity occurs.

EVIDENCE BASE
FOR THE DIR/FLOORTIME APPROACH

Evidence-based practice is an approach to treatment rather than a specific treatment. This understanding promotes and integrates the best available scientifically rigorous research, clinical expertise, and the therapist's characteristics to ensure the quality of clinical judgments and delivery of the most cost-effective care (Weisz & Gray, 2007). A starting point to measure the effectiveness of intervention is to determine the factors to be measured. This is a major challenge in the field of developmental disabilities. Generally, behavioral approaches measure specific targeted behaviors. More recently, there has been a focus on measuring spontaneous interactions and generalization of skills, which presents new challenges in measurement. Developmental play therapy programs like DIR/Floortime, in contrast to behavioral approaches that tend to measure specific targeted behaviors, target underlying capacities or "core deficits" as the focus of intervention, with progress made evident in a complex array of changes in interactive behavioral patterns (Cullinane, 2011).

Developmental approaches seek to measure changes in an individual's capacity for:

- Shared attention.
- Ability to form warm, intimate, and trusting relationships.
- The ability to *initiate* (rather than respond), using intentful actions and social engagement; spontaneous communication.
- The ability to participate in *reciprocal* (two-way, mutual) interactions while in a range of different emotional states.
- Problem solving through a process of coregulation, reading, responding, and adapting to the feelings of others.
- Creativity.
- Thinking logically about motivations and the perspectives of others.
- Developing an internal personal set of values.

Additionally, developmental models emphasize individual processing differences and the need to tailor intervention to the unique biological profile of children as well as the characteristics of the relationship between parent and child. Because both the factors being measured are complex and because of the wide range of individual neurological processes in the population, research on the effectiveness of a developmental framework has progressed by examining the subcomponents of the overall approach. As previously mentioned, the subcomponents can be summarized by looking at the three major aspects of the DIR/Floortime approach: D—the developmental framework; I—the individual underlying neurological processing differences of a child; and R—relationship and subsequent affective interactions.

D: The Developmental Framework

A developmental approach is founded on work by major developmental theorists such as Piaget, Vygotsky, Erikson, and Kohlberg. A developmental approach considers behavior and learning in the greater context of a developmental or changing process. In 1987, evidence first showed the promise of the DIR/Floortime approach when Dr. Greenspan and his partner Dr. Wieder reviewed 200 charts of children who were initially diagnosed with ASD. The goal of the review was to reveal patterns in presenting symptoms, underlying processing difficulties, early development, and response to intervention in order to generate hypotheses for future studies. The chart review suggested that a number of children with ASD diagnoses were, with appropriate intervention, capable of empathy, affective reciprocity, creative thinking, and healthy peer relationships (Greenspan & Wieder, 1987). The results of the 200 case series (Greenspan & Wieder, 1997) led Greenspan and Wieder to publish in 2000 the full description of the DIR/Floortime model (ICDL, 2000). In 2005, Greenspan and Wieder published a 10- to 15-year follow-up study of 16 children diagnosed with ASD who were part of the first 200-case series. The authors described that 10 to 15 years after receiving DIR/Floortime as a treatment method, these children had become significantly more empathetic, creative and reflective adolescents with healthy peer relationships and solid academic skills (Greenspan & Wieder, 2005). Previous approaches using behavioral principles relied upon outside motivators on the premise that children with autism did not have their own motivation to participate in social interaction or to learn (Mastrangelo, 2009). In contrast, the DIR/Floortime approach revealed that all children will show purpose and initiative, and will seek close social relationships, when provided with interactions that respect their interests and are tailored to their individual underlying neurological differences.

The DIR/Floortime model has provided a developmental framework that has been studied and found to be accurate in understanding behavior. A common pediatric assessment tool, the Bayley Scales of Infant Development, has adopted the DIR milestones, specifically configured as the Greenspan Social–Emotional Growth Chart (SEGC) as the measure by which social and emotional development is measured (Greenspan, 2004). In 2007, Solomon, Necheles, Ferch, and Bruckman published an evaluation of the Play Project Home Consultation (PPHC), an in-home based version of the DIR/Floortime model that trains parents of children with ASD in the DIR/Floortime model. The results showed significant increases in the reciprocal relationship capacity as scored on another pediatric assessment tool, the Functional Emotional Assessment Scale (FEAS; Greenspan & DeGangi, 2001), after an 8- to 12-month program using DIR/Floortime (Solomon et al., 2007). In June, 2011, Pajareya and Nopmaneejumruslers published a pilot randomized controlled trial of DIR/Floortime with preschool children with ASD. Results showed improvements in the FEAS, the Childhood Autism Rating Scale (CARS), and the functional emotional questionnaires, confirming the results of the Solomon et al. study.

I: Individual Underlying Neurological Processing Differences

Keeping playful interactions "alive" and fun actually requires a lot of attention to the play partner's nonverbal communication and the ability to make rapid adjustments in response to these cues, while also regulating emotional intensity to stay on the "right frequency" for sustaining this pleasurable connection. Shifts in this frequency, much like changes in prosody in humans, can bring play to a halt instantly, along with a shift into freeze mode of mobilized defense. In short, free play is actually a very creative process requiring a lot of people reading and emotion regulation skills, a lot of "emotional intelligence." When playfulness is suppressed in a parent–child relationship, both parent and child are robbed of one of the most powerful processes for strengthening their connection (Hughes & Baylin, 2012).

In 1979, occupational therapist Jean Ayres pioneered discoveries about the ways in which a child's sensory-processing capacities could impact the manner by which children learned and integrated themselves into their worlds. This revolutionary idea provided a new way to understand the importance of movement and regulatory behaviors in children and began to offer explanations for some of the more worrisome behaviors impacting children with developmental concerns like autism. Over the last 40 years, a large body of research has further illuminated the impact of biologically based differences in regards to both sensorimotor processing and the impact on emotional regulation. This provided a new way of understanding movement and regulatory behaviors. In addition, this work showed that these biological differences could be influenced and changed by specific therapeutic interventions.

Developmental models emphasize individual differences and the need to tailor intervention to the unique biological profile of the child *and* to the unique characteristics of the parent–child interaction. In 2001, the National Research Council of the National Academy of Sciences published a report entitled *Educating Children with Autism* that called for the tailoring of treatment approaches to fit the unique biological profile of the individual child (Committee on Educational Intervention for Children with Autism, 2001). Lillas and Turnball (2009) describe how all behavior is influenced by the sensory systems in the brain. They indicated that an infant's sensory capacities are genetically prepared to respond to human interaction and shift in direct relationship to the parent's touch, facial, vocal, and movement expressions. Child–parent interactions and sensory activities create nerve cell networks and neural pathways in the development of the child's brain. The exchange that takes place during child–parent play interactions are seen as an ongoing loop of sensorimotor transformations (Lillas & Turnball, 2009).

Because of the wide range of individual differences in autism, there is more interest in using single-subject research designs. Dionne and Martini (2011) created a single-subject study design used to evaluate the effectiveness of Floortime play with a 3½-year-old boy with autism. The study used an observation and intervention phase, and utilized circles of communication as the measure of change. Results showed a significant improvement using Floortime play strategies and mother's journal, which included insights on the changes observed. Additionally, Pajareya and Nopmaneejumruslers (2011) conducted a pilot control study where their randomized findings showed the effectiveness of sensory integration treatment for children with autism. Results showed improvement in social responsiveness, sensory processing, functional motor skills, and social–emotional factors, with a significant decrease in autistic mannerisms.

R: Relationship and Affect

Developmental models have evolved from many years of discovery in the field of infant mental health. Beginning in the 1950s, there was a new understanding of the importance of parent–child interaction (Bowlby, 1951). Building on these years of research in developmental psychology that underscores the importance of early relationships and family functioning, Dr. Stanley Greenspan and his partner Dr. Serena Wieder began their work together studying the interaction of mothers and their babies in the context of infants who were at high risk for attachment problems (National Center for Clinical Infant Programs, 1987). Subsequently, numerous research studies have confirmed the importance of parent–child interaction and the value of intervention programs that focus on supporting the parent–child relationship, particularly in the areas of joint attention and emotional attunement (Mahoney & Perales, 2004). In 2006, Gernsbacher published a paper that showed how intervention itself between a parent and child could change the way in which parents interact, in turn increasing reciprocity, and that these changes correlated to positive changes in social engagement and language. In 2008, Connie Kasari and colleagues at the University of California at Los Angeles (Kasari, Paparella, Freeman, & Jahromi) used a randomized controlled trial to look at joint attention and symbolic play with 58 children with autism. Results indicated that expressive language gains were greater for treatment groups where a developmental model was utilized as compared with a control group that was based on exclusive behavioral principles.

SUMMARY AND CONCLUSIONS

ASD is now recognized as a disorder of integration among various distinct brain functions. Research investigation is currently focused on understanding deficits in neuronal communication as a basis of the wide array of behavioral manifestations of the disorder (Cullinane, 2011). Developmental intervention has advanced to incorporate the use of affect to enhance integration of sensory–regulatory, communication, and motor systems. With that in mind, neuroimaging research is beginning to provide a deeper understanding as to how emotional experiences are actually impacting developing brain growth. Siegel (2001) showed how attuned relationships in infancy change brain structure in ways that later impact social and emotional development. To further investigate the efficacy of the DIR/Floortime, researchers Casenhiser, Stieben, and Shanker (2011), through the Milton and Ethel Harris Research Initiative, at York University in Canada, conducted a randomized controlled trial study. The specific aims of this preliminary study were to assess (1) the efficacy of 12 months of intensive DIR Floortime treatment; (2) the magnitude of the gains made by children receiving 24 months of DIR Floortime treatment; and (3) the neurophysiological changes that occur as a result of intensive treatment for autism. Recently, Casenhiser et al. (2013) updated the findings of their preliminary investigation showing behavioral and neurophysiological outcomes of intensive DIR/Floortime intervention, using both event-related potential and electroencephalographic measurements. They found significant improvements in attention, joint attention, enjoyment, involvement, social interaction, and language after 2 hours a week of DIR-based therapy for 1 year. Results of imagining studies are in publication. Discussion is also continuing on ways to apply the basic principles of DIR/Floortime toward an adult developmentally delayed population (Samson, 2013).

Efforts continue to deepen our understanding of the complexities of autism. The alarming increase in the diagnosis of ASD worldwide (Kogan et al., 2009), as well as the lack of specific information about the etiology of the disorder, demands that play therapists and most importantly parents increase their knowledge and understanding of how a child's development is impacted by individual underlying neurological processing differences and the interaction of the relationships that the child has in the world (Greenspan & Wieder, 2005). In September 2009, the journal *Zero to Three* focused an entire issue on the importance of play, specifically on the role of spontaneous, child-led, social play experiences that support social, emotional, and cognitive growth (Hirschland, 2009). The Bridge Project 2009 is a joint effort of the Bridge Collaborative, a group comprised of clinicians from the University of California at San Diego, Rady Children's Hospital, the San Diego Regional Center, the Harbor Regional Center (Torrance, Long Beach), Kaiser Permanente, and parents. They were awarded a $250,000 National Institute of Health R01 grant for a pilot study, with a clear path toward a $2,500,000 grant, to implement evidence-based screening and intervention in Southern California. They have chosen Project ImPACT and added components of engagement, individual differences, and reflective process. Dr. Richard Solomon is doing a randomized control trial study on the Play Project. The National Institute of Mental Health has granted $1.85 million to execute a Phase II study. The Play Project has partnered with Easter Seals and Michigan State University to conduct this 3-year-long study (Cullinane, 2011).

In 2010, Wallace and Rogers published a review of controlled studies that identified four factors that were most important for effective intervention for infants with autism: (1) parent involvement in intervention, including ongoing parent coaching that focused on parental responsivity and sensitivity to child cues and on teaching families to provide the infant interventions; (2) individualization to each infant's developmental profile; (3) focusing on a broad rather than a narrow range of learning targets; and (4) temporal characteristics involving beginning as early as the risk is detected and providing greater intensity and duration of the intervention. Although research continues, it is imperative that developmental approaches like DIR/Floortime remain a viable short-term play therapy intervention for parents and their children with developmental delays. DIR/Floortime, implemented as a short-term therapy for children impacted by ASD, requires parents to appreciate the polarity between following the child's lead and entering his or her world. Only then can children be "pulled" into a shared world, by finding their pleasures and joys while continually challenging them to master each of the functional developmental capacities. That means paying attention to the child's underlying individual neurological differences in such a way that they process sound, sights, movements, and sensations. Additionally, each time parents fine-tune their own interactions with their children with need, they are creating the potential for that "great date" a mutually emotionally validating play experience for all.

REFERENCES

Ayres, J. A. (1979). *Sensory integration and the child.* Los Angeles: Western Psychological Services.

Boucher, E. E., & Wolery, M. (2003). Editorial. *Autism, 7*(4), 339–346.

Bowlby, J. (1951). *Maternal care and mental health* (World Health Organization Monograph Series, No. 51). Geneva, Switzerland: World Health Organization.

Casenhiser, D. M., Shanker, S. G., & Stieben, J. (2013). Learning through interaction in children with autism: Preliminary data from a social-communication-based intervention. *Autism, 17*(2), 220–241.

Committee on Educational Interventions for Children with Autism. (2001). *Educating children with autism.* Washington, DC: National Academies Press.

Cullinane, D. (2011). Evidence base for the DIR®/Floortime approach. Retrieved from *www.drhessautism.com/img/news/EvidenceBasefortheDIR®Model_Cullinane090111.pdf.*

De Faria, L. (2010). Providing parental support with floor time. *Best Practices Newsletter of the Interdisciplinary Council on Developmental and Learning Disorders, 6,* 7–10.

Dionne, M., & Martini, R. (2011). Floor time play with a child with autism: A single-subject study. *Canadian Journal of Occupational Therapy, 78*(3), 196–203.

Greenspan, S. I. (2004). *The Greenspan Social Emotional Growth Chart: A screening questionnaire for infants and young children.* Bethesda, MD: PsychCorp (Hartcourt Assessment).

Greenspan, S. I. (2010). Floor Time™: What it really is, and what it isn't. Retrieved from *www.icdl.com/dirFloortime/newsletter/FloortimeWhatitReallyisandisnt.shtml.*

Greenspan, S. I., & DeGangi, G. (2001). Research on the FEAS: Test development, reliability, and validity studies. In S. Greenspan, G. DeGangi, & S. Wieder (Eds.),

The Functional Emotional Assessment Scale (FEAS) for infancy and early child-hood: Clinical and research applications (pp. 167–247). Bethesda, MD: Interdisciplinary Council on Developmental and Learning Disorders.

Greenspan, S. I., & Wieder, S. (1987). Developmental patterns of outcome in infants and children with disorders in relating and communicating: A chart review of 200 cases of children with autistic spectrum diagnoses. *Journal of Developmental and Learning Disorders, 1*(87), 87–141.

Greenspan, S. I., & Wieder, S. (1999). A functional developmental approach to autism spectrum disorders. *Journal of the Association for Persons with Severe Handicaps, 24*(3), 147–161.

Greenspan, S. I., & Wieder, S. (2005). Can children with autism master the core deficits and become empathic, creative and reflective?: A ten to fifteen year follow-up of a subgroup of children with autism spectrum disorders (ASD) who received a comprehensive developmental, individual-difference, relationship-based (DIR®) approach. *Journal of Developmental and Learning Disorders, 9*, 39–61.

Habermas, T., & Bluck, S. (2000). Getting a life: The emergence of the life story in adolescence. *Psychological Bulletin, 126*, 748–769.

Hess, E. (2009, August). *DIR®/Floor Time™: A developmental/relational approach towards the treatment of autism and sensory processing disorder.* Paper presented at the annual conference of the American Psychological Association, Toronto, Canada.

Hess, E. (2012). DIR Floortime: A developmental/relational play therapy approach for treating children impacted by autism. In L. Gallo-Lopez & L. C. Rubin (Eds.), *Play-based interventions for children and adolescents with autism spectrum disorders.* New York: Routledge Taylor & Francis Group.

Hirschland, D. (2009). Addressing social, emotional, and behavioral challenges through play. *Zero to Three, 30*(1), 12–17.

Hughes, D., & Baylin, J. (2012). *Brain-based parenting: The neuroscience of caregiving for healthy attachment.* New York: Norton.

Interdisciplinary Council on Developmental and Learning Disorders (ICDL). (2000). *ICDL clinical practice guidelines: Redefining the standards of care for infants, children and families with special needs.* Bethesda, MD: Author.

Kasari, C., Paparella, T., Freeman, S., & Jahromi, L. B. (2008). Language outcome in autism: Randomized comparison of joint attention and play interventions. *Journal of Consulting and Clinical Psychology, 76*(1), 125–137.

Kasari, C., Gulsrud, A. C., Wong, C., Kwon, S., & Locke, J. (2010). Randomized controlled caregiver mediated joint engagement intervention for toddlers with autism. *Journal of Autism and Developmental Disorders, 40*(9), 1045–1056.

Kogan, M. D., Blumberg, S. J., Schieve, L. A., Boyle, C. A., Perrin, J. M., Ghandour, R. M., et al. (2009). Prevalence of parent-reported diagnosis of autism spectrum disorder among children in the US (2007). *Pediatrics, 10*, 1522–1542.

Lillas, C., & Turnball, J. (2009). *Infant/child mental health, early intervention and relationship-based therapists: A neuro-relationship framework for interdisciplinary practice.* New York: Norton.

Mahoney, G., & Perales, F. (2004). Relationship-focused in early intervention with children with pervasive developmental disorders and other disabilities: A comparative study, *Journal of Developmental and Behavioral Pediatrics, 26*, 77–85.

Mallach, S., & Trevathen, C. (2009). *Communicative musicality: Exploring the basis of human companionship.* London: Oxford University Press.

Mastrangelo, S. (2009). Harnessing the power of play: Opportunities for children with autism spectrum disorders. *Teaching Exceptional Children, 42*(1), 34–44.

Myers, S. M., & Johnson, C. P. (2007). Council on Children's Disabilities. *Pediatrics*, *120*, 1162–1182.

National Center for Clinical Infant Programs. (1987). Infants in multi-risk families: Case studies in preventative intervention. In S. I. Greenspan, S. Wieder, R. A. Nover, A. Lieberman, R. S. Lourie, & M. E. Robinson (Eds.), *Clinical Infant Reports, Number 3*. New York: International Universities Press.

Pajareya, K., & Nopmaneejumruslers, K. (2011). A pilot randomized controlled trial of DIR/Floortime parent training intervention for pre-school children with autistic spectrum disorders. *Autism*, *15*(2), 1–15.

Samson, A. (2013). *Applying DIR®/Floor Time principles to a developmental disabled adult population*. Paper presented at the meeting of the California Association for Disabilities, Los Angeles, CA.

Siegel, D. (2001). Toward an interpersonal neurobiology of the developing mind: Attachment relationships, "mindsight," and neural integration. *Infant Mental Health Journal*, *22*, 67–94.

Solomon, R. S., Necheles, J., Ferch, C., & Bruckman, D. (2007). Pilot study of a parent training program for young children with autism: The P.L.A.Y. Project Home Consultation Program. *Autism*, *11*(3), 205–224.

Wallace, K. S., & Rogers, S. J. (2010). Intervening in infancy: Implications for autism spectrum disorders. *Journal of Child Psychology and Psychiatry, 51*(12), 1300–1320.

Weisz, J., & Gray, J. S. (2007). Evidence-based psychotherapy for children and adolescents: Data from the present and a model for the future. *ACAMH Occasional Papers*, *27*, 7–22.

Chapter 13

᪣

Short–Term Play Therapy
for Adoptive Families

*Overcoming Trauma, Facilitating Adjustment,
and Strengthening Attachment
with Filial Therapy*

Risë VanFleet

One of the most important functions that families play is to provide a physical and emotional safe haven for family members. The attachment relationships within a family can make a difference in how individual family members, as well as the family as a whole, adjust and adapt to the stresses and strains of daily life. Adoptive families are no different, but they face unique challenges in creating this safe, secure environment, which permits everyone in the family to thrive. This chapter outlines some of these challenges and illustrates how Filial Therapy (FT) facilitates the adjustment process while meeting the needs of everyone in the family.

When couples decide to adopt a child, they are embarking on a journey that is both exciting and daunting. Whereas adoption often fulfills the couple's long-time desire for a child, it also introduces significant adjustments and potential problems for the family to overcome. Older adoptive children may have longed for the adoption as much as their parents have, yet they bring years of turbulent history with them that is not so easily set aside. When an adoption is finalized by the court, it is a joyous occasion, but considerable patience, flexibility, and hard work are needed to integrate the child fully into the family's life from that point forward. Perhaps the most important developmental task of adoptive families is to create healthy, secure attachments within the family. Trusting, reliable relationships provide the base from which children and adults alike can explore and enjoy their lives fully.

This chapter describes the challenges faced by adoptive families and the importance of secure attachments for all family members. The use of FT to assist the adjustment of adoptive children and families is discussed, including its use as a prevention/family enhancement method as well as an intervention for very difficult trauma and attachment problems.

COMMON CHALLENGES
FACED BY ADOPTIVE FAMILIES

There are many reasons that parents make the decision to adopt, just as there are many reasons that children become available for adoption. A "typical" adoptive family does not really exist. Although there are similarities among adoptive families, there is also tremendous diversity. A family's postadoption adjustment can be influenced by many factors. Some of the common characteristics and needs of adoptive families are outlined in the following discussion, but readers should bear in mind that each child, each parent, and each family is unique.

Adoptive Children

Adoptive children vary widely in their psychosocial characteristics, as well as in their needs. Age at adoption, temperament, coping abilities, history of abuse or neglect, involvement in the foster care system, prior attachment experiences, and general life experiences all play a profound role in children's adjustment to adoption. A shared characteristic of adoptive children is the major disruption that has occurred in their normal development, including the development of attachment relationships. This disruption can interfere with children's individual development at many levels and their capacity to form satisfying, secure, intimate family relationships (Ginsberg, 1989; VanFleet, 1994, 2003).

The challenges presented by adoptive children include anxiety, behavior problems, impulsivity, attachment difficulties, unresolved reactions to past abuses, losses or rejections, confused personal boundaries, posttraumatic stress disorder, insecurity about the family environment, and an inability to conceive of or plan for the future. Some adoptive children have lived with a long line of family members or foster families, and it may be difficult for them to believe that an adoption is "final." Sometimes they have been moved at a moment's notice, placed with a new family in a new town, and then penalized for having negative reactions to these sudden and unpredictable changes. Such experiences can intensify their feelings of rejection and helplessness and exacerbate their emotional and behavioral reactivity.

Adoptive children, especially those who come from foster placements, have sometimes been separated from the support of their siblings, and they may have many questions about their biological families. It can be difficult for them to determine their roles in the adoptive families when they have so much confusion about their biological families.

These potential problems do not appear in all adoptive children, but the disruptions in these children's lives place them at greater risk for developmental, learning, social, emotional, and behavioral difficulties.

Adoptive Parents

Adoptive parents have usually endured many stresses prior to actually adopting a child. Inability to conceive can result in feelings of loss, guilt, and anger, as well as marital stress. The adoption process can be long and frustrating, and most adoptive parents have heard horror stories of children being placed in loving adoptive homes only to be reclaimed by biological parents at the last minute. Uncertainties prevail.

When a child is placed, it is typically a happy occasion, yet it is fraught with stress. Sometimes the placement occurs suddenly and unpredictably, and the family's lifestyle is changed almost overnight. When adoptive parents are faced with the actual infant or child, self-doubt about their ability to parent him or her often arises.

Adoptive parents sometimes express concern about the role of the biological parents in the child's life. They need information about how, what, and when to tell the child about the adoption and his or her biological parents.

Adoptive parents also need as much information as possible about the child's medical and psychosocial history. For infant or toddler adoptions, parents want to know what to expect in their child's development and any potential problems to watch for. With adoptions of older children, parents may have some idea of the problems experienced by the child, yet still be at a loss as to how to handle problematic emotions, behaviors, or medical conditions. Sometimes attachment problems emerge in a totally unexpected manner. The first few months in the family home may go smoothly, referred to sometimes as the "honeymoon period," followed by the sudden eruption of disturbance. Parents need to be prepared for these possibilities and how to find assistance if needed.

Other Children in the Family

If there are other children in the family, the adoption can pose some challenges there as well. They might be biological or adoptive children, but the addition of a new child can trigger sibling rivalry, acting out, withdrawal, or other forms of interpersonal distress. Families report that their attentions shift, temporarily, to the newcomer in the family, ensuring that the newly adopted child feels welcome and comfortable. At the same time, children already in the family might perceive this as favoritism and feel slighted by this shift of attention away from them. If other children in the family have been adopted themselves, parents might be surprised when they react negatively, expecting them to be more understanding of the new child's position. What might be overlooked are the attachment needs of the previously adopted children that can be triggered with the new child's adoptive process. There are many families in which the other children are happy to welcome the adoptive child, but once again, there is increased risk of some sibling issues arising.

RATIONALE AND DESCRIPTION OF THE APPROACH

This section explores the importance of building secure attachment relationships within adoptive families, a detailed description of FT, information about why FT is so relevant and beneficial for adoptive families, and a model of implementing FT that helps stabilize placements and provides adoptive families with the tools needed to help their children cope with and overcome trauma and attachment difficulties that they bring with them. FT is a fully integrated form of family therapy and play therapy that offers a unique way to meet the needs of all family members before, during, and after an adoption.

The Importance of Attachment

One of the primary functions of a family is to provide a safe, secure environment in which all members can develop in positive ways. This is particularly important for adoptive families, in which normal developmental processes of attachment have usually been disrupted. Secure attachments and healthy parent–child relationships are associated with psychosocial health, whereas insecure or damaged attachments are linked to a wide range of difficulties (Belsky & Nezworski, 1988; Brodzinsky & Schechter, 2006; Clark & Ladd, 2000; Humber & Moss, 2005; Ladd & Ladd, 1998; Leathers, Spielfogel, Gleeson, & Rolock, 2012; Youngblade & Belsky,

1992). Healthy attachments provide a protective shield for family members when they face and cope with life difficulties (Figley, 1989; Hart, Shaver, & Goldenberg, 2005; La Greca, Silverman, Vernberg, & Roberts, 2002; Nilsson et al., 2011; Sroufe, 1983, 1988; Sroufe & Rutter, 1984). Family psychologists, therapists, and researchers have paid increasing attention to the implications of developmental attachment processes for family relations (Bifulco & Moran, 1998; Bifulco, Moran, Ball, & Lillie, 2002; Bifulco & Thomas, 2013; Cheung & Hong, 2005; Johnson, 2005; Marvel, Rodriguez, & Liddle, 2005). Such implications are relevant to the way in which practitioners work with adoptive families in prevention and intervention programs.

Attachment disruptions in children arise from separations from parents, temperamental factors, anxiety of parents, traumatic events, lack of physical or emotional safety, unpredictability in the child's environment, abuse, neglect, frequent changes in living conditions, institutional placements, and so on (VanFleet & Sniscak, 2003a). When children lack a strong connection with their parents, or, worse, are abused by those entrusted with their care, they often feel insecure, frightened, helpless, and angry. When poor attachment arises from traumatic conditions in which their needs are ignored or violated, children can become mistrustful of all people. James (1994) has clearly described the dynamics through which attachment trauma problems are created and manifested, and Terr (1990) has documented the long-term negative impact of trauma on children. Even the very system developed to protect abused children has been responsible for new abuses and victimization (Bernstein, 2001). Most child therapists can describe situations in which "the system" has failed the children in its care, sometimes miserably.

The impact of attachment disruptions on children's lives can be devastating and far-reaching (Bifulco & Thomas, 2013). Children who have not experienced healthy attachments, or whose attachments have been weakened or broken, develop a wide range of difficult behaviors, including rage and explosiveness, numbness and detachment, dissociation, trauma reactions, unhealthy trauma bonds, depression, self-injury, intense fears, isolation, unhealthy relationships, sexualized and/or violent behaviors, and poor self-regulation (James, 1994; Ziegler, 2000). The scope and intensity of attachment problems sometimes lead to frequent changes in placement and repeated life experiences of failure and rejection. The attachment styles of caregivers can aid or exacerbate these difficulties (Bifulco & Thomas, 2013). Because many children who are adopted have had attachment disruptions of varying degrees, it is important for parents and professionals involved with adoption to be familiar with attachment relationships and know the resources available to strengthen them.

An understanding of how healthy attachment relationships develop can inform the education and treatment of adoptive families grappling with trauma and attachment-related problems. Much has been written on the process of attachment (Ainsworth, 1982; Belsky & Nezworski, 1988; Bifulco & Thomas, 2013; Bowlby, 1982; Brazelton & Cramer, 1990), and this work can guide the interventions we employ to establish it in adoptive families. FT, the treatment approach emphasized in this chapter, aims to help adoptive children and parents develop healthy attachments, while encouraging children to work through their trauma issues in a safe, accepting environment. Furthermore, this approach is noncoercive and emphasizes the reciprocity important in healthy bonds. Although the treatment of attachment-related problems is not always short term, it can be, and the use of the approaches defined here can substantially reduce the amount of therapy time required. Such treatment is accomplished through the involvement of adoptive parents as the primary change agents for their own children. FT, with its use of nondirective play sessions, re-creates parent–child interactions similar in many ways to those that lead to healthy attachment in infancy (Ryan & Wilson, 1995).

Bifulco and Thomas (2013) have described the role of FT in strengthening attachment as follows:

> Because Filial Therapy encourages working with both parents to effect change and promote secure parent–child relationships, it has a strong focus on parental attachment and behaviour, as well as on the whole family system and its dynamics so that the target child is not singled out. Its approach recognises the need for parents to be directly involved in building emotional bonds and thus become the stress moderators and behaviour managers. (p. 203)

Prevention and Intervention

FT is a relatively short-term, time-limited intervention that effectively strengthens attachment within adoptive families. It is a psychoeducational approach that combines family therapy and play therapy, with the goals of building secure attachments, strengthening families, and treating a wide range of child and family problems. Rather than focusing on dysfunction and an expert model of treatment delivery, however, psychoeducational models emphasize the development and application of skills in a supportive environment that will promote adaptation and adjustment. FT favors a collaborative model of working with clients.

In FT, the therapist trains the parents to conduct special child-centered play sessions with their own children. The therapist then observes the initial parent–child play sessions and provides constructive feedback to facilitate the parents' skill development. Discussions of the possible meanings of the child's play themes within the context of family and community life help the parents to understand their children better and to respond to their needs more satisfactorily. Parents invariably have their own reactions to the play sessions and the child's play themes, and the therapist helps them process their reactions in a manner that often results in parent changes as well. As the parents develop competence and confidence in conducting the play sessions, they eventually hold them more independently in the home setting. In the final stage of FT, the therapist helps the parents generalize and maintain the use of the skills they have learned during the play sessions. FT has been used for many years with adoptive families with notable success.

Overview of FT

FT, developed by Bernard and Louise Guerney (B. G. Guerney, 1964; L. F. Guerney, 1983, 2003; Guerney & Ryan, 2013; VanFleet, 2014), is a theoretically integrative and evidence-based approach that combines play therapy and family therapy. It is a highly effective intervention that can be very beneficial for adoptive families (VanFleet, 1994, 2003). In FT, the therapist trains and supervises parents as they conduct special child-centered play sessions with their own children. With appropriate training and supervision, parents eventually are able to conduct these special play sessions at home without the therapist's direct supervision.

The goals of FT are to help parents create an accepting, safe environment in which their children can express their feelings fully, gain an understanding of their world, solve problems, and develop confidence in themselves and their parents. The therapy process is designed to help parents become more responsive to their children's feelings and needs, to become better at solving child- and family-related problems, and to become more skillful and confident as parents. Families who participate in FT are expected to emerge with better communication skills, problem-solving and coping skills, and stronger family relationships. FT helps the family create a network of healthy, secure attachment relationships. It is usually an enjoyable process for the entire family, and many families incorporate it into their lifestyles after formal therapy has ended (VanFleet, 1998).

Because of its educational and strengths-based nature, FT has never been a lengthy therapeutic approach. Families with mild-to-moderate problems typically require 15–20 one-hour sessions before discharge. It can be provided in as few as 10 sessions, however, and there are a number of relatively short-term group formats for its use as well.

Filial Play Session Skills

Parents learn four specific skills in order to conduct the special play sessions with their children. After the parents have mastered these skills during the play sessions, their use can be generalized to everyday parenting situations. The four skills, detailed in VanFleet (2006, 2012, 2014) and in VanFleet, Sywulak, and Sniscak (2010), are briefly described here:

1. The *structuring skill* helps children understand how the play sessions work. Parents learn how to explain the sessions to their children, what to say when starting the play session, and how to handle departure from the room and the ending of the play session. The therapist prepares parents to handle resistance from a child, particularly when the play session ends.

2. The *empathic listening skill* enhances parents' attunement to the child, helping them show greater understanding and acceptance of their child's feelings, motivations, and needs. The therapist teaches parents to rephrase aloud the child's main activities and emotions and to convey interest in the child by their nonverbal behavior. Parents learn to refrain from leading, teaching, questioning, or directing the child's play.

3. The *child-centered imaginary play skill* is actually another form of attunement and empathy. The parents engage in pretend play when invited by the child, and in a manner consistent with the child's wishes. They learn to act out different roles the child might assign. Parents follow the child's ideas for the direction of the play so that themes of importance to the child can emerge.

4. The *limit-setting skill* creates safety within the play sessions as parents set and enforce the rules when needed. The number of limits is minimized, but they are important to help children understand their boundaries and figure out how to redirect their energies if their behavior becomes unsafe or destructive. The therapist teaches parents a three-step limit-setting process: (1) state the limit clearly and specifically when it is first broken and redirect the child in a general way; (2) give the child a warning on the second infraction of the same limit, informing the child that the play session will end if he or she tries it a third time; and (3) enforce the consequence for the third infraction of the same limit by ending the play session.

The Process of FT

VanFleet (2006, 2014) has detailed the methods and process of FT, as follows:

1. The therapist explains the rationale and methods of FT, answering parents' questions and engaging them as partners in the process.

2. The therapist then demonstrates the play sessions individually with the children in the family as the parents watch and record their observations and questions. The therapist fully discusses the play session demonstrations with the parents afterward.

3. The therapist trains the parents in the four basic play session skills: structuring, empathic listening, child-centered imaginary play, and limit setting. A variety of training approaches can be used, but this phase culminates in mock play sessions in which the therapist pretends to be a child and the parents practice the four basic skills in a role play. The therapist provides ongoing feedback during the mock session to help shape the parent's use of the skills, and then discusses the experience fully with the parents at the end, providing feedback on their skills and expectations of how the process will work with the children in the family. The feedback offered to parents throughout FT focuses heavily on their strengths and offers suggestions for improvement.

4. The parents begin play sessions with their own children under the supervision of the therapist. The play sessions involve one parent and one child at a time, and the sessions can be alternated to include all family members (VanFleet, 2006, 2014). The therapist provides feedback to the parents on their play session skills, helps them understand their children's play, and discusses a variety of family dynamics issues that emerge from the play sessions.

5. After parents develop confidence and competence in conducting the play sessions, they begin to hold them independently at home. The therapist and parents meet periodically to discuss the home play sessions, problem-solve family issues that arise, and generalize the skills beyond the play sessions to daily life.

The Value of FT for Adoptive Families

FT is particularly useful for adoptive families. Because FT builds healthy attachments while simultaneously permitting children to work through problems or traumatic reactions, it provides adoptive families with the tools needed to resolve problems and to create a satisfying home environment. It also assists adoptive parents in understanding the complex needs of their adopted child so that they are more likely to know how to address those needs in constructive ways. There are many reasons why FT is applicable, and often the treatment of choice, for adoptive families (VanFleet & Sniscak, 2003a):

1. FT creates a physically and emotionally safe environment for the child. Physical safety is ensured by the structuring and limit-setting skills, and emotional safety is demonstrated by the parent's/caregiver's empathic acceptance and child-centered imaginary play skill (another form of empathy and attunement).

2. FT offers the child acceptance of *self* by primary caregivers, and this in turn can strengthen the child's own sense of self.

3. Children in FT are free to explore their own interests, motives, struggles, wishes, and so on, and this can help strengthen identity.

4. The nondirective nature of the play sessions fosters the development of trust, as the child learns from repeated exposure during the play sessions that all of his or her feelings and expressions are accepted unconditionally.

5. Children in FT learn better emotional and behavioral regulation through the combined use of play session skills that can eventually be employed by parents in daily life. This is accomplished by providing the child with much-needed nurturance and acceptance while simultaneously and firmly limiting inappropriate behaviors.

6. The FT play session skills help build attunement between parent and child. It helps parents to understand their children better and, consequently, to focus on and meet their needs better.

7. FT is a developmentally sensitive intervention. It uses play as the primary means of building attachment, and the child can work through clinical, developmental, and relationship issues simultaneously.

8. FT allows adoptive children to express and master their trauma issues in a nonthreatening and facilitative environment.

9. FT recognizes the reciprocity of relationships. It helps parents help their children, and parents model for their children the healthier attitudes and behaviors that they wish their children to adopt. FT encourages the interplay of parent and child as they appreciate each other, learn about each other, and have fun together.

10. FT provides parents with the empathy, encouragement, and support to use (a) the play session skills, (b) their clearer understanding of their child, and (c) insight about their own feelings and reactions to change their own attitudes and behaviors, resulting in more satisfying relationships with their children.

11. Because the entire family is involved in the process, FT helps strengthen family identity, trust, and cohesion. As parents and children together work through their dynamic issues and develop stronger bonds, their joint sense of belongingness and attachment is forged.

12. FT involves other children already in the family, whether they are biological or previously adopted children. It helps to prevent or reduce sibling rivalries that may arise. Siblings have their own play sessions so they are less likely to resent the newly adopted child's special times with the parents. It helps the family appreciate the uniqueness of all the children and facilitates family cohesion rather than competition.

13. The FT process enables parents to "take the therapy home," often reducing the amount of office-based therapy needed.

14. FT provides parents with lifelong skills that can be used long after therapy ends and adapted as the child's developmental level changes.

15. FT is transportable and can be used in many different settings with a variety of caregivers. It can be used to facilitate difficult transitions for children, such as from foster care into adoptive placement, and to serve as a template for healthy relationships along the way.

FT Models for Use with Adoptive Families

The needs of adoptive families are varied, and FT has the flexibility to adapt to those needs. The strength of FT lies in its training methods, its positive strengths-based focus, its use of play as a means of connecting parents and children, and its collaborative trust and involvement of parents as the primary change agents for their own children. When these essential ingredients are incorporated, the actual format for treatment can take many forms and remain effective. Descriptions of different individual and group formats are available (Caplin & Pernet, 2005; Ginsberg, 2004; Guerney, 1983; Guerney & Ryan, 2013; Landreth, 2012; Landreth & Bratton, 2006; VanFleet, 2014; VanFleet & Guerney, 2003; VanFleet, Sniscak, & Faa-Thompson, 2013; Wright & Walker, 2003). Three general options for the use of FT with adoptive families are included in the following discussion.

Filial Therapy as a Prevention Program

Many adoptive families adjust well to the changes in their lives. Adopted infants and adopted children with less traumatic histories often adjust smoothly. Even children with backgrounds of abuse and neglect sometimes settle into life with their adoptive families rapidly and without undue strain. Even so, it is desirable for adoptive families to strengthen their attachments and to prevent at-risk children from developing difficulties at a later date. FT can help them do this. Furthermore, the FT play sessions are very enjoyable and offer a unique way for parents and children to connect, and for parents to feel confident in their parenting approach. Therefore, FT can be offered to some adoptive families simply as a prevention program to facilitate their development as a family.

In this case, FT can be offered as a very short-term program, perhaps in a 10- to 15-week individual family format, or a 10- to 15-session small-group format. A session-by-session sample of such a program for individual families is outlined here. Asterisks show points in the process where sessions can be added or deleted, as needed by the family. Furthermore, Sessions 1 and 2 can be combined if a full assessment of the family is deemed unnecessary.

Session 1:

- Intake with parents
- Discussion of adoption and attachment issues
- Explanation of the importance of play
- Preliminary information about FT
- Premeasures

Session 2

- Family play observation
- Discussion of family play observation with parents only
- Recommendation for FT
- Overview of FT process and skills

Session 3

- Therapist–child play session demonstration; parents watch
- Discussion of play session
- Introductory training in the four play session skills

Sessions 4–5*

- Training of parents in play session skills
- Mock play sessions

Sessions 6–10*

- Filial play sessions, directly supervised
- Discussion and feedback with parents alone

Sessions 11–15*

- Home FT play sessions
- Reports on home sessions and discussion
- Generalization and maintenance of skills
- Postmeasures

To accommodate a number of children and as many as two parents in this format, the FT play sessions that are directly observed by the therapist in Sessions 6 through 10 are held for 20 minutes each. Each parent holds one session for 20 minutes, and the therapist uses the remaining 20 minutes for discussion and feedback. When the parents begin their home sessions, they are each asked to hold a 30-minute play session with each of their children each week, if possible.

The original group FT model (Guerney & Ryan, 2013) as well as several short-term group adaptations are also appropriate for adoptive families as prevention programs. Landreth and Bratton (2006) have developed and researched a 10-week group filial training format that teaches parents the basic play skills and provides a small amount of direct observation of the parent–child play sessions. Descriptions of this format are also available in Landreth (2012) and in several chapters in VanFleet and Guerney (2003).

Caplin and Pernet (2005) have developed a 12-session group format for the use of FT with impoverished and at-risk families; they and their colleagues have used it in Philadelphia for more than 10 years. It was also implemented in New Orleans with displaced families after Hurricane Katrina. Their format can work very well with adoptive families. Two therapists lead a group of 10 or 12 parents. The didactic material is covered with the entire group together. When parents practice the skills and hold their play sessions with their children, the group divides, each half meeting with one of the therapists. Play sessions are shortened to 10–15 minutes to permit more opportunities for supervised practice. This approach permits the parents to obtain considerable individualized feedback and support from the therapists, and it allows other children in the family to be involved in the process too. Home play sessions are reported during the final weeks of FT, with the entire group intact once more.

Wright and Walker (2003) have developed a similar approach with Head Start families that incorporates the strengths of the original Guerney FT group model (Guerney & Ryan, 2013) and the Landreth–Bratton 10-week group training format (Landreth & Bratton, 2006). Two group leaders divide the group for the practice sessions and for observations of the actual parent–child play sessions, yet meet with the entire group jointly to cover didactic material, hold toy-making sessions, and discuss progress. They provide additional innovative interventions to ensure group attendance and involvement. The Wright and Walker (2003) format entails 12 sessions of a core program, followed by one or two "reunion sessions" held several months after the core sessions have ended. This approach, too, seems very applicable to adoptive families.

In the VanFleet, Sniscak, and Faa-Thompson (2013) short-term group model, the meetings are extended to 3 hours, during which the entire group meets for didactic sessions, and then divides for skills practice and play sessions. The play sessions are usually held for 20 minutes each following the skill-building and mock play sessions with the parents, and are supervised directly before parents begin their home sessions. The group continues to meet to go over the progress being made at home. This model can be run from 14 to 18 sessions, depending on the needs of the children and families involved.

FT for Adoptive Families Experiencing Problems

When adoptive families experience problems, often due to the child's traumatic past or the additional strains on family life, FT may be a beneficial intervention. Other play therapy and behavioral interventions may be needed as well, but because FT typically addresses emotional, social, behavioral, and parenting issues, it can often be used as a single systemic intervention. The form of therapy offered to an adoptive family varies greatly, depending on specific child and family needs. It is not always short term, but FT, with its involvement of the parents and the entire family system, tends to reduce significantly the amount of therapy time needed.

There are instances when other interventions may be required prior to the start of FT, such as the following: (1) if the parents have exhausted their physical and emotional reserves prior to seeking therapy, (2) if the child's behaviors are so extreme that crisis intervention is needed, or (3) if the parents are unlikely to be able to accept the potentially intense emotional content of the child's play (e.g., sexualized play related to molestation or play related to other traumas). Decisions about the course of therapy, with these factors in mind, are made with full input of the parents.

For example, an adoptive mother of a child with reactive attachment disorder was exhausted after 2 years of attempts to tame the child's behavior and unsuccessfully seeking treatments that would work. She had been told that play therapy would not work for her daughter, and she and her child had been traumatized by a coercive holding method recommended and conducted by another professional. Her child had been placed in therapeutic foster care for the safety of other children in the family. The skeptical adoptive mother requested that the therapist work with the adopted girl first to see if interventions would be successful, and if so, she would become involved in FT at a later date. The therapist conducted child-centered play therapy and more directive trauma interventions with the child, while working with the foster mother and the adoptive mother on consistent behavior management approaches. During 35 play sessions, the child worked on intense trauma and attachment issues and showed behavioral improvements in her daily life with her foster parents and on weekend visits with her adoptive family. The adoptive mother then learned to conduct the FT play sessions, and after 10 such sessions, the child returned home. The adoptive mother had been given a much-needed respite and the daughter's intensity had diminished. The FT play sessions continued at home while the child participated in a small play-based social skills group. FT, combined with a variety of play therapy and parenting interventions, was successful in helping the adoptive family establish more secure attachment relationships that have continued for several years posttreatment (VanFleet & Sniscak, 2003a).

Other child-oriented therapies that may be considered as an adjunct to FT with adoptive families include cognitive-behavioral play therapy (Kaduson, 1994; Knell, 1993), release play therapy for trauma (Kaduson, 1994; Schaefer, 1994), identity activities, sandtray interventions, thematic play therapy (Benedict & Mongoven, 2000), dramatic play therapy (Gallo-Lopez & Schaefer, 2005), bibliotherapy (e.g., *Brave Bart* by Sheppard, 1998), and the use of educational workbooks (e.g., *When Something Terrible Happens* by Heegaard, 1991), developmental play therapy (Brody, 1993), and animal-assisted therapies (Chandler, 2012; Fine, 2010; Levinson & Mallon, 1997; VanFleet, 2008; VanFleet & Faa-Thompson, 2010). These interventions can help children address the legacy of their prior traumas and develop a clearer understanding of themselves; they can also reduce levels of emotional arousal and anxiety and enhance social skills and adjustment. Of course, children should also be referred for appropriate physiological/biological interventions as needed, such as medical/psychiatric treatment, physical therapy, occupational therapy/sensory integration, and speech/hearing services.

Other family-oriented therapies can be useful as well. These include training in behavior management and parenting skills (although these are also built into the FT process), Theraplay (Booth & Lindaman, 2000; Jernberg & Booth, 1999; Munns, 2000), the Circle of Security program (Marvin, Cooper, Hoffman, & Powell, 2002), the Watch, Wait, and Wonder program for infants (Cohen et al., 1999; Muir, Lojkasek, & Cohen, 1999), parental involvement in therapist-directed activities (as in Hughes, 1997), and other family collaborative play activities.

Whether FT is used alone or in conjunction with other therapeutic interventions, some adjustments may be needed to assist adoptive families. Possible adaptations of the FT method are described in detail elsewhere for trauma issues (VanFleet & Sniscak, 2003b) and attachment-related problems (VanFleet & Sniscak, 2003a), both areas that intersect with adoptive families. Adaptations of the method are briefly discussed in the following paragraphs.

First, where relevant to the child's history, adoptive families need to understand the impact of attachment/trauma problems on the child. Internet chat rooms are full of dire predictions and punitive "solutions" that can exacerbate tensions at home. Therapists need to educate parents about trauma, attachment, affective, and relationship issues; how their child's behavior is related to such issues; and how they and their children discharge distress (Jackins, 1994; James, 1994; VanFleet et al., 2013; Ziegler, 2000).

Second, when the adoptive family comes to treatment in crisis mode, parenting skills and behavior management interventions may be required immediately to reduce the level of emotional arousal in the family. Guerney's (1995) parenting skills program, consistent with FT, is useful here.

Third, adoptive parents sometimes need a bit more time spent in the training phase of FT. This is true when the child exhibits extreme conduct problems or intense posttrauma reactions. After parents learn the basic play session skills during the normal FT process, they may benefit from additional observations of therapist-conducted play sessions with their child and/or a third mock play session during which the therapist prepares them for the more difficult child behaviors that may emerge during play sessions.

Fourth, adoptive parents may need extra encouragement and support as they conduct the play sessions with their children. Although always an integral part of the FT process, therapists may need to provide considerable empathy, patience, and practical guidance for parents as they conduct the play sessions, discuss the play themes, explore their own feelings, and decide how to handle problematic situations at home. Sometimes, with severely distressed children, the therapist and adoptive parents may decide to continue play sessions under the therapist's supervision for a longer-than-usual time before starting the home play sessions.

Additional child and family interventions and adaptations to the FT method are not always needed for adoptive families. The systemic FT process is powerfully effective as a short-term intervention, and it often ameliorates adoptive family problems readily. An advantage of the systemic nature of FT is that it reduces the amount of therapy that an adoptive family needs. Additions and adaptations are made only on a case-by-case basis.

FT Model for Successful Transition from Foster Care to Adoption

Children who have been involved in the foster care system sometimes have difficulty in making the transition from home to home, and the move into adoption is no exception. Although most of these children desperately want to be part of a family, the abuse or neglect they suffered in their biological families, coupled with frequent and unexpected moves from placement to placement, leave them suspicious that the adoptive placement is "for real." FT can help stabilize foster placements and provide an excellent transition tool to ease the move into adoption. In this model, the therapist trains and supervises foster parents or kinship caregivers as they hold FT play sessions with the child. When adoptive parents are identified, the therapist trains them as well, and through a series of alternating FT play sessions with caregivers and adoptive parents helps the child move from an emotionally safe placement to a secure adoptive home.

FT has been used successfully with foster parents (Sweeney, 2003), kinship caregivers (Malon, 2003), and adoptive families (Ginsberg, 1989; VanFleet, 1994, 2003). This FT transition model combines these approaches in a continuous, but relatively short-term intervention across the systems in which the child lives (VanFleet et al., 2013).

Mental health professionals sometimes worry about a child forming an attachment to foster parents or temporary kinship caregivers, fearing that it will be damaging to the child to have that attachment broken when the child moves into adoption. This FT transition model encourages healthy attachments with foster or kinship caregivers for several reasons.

First, many children in the care system have little or no experience with healthy attachments. Their only experiences are with insecure attachments and hurtful relationships. If they can experience a healthy relationship with their caregivers, then it adds a "template" of secure attachment to the child's frame of reference. This can help increase the child's eventual ability to discern healthy from unhealthy relationships. Even for parents, the experience of connection during their own life histories can provide this template for future relationships. An adoptive mother reported, during FT, "When I was growing up myself, I wasn't very close to my parents. They were always too busy or very critical. But my grandmother saved the day. I could talk with her about *anything*, and she really listened and understood. That's the kind of mother I want to be for Brad."

Second, FT play sessions provide foster children with perhaps their first experience of empathy from another person. It is difficult for a person to have empathy for another person if he or she has not experienced it first.

Third, foster children develop bonds with their caregivers by virtue of living with them. Using FT can help ensure that the bonds are healthy ones. It is not unusual for foster children to begin immediately calling new foster parents "Mom" and "Dad" and saying "I love you" to them. This demonstrates their need and desire for engagement. Foster children can also behave in provocative ways that result in relationships that mimic the abusive relationships of their past. FT can prevent this from happening, and it can deepen the relationship so that the child's needs for security and attachment are better met. This, in turn, can reduce problematic behaviors of the child, which in turn can reduce or eliminate changes in the child's placement.

Fourth, children sometimes remain in foster placement or kinship care for extended periods of time. Because healthy relationships are so critical to children's well-being, it may be a disservice to children to "wait" until they are adopted before facilitating their healthy attachment with caregivers. To counteract feelings of rejection, isolation, and low self-esteem, these children also need to feel valued. FT helps foster or kinship caregivers *show* children how valued they are by their acceptance during the play sessions.

Fifth, most people's lives are populated with a variety of relationships, of varying degrees of connection and health. In all lives, some of the attachments (e.g., friendships, family relationships, intimate relationships) are broken or left behind. When the relationship of best friends is disrupted by one child's move to another city, their friendship may endure through e-mails and visits, or it may dissolve, but the experience of that friendship stays with the children throughout their lives. Moreover, most people have a number of attachment relationships at any given time, with some closer than others. Therefore, it is a relatively normal experience to have multiple attachments, some of which change or end, and it is a developmental task to adjust to such changes. The transition model that follows helps children engage in healthy relationships and then adjust to changes in those relationships.

For many children awaiting adoption, the transition from the foster home to the adoptive home is relatively abrupt. The child meets the pre-adoptive parents, has several visits with them, including some overnight visits, and then moves in with them permanently. This entire process is sometimes completed in 1–2 months. Although the visits help alleviate the anxieties the adoptive child and parents are likely to feel, this process does not always permit true relationships to develop. A 16-year-old adoptive boy commented on his adoption at age 12: "I met them a few times and liked them, but we were all on our best behavior. I didn't really know them. I liked my foster family and knew them pretty well, so it was pretty scary to just leave and move in with my adoptive parents, knowing that it was supposed to be forever, and I hardly knew them!"

Some placement agencies have espoused the view that children should leave their foster homes and "move on with their lives." A prevalent belief is that the fostering relationship must end in order for the adoptive relationship to start. For the reasons stated earlier, this belief seems misguided. It is difficult for children to leave a predictable, safe relationship with a foster family to enter the unknown world of an adoptive family. Instead, it can be much easier for children to make a transition from the foster family when they are moving toward another family with whom they have already forged some very positive bonds.

FT has been used successfully to help adoptive families establish meaningful relationships *during* the visitation process, thereby reducing transition anxieties. The adoptive child is moving from one healthy attachment
relationship to another. This process provides adoptive families with specific activities to get their new relationships off on the right foot.

The FT transition model (VanFleet, 2005; VanFleet et al., 2013)
includes training both foster parents/kinship caregivers and preadoptive
parents to hold FT play sessions with the children involved. The process
weans children from the play sessions in the foster home to regular play
sessions in the adoptive home. FT serves as a core intervention that follows
the child through all transitions until the need for treatment has ended.

While the child is in foster or kinship placement, the therapist employs
FT to stabilize the placement and to create healthy relationship patterns
for the entire family. The children often use these play sessions to work on
a variety of issues, including their trauma experiences, anxieties, past and
current relationships, hopes for the future, and so on. The foster parents
learn a set of skills they can use with other foster children in the future,
although a therapist fully trained in FT should monitor that use when
it occurs. Overall, the placement can be stabilized and the child has an
opportunity to work through a variety of issues with weekly play sessions.
The foster parents are supported and supervised on a weekly or biweekly
basis by the therapist. Other interventions, such as therapist-conducted
play therapy, behavior management, or other family/parent consultations
are added as needed.

Immediately after a match has been found for the adoptive family, the
therapist meets with the preadoptive parents to provide them with (1) an
overview of what to expect, good and bad, from the child's behavior; (2)
education about trauma, its impact on emotions and behaviors, and the
importance of healthy attachments; (3) tips on interacting with the child,
including some basic positive parenting and behavior management skills, if
needed; and (4) training in the FT play session skills. This takes approximately three or four sessions. During this training phase, the preadoptive
parents observe a play session conducted by one of the foster parents or the
therapist, with the child's advance knowledge and agreement.

Next, a series of day visits and overnight visits are accompanied by FT
play sessions with the already-trained adoptive parents. Initially, these take
place at the therapist's office, in coordination with the visits, and then shift
to home play sessions when the adoptive family is ready. During this visitation period, the play sessions continue in the foster home as well.

After the child has moved permanently to the adoptive home, there
are several visits with the foster parents, during which play sessions are
held, terminating in a final visit, play session, and "farewell" activity. The
parent–child play sessions continue in the adoptive home as long as they

are needed, and parents hold play sessions with any siblings as well. The therapist monitors and supports these play sessions until a satisfactory adjustment and attachment have been made, helping the adoptive parents to generalize the use of the play session skills to daily life. The FT play sessions can be augmented with other family interventions, such as family storytelling for sharing histories and creating a new combined history, special family rituals including enjoyable times, the creation of a special scrapbook and/or photo album for the child and family, and the like.

The FT transition model has been used in transitions from foster care to adoption with more than 50 families to date, where appropriate funding could be secured. In all cases where the foster and adoptive parents and the child placement and adoption agencies cooperated fully with the therapy plan, successful, smooth adoptions took place. Although some of the adoptive children exhibited serious trauma and attachment problems while in care, their adjustment to adoption was facilitated by the use of FT. One adoptive father put it this way:

> "We knew we wanted to add this boy to our family, and we liked him. What we didn't expect was how traumatized he was. Filial Therapy gave us the tools we needed to help him adjust to us and for us to understand what was going on for him. The foster mom helped him settle down to a point where he was ready for us, and then when we took over the play sessions, he just seemed to hit his stride and keep on going. It was great for us, and we still do the play sessions 2 years later!"

Although FT has a strong empirical history, this specific model of transitioning children from foster care to adoption using FT as a bridge has not yet been researched fully. Initial results from in-depth case studies and small pre- and postevaluations are promising.

CASE ILLUSTRATION

Identifying information about the following case has been disguised in order to protect the privacy of the children and families. The case illustration reflects a composite of several families, but it accurately represents the course of treatment using FT.

History

Polly had been in foster care from the time she was 5 years old. Both of her parents had been involved in selling drugs, and her mother abused cocaine.

Polly had been exposed to all aspects of the drug trade, and she witnessed domestic violence on numerous occasions. She was badly neglected at times, and her father had beaten her on several occasions when he became frustrated with her crying. When her mother was arrested, her situation came to light and she came into care. Little else was known about her early years with her parents.

Polly had been through numerous foster placements because of her extreme behaviors. She was easily triggered by seemingly innocuous comments or events, and she flew into rages, deliberately breaking anything in her path. The foster families with whom she was placed were ill-equipped to deal with her destructive, out-of-control behaviors. In two of her placements, the foster parents implemented behavior management plans with the aid of an in-home support program, but they had little impact when she went into one of her rages.

By the time she was referred to me, she had been in 12 different homes. She was now 10 years old. Her current foster mother, Jane, told me that she was a bright, sweet girl "when she wanted to be," but that she had seen three of her "episodes" where she seemed "completely out of her mind." Jane had already tried talking with her to no avail. Jane had also attempted to put her into time-out, but that had become a physical tussle, and even though Polly was small, she was strong and it had been potentially dangerous to both of them. Jane expressed interest in trying to work with her and help her with her problems. She had not yet burned out.

Fortunately, Polly did well in school and seemed to like it. Her current teacher had reported moments when she seemed to "space out," however, which no one had reported from the school before. To date, Polly had responded when the teacher called her name. She had no medical problems of note. She had a few friends whose homes she occasionally visited, but she did not appear to be particularly close to anyone.

The Start of FT

I decided during the intake that FT could be started right away with Jane and Polly. Jane was motivated and interested, and I thought that Polly might respond well to the acceptance she would experience in the FT play sessions.

I first wanted to provide some education to Jane about trauma and attachment problems, so I met with Jane alone to provide an overview of some of the dynamics that often are at play. We discussed how triggers were developed through associations made during traumatic times, and how Polly's rages were probably related to her emotional dysregulation in general. Jane was thoughtful and asked questions that showed she truly was trying to understand the information. I provided some basic ideas that Jane could follow at home to avoid triggering Polly's rages, and also how she could respond when she saw the first signs of them. I then discussed the basics of FT with her and suggested that she bring Polly in for a play session demonstration the next meeting.

During the play session demonstration, I conducted a child-centered play therapy session with Polly while Jane watched and jotted down her observations and questions. Polly quickly engaged with the toys and explored the playroom. She talked animatedly and moved throughout the playroom touching or playing briefly with many different items there. I empathically listened as she did this, "You're checking out those costumes. Ah . . . you like that lacy yellow one. . . . Trying it on. . . . " She stood in front of the mirror and made a gesture, which I reflected, "Oooo, you're feeling very fancy in that!" For a brief time after exploring the costumes, she invited me to try on some items as well. She wrapped a boa around my neck and laughed when I tossed the loose end back over my shoulder. She announced we would have a fashion show and we both had to parade around the playroom like models. She showed me the exaggerated strut of a model and told me to follow her, which I did. Since I couldn't quite pull it off as smoothly, she laughed heartily at me, and I reflected, "You think that's pretty goofy. I can't seem to pull it off." She told me that I might have to go back to "model school." She then shifted her attention back to exploring other toys and I returned to empathic listening. No limits were needed during this session.

I met briefly with Jane afterward while Polly stayed in the waiting room, and Jane asked a few questions and I pointed out some of the things I was doing. We both discussed how Polly presented as if she were 8 rather than 10, and I explained that was common in children with histories such as hers. At the end of the meeting, Jane agreed to proceed with FT and we arranged for her training sessions.

FT Parent Training Sessions

It took the usual three sessions to prepare Jane for the FT play sessions. She learned quickly and could use the basic skills quite well during the mock play sessions that I held with her. During the second mock session, I challenged Jane a little more to ensure that she knew how to handle limits, "cranky" comments, and other things that Polly might do. Throughout the training, I offered in-the-moment positive feedback to Jane, and then more in-depth feedback at the end of each skills practice segment.

Supervised FT Play Sessions with Polly and Jane

At home, the situation had deteriorated somewhat. Jane reported that there had been two more rage situations where she tried to implement the things we had talked about. This had gone reasonably well, but the incidents had been unsettling for both her and Polly. I suggested we continue with the FT play sessions as planned, as I thought that had the best chance of creating the type of connection and safety that Polly needed to gain better self-regulation.

In her first play session, Polly again explored the playroom for a few minutes, and then returned to the dress-up clothes. She again donned the lacy item and told Jane that she would be the "judge of the models." Polly again strutted around as if she were a model, occasionally turning to Jane for her judging reaction. Jane applauded, which seemed just what Polly had wanted. Polly went back to solitary play, and Jane tracked her behaviors very well. She was able to reflect a few of the feelings, but missed some as well. Polly went to the sandtray and began placing houses in it. Jane reflected, "You put in a house. Another house. Three houses." Polly seemed particularly intent as she did this. At one point, she selected a dark-colored house, put it in the sandtray, and said, "This is the evil house." Jane commented, "That's the evil house." Polly's play again changed quickly after that. In general, her play showed themes of exploration, identity and self-esteem (the dress-up play), control, and the short play in the sandtray that seemed to reflect something of her formative or foster care experiences.

At the end of the session, I met alone with Jane to discuss how it went. Jane had been nervous about "getting it right," and as is quite typical of early FT sessions, she had been concentrating so hard on the skills that she had missed seeing some of Polly's emotions. She was pleased with herself overall though. I highlighted many of the specific things she had done very well with her empathic listening and brief child-centered imaginary play as the judge. The one suggestion for improvement that I gave her was to watch more for the feelings and to empathically listen to them. I gave several examples of this so she understood what I meant.

In their second play session, Polly seemed much more relaxed and immediately decided to play school. She was the teacher and Jane was to be her pupil. Polly portrayed a demanding and bossy teacher who found fault with all of Jane's work. Jane played the expected role well, commenting under her breath (in role) how she just couldn't seem to get it right and that her teacher was very hard to please. Polly thoroughly enjoyed the way Jane played the role, giving a few suggestions now and then about what Jane should say or do. Play themes for this session included power and control, meeting expectations of others, and feelings of inadequacy. During the discussion I had with Jane at the end, Jane seemed pleased with herself, and I reinforced the many things she had done very well. When we discussed play themes, Jane was worried that it might not be such a good idea to allow Polly to be so bossy in her play. I listened empathically to her concerns, and then I provided an explanation of how Polly might be telling us some very important things about her life and her perceptions, and that we needed to be accepting of them and to hear them. I reassured her that typically the controlling or demanding play rarely spilled over into daily life, but if she thought things became worse at home, she could call me. She seemed satisfied with that.

When they arrived the following week, Polly continued with her controlling and demanding play, although she selected different roles and ways to express them. At one point, she pretended to have an angry fit and threw a block toward Jane. Jane set the limit as she had been taught. Polly retorted, "I wasn't throwing it *at* you—it just bounced over that way!" Jane replied, "You want me to know that you didn't do that intentionally. Even so, the blocks can't be thrown anywhere in my direction. You can do just about anything else." She had handled that challenging moment just as we had discussed. Polly accepted it at that point and moved on to other play. During the postsession discussion with just Jane, Jane told me that Polly had not been bossy or demanding after the last session. We discussed Jane's brilliance in handling the limit-setting situation and how important that was for Polly's ultimate feelings of security, even if she didn't like it in the moment. Jane and I both were feeling good about her skill development, and most of our discussion centered on the play themes and Jane's feelings.

I watched two more live play sessions between Jane and Polly. Jane continued to use the skills better and better, and she became more adept at recognizing play themes. Polly continued to play themes of power and control, which is common for children who feel powerless in their lives. At times she engaged in aggressive play, mostly using the bop bag, but she never did anything that required Jane to set another limit. She began to play more family and nurturance themes, where she asked Jane to play a mother animal and she played a baby animal. The mother animal always had to take care of the baby animal. At the end of the fifth supervised play session, Jane said that things had seemed quite stable at home. There had been no further displays of rage, and Jane had become better at recognizing when Polly felt out of sorts. Jane also said that she was able to intervene when Polly showed the earliest signs of being triggered, and she helped Polly take a break, sit down, and they would then either talk or simply cuddle, if Polly felt like doing that.

Home Play Sessions with Polly and Jane

Jane began holding the FT play sessions at home and met with me regularly to discuss them. On occasion, she made a video of their play session and showed me parts of that as well. In many ways, our meetings resembled those when I provide supervision or case consultation with therapists. Jane reported on the session, and we discussed her use of skills, what went well, what did not go well, questions that she had, play themes that emerged, and how she felt about it all.

Jane was excited when she arrived to report on her first home session. "You're not going to believe this!" she said. She told me how their first session at home had started with exploration of the somewhat different toys that she had there, and then had proceeded into some limit-testing behaviors. Polly pretended that she was going to throw things at Jane, but she didn't actually throw them. Jane was able to empathically listen to most of this: "You're thinking about throwing that at me. . . . You're ticked off and want me to know it. . . . You want to see what you can get away with now that we're here at home." These were all excellent reflections of Polly's feelings and her intentions. At no time did Polly actually break any limits. I was able to praise Jane for being able to make the discrimination between Polly's feelings and posturing and an actual limit-setting situation. After the more aggressive, limit-testing play, Polly had poured water into the baby bottle and began sucking it as she wandered around the room. Jane was sitting in a corner, reflecting. Polly eventually sat down next to Jane and leaned against her, still sucking the baby bottle. Jane recognized the important connection that Polly had initiated. She saw this as a major breakthrough because Polly had typically been unable to express much affection or need for affection.

Their play sessions continued at home and I met with Jane weekly at first, and then biweekly to monitor them. I occasionally saw Polly for some directive animal-assisted play therapy with my dog in order to build some specific skills and coping strategies. We worked on an understanding of relationships, feelings, and some nurturance activities. I also used other directive play therapy techniques, again to help her develop her ability to cope with her trauma reactions and some bullying issues that had come up at school. She was actively working through her trauma with the FT play sessions, so I used our sessions to focus on more specific skills that she needed.

During their home sessions, Polly interspersed themes of power and control, family relationships, nurturance, and safety. She often created imaginary scenes with Jane in which there was vulnerability followed by safety. It was clear that she was working through the many difficult experiences in her life, and she was learning to trust Jane more fully with her feelings. At the same time, her behavior in daily life had improved considerably. Her teacher reported that the "space out" times at school had disappeared.

FT during Polly's Preadoptive Transition

After 6 months, it was clear that the FT had helped stabilize Polly's placement with Jane. She had shown signs of progress in all areas. Plans moved forward for her adoption, and a couple was identified as a match for her. I met with them, Rob and Carrie, before they met Polly, telling them about the work we had been doing and suggesting that they learn and use FT as part of their transition process. This had full agency support, including funding. They agreed and immediately began the training phase of FT.

They met Polly and Jane at the adoption agency, and by the time they were ready for their second meeting, they had nearly finished their FT training. Polly, Jane, Rob, and Carrie had met for ice cream at a local shop prior to coming to see me. Polly and Jane had agreed to provide a demonstration of one of their play sessions for Rob and Carrie to watch. Polly was excited about the adoption and the idea that they would have special play sessions with her too. Polly played cautiously and occasionally glanced at Rob and Carrie during the play session. They thanked her and stayed after Polly and Jane had left to discuss it with me. We finished their training that night as well.

Polly and Jane continued their home sessions throughout the transition phase. Rob and Carrie took turns holding play sessions with Polly on nearly all of their visits. During this time period, Polly's play was more "conservative" than it was with Jane, mostly likely because she was concerned with making a good impression so the adoption would go through. Her play with Jane continued to have themes of vulnerability and safety, nurturance and connection, and a newly emerging theme that seemed to be about uncertainty. This mirrored what was happening in her own life. Rob and Carrie both did well, and they were able to demonstrate acceptance of Polly's feelings during the play sessions so that she gradually relaxed with them and seemed more herself. She went through aggressive play and attempted to "trick" Carrie into closing her eyes so she could dump water on her during their third play session together. Carrie realized what was happening and set a limit just as the water began to pour. She laughed with surprise as some of the water hit her, but she then firmly set the limit. Soon, Polly began playing family themes and relationship building with Rob and Carrie. They were able to respond using their FT play session skills, and the early sessions helped everyone relax as they faced this big event in their lives.

Just before Polly was slated to move into Rob and Carrie's home, I held a meeting with Jane, Rob, and Carrie to discuss some of Polly's prior trauma- and attachment-derived problematic behaviors. Jane shared strategies that had worked for her, and I discussed some of the same information I had shared with Jane. I was careful to provide honest and practical information without scaring them. The message was one of "you might encounter some tough times here and there, but you are gaining the skills to deal with them, and I'll be here to help you get through the rough spots." Jane also offered her assistance at any time.

Polly had a final play session with Jane at my office, after which we had a little celebration of their time together. Jane promised to keep in touch from time to time. Polly then moved in permanently with Rob and Carrie.

FT Sessions in Polly's Adoptive Home

Rob and Carrie held their separate play sessions with Polly in the first few days after she moved into their home. Using the miniatures, Polly showed Carrie how the baby dinosaur had to leave the mommy dinosaur and go live with another family. Because she had been prepared for this potentially difficult material, Carrie reflected, "The baby dinosaur is scared about moving away." Polly had responded, "Not really scared, but just sad." Carrie had further reflected, "The baby is sad about leaving the mom she cared about." Polly nodded in agreement and moved on to other play. After several minutes, she returned to the baby dinosaur and the new family (a rhino and a gorilla miniature) and played them all going to a swimming pool to have fun. With Rob, Polly mostly played hide and seek where she hid and he had to find her. When Rob and Carrie came in to discuss their home sessions with me, we talked about how well they had helped her handle those feelings of uncertainty and the loss of her secure foster placement in her play, and how her play themes also reflected her hopes for her new life with them.

Rob and Carrie each held weekly play sessions with Polly for the first 2 months. After that, they took turns holding a single play session with her each week. Although her transition was not completely smooth—she did experience a couple meltdowns with them—Rob and Carrie were able to be more attuned to her needs and were able to head off a number of potentially traumatic and dramatic conflicts. In the play sessions, Polly continued to play out themes related to her trauma-related feelings, gradually showing more empowerment of the previously vulnerable characters. Much of this was done through role play using the costumes.

After Polly had had 10 sessions with either Rob or Carrie, she had a particularly notable session in which she told Carrie that she, Carrie, was pregnant. Carrie had to walk around the playroom with a pillow under her costume, waddling and having trouble sitting down and getting up. Polly directed all of this play and laughed as Carrie did as she asked. Polly then told Carrie, "It's time! You have pains and you scream!" Carrie gave a short scream as Polly wanted, but Polly insisted that she had to scream very loudly. "It's a very very very very very big baby!" Carrie did as she was asked. Next, Polly went and sat at Carrie's feet and said, "Now I'm your baby. Feed me!" Carrie took the bottle of water and fed Polly. Carrie was very moved by this play, clearly seeing the connection with the adoption.

Rob also had a special session that moved him. Polly had been quite bossy during the first part of the play session, with a reemergence of the school teacher and pupil theme. She then told Rob that he was going to be her friend and he was coming to a special dinner. They enacted the scene as Polly wished, and she served him a dinner of plastic food, naming each item that she had prepared. "This is a very special starter. I made it just for you. . . . Now here's my special sauce for spaghetti. It is very hard to make, and I had to cook it all day. I hope you like it. . . . This dessert is my favorite and you are going to love it." The theme was obviously one of giving him things to please him and make him happy, and he recognized her desire to connect further with him.

Polly handled the transition very well, and in fact, much better than she had handled any of her prior transitions from foster home to foster home. She had acquired a sense of safety and security from Jane initially, and then during the early FT sessions with Rob and Carrie.

Outcomes

Polly continued to do well with Rob and Carrie. I saw them for a total of 20 sessions, which was relatively short term considering the level of seriousness of Polly's trauma and attachment problems. The early sessions were held during visits; the middle sessions occurred on a biweekly basis as they reported on their home sessions; and we used a phased-out discharge near the end where I saw them once every 3–4 weeks to ensure that progress was continuing and to help them generalize the use of the skills to everyday life.

We held planned follow-up phone calls 3 and 6 months after discharge, and Carrie told me that everything was still going well. They were still holding play sessions and marveling at what they had been able to learn about Polly through that process. They believed that Polly had increasingly opened up to them, and that they were well equipped to deal with most of her problems, even the intense ones. They knew they were welcome to come back at any time should problems arise in the future.

EMPIRICAL SUPPORT FOR FT

FT has been researched steadily since its inception in the early 1960s. Studies of its process and efficacy have increased through the years, and research has been or is being conducted with a variety of problem areas and in different settings, cultures, and countries. A meta-analysis of play therapy included 34 studies of FT that met the criteria for inclusion (Bratton, Ray, Rhine, & Jones, 2005). This clearly demonstrated that FT is very effective as a treatment modality. VanFleet, Ryan, and Smith (2005) have provided a critical review of the empirical basis of FT, noting its consistently positive outcomes and robustness as a therapy useful in addressing a wide range of problems. Guerney and Ryan (2013) have summarized the research in their book as well. Controlled studies have demonstrated its effectiveness in (1) improving children's presenting problems and behaviors, (2) developing parental acceptance and understanding of their children, (3) strengthening parents' skills, (4) decreasing parents' stress levels, and (5) improving parents' satisfaction with outcomes. Follow-up studies have shown that family gains are maintained 3 and 5 years after therapy has ended. More recently, a study of 27 families designed to predict FT outcomes (Topham, Wampler, Titus, & Rolling, 2011) found that children with poorer self-regulation and parents with higher levels of distress showed the greatest gains in a FT program. Children with poor emotional regulation had the greatest reductions in problem behaviors. Parents with poor emotional regulation showed greater increases in acceptance of their children. This exciting line of research is continuing.

These quantitative outcomes are augmented by qualitative information and compelling case studies (VanFleet & Guerney, 2003). The use of FT has grown dramatically during the past decade, largely because of its effectiveness. More controlled studies are needed, but the empirical foundations of FT show it to be an effective way to treat the types of problems experienced by many adoptive families.

SUMMARY AND CONCLUSIONS

Adoption poses many challenges for children and parents alike. The primary task is to provide healthy, strong relationships within the family that meet everyone's needs as fully as possible. This can be challenging, especially when the adopted children have histories of attachment disruption. FT is a relatively short-term evidence-based intervention that fully integrates play therapy with family therapy. It simultaneously allows children to work through salient emotional, social, behavioral, and trauma-related issues while establishing secure attachments with adoptive parents. It can be used as a prevention program to provide an avenue for secure attachment, or it can be used to intervene in extremely difficult problems of the child and family. Finally, it holds great promise as a mechanism through which the transition from foster care to adoption can be facilitated, allowing the child to have several experiences of genuine, healthy engagement along the way and culminating in strong, satisfying adoptive relationships for everyone involved.

REFERENCES

Ainsworth, M. D. S. (1982). Attachment: Retrospect and prospect. In C. M. Parkes & J. Stevenson-Hinde (Eds.), *The place of attachment in human behavior* (pp. 3–30). New York: Basic Books.

Belsky, J., & Nezworski, T. (Eds.). (1988). *Clinical implications of attachment.* Hillsdale, NJ: Erlbaum.

Benedict, H. E., & Mongoven, L. B. (2000). Thematic play therapy: An approach to treatment of attachment disorders in young children. In H. Kaduson, D. Cangelosi, & C. E. Schaefer (Eds.), *The playing cure* (pp. 277–315). Northvale, NJ: Jason Aronson.

Bernstein, N. (2001). *The lost children of Wilder: The epic struggle to change foster care.* New York: Pantheon Books.

Bifulco, A., & Moran, P. (1998). *Wednesday's child.* London: Taylor & Francis.

Bifulco, A., Moran, P. M., Ball, C., & Lillie, A. (2002). Adult attachment style: Its relationship to psychosocial depressive-vulnerability. *Social Psychiatry and Psychiatric Epidemiology, 37,* 60–67.

Bifulco, A., & Thomas, G. (2013). *Understanding adult attachment in family relationships: Research, assessment and intervention.* London: Routledge.

Booth, P. B., & Lindaman, S. L. (2000). Theraplay for enhancing attachment in adopted children. In H. G. Kaduson & C. G. Schaefer (Eds.), *Short-term play therapy for children* (pp. 194–227). New York: Guilford Press.

Bowlby, J. (1982). *Attachment* (2nd ed.). New York: Basic Books.

Bratton, S. C., Ray, D., Rhine, T., & Jones, L. (2005). The efficacy of play therapy with children: A meta-analytic review of treatment outcomes. *Professional Psychology Research and Practice, 36*(4), 376–390.

Brazelton, T. B., & Cramer, B. G. (1990). *The earliest relationship: Parents, infants, and the drama of early attachment.* Cambridge, MA: Perseus Books.

Brody, V. (1993). *The dialogue of touch: Developmental play therapy.* Treasure Island, FL: Developmental Play Training Associates.

Brodzinsky, D. M., & Schechter, M. D. (Eds.). (1990). *The psychology of adoption.* New York: Oxford University Press.

Caplin, W., & Pernet, K. (2005). *A 12–session group model of filial therapy.* Boiling Springs, PA: Play Therapy Press.

Chandler, C. K. (2012). *Animal assisted therapy in counseling* (2nd ed.). New York: Routledge.

Cheung, S., & Hong, G. K. (2005). Clinical application of attachment theory: Cultural implications. *Family Psychologist, 21*(2), 15–16.

Clark, K. E., & Ladd, G. W. (2000). Connectedness and autonomy support in parent–child relationships: Links to children's socioemotional orientation and peer relationships. *Developmental Psychology, 36*(4), 485–498.

Cohen, N. J., Muir, E., Lojkasek, M., Muir, R., Parker, C. J., Barwick, M., et al. (1999). Watch, Wait, and Wonder: Testing the effectiveness of a new approach to mother–infant psychotherapy. *Infant Mental Health Journal, 20*(4), 429–451.

Figley, C. R. (1989). *Helping traumatized families.* San Francisco: Jossey-Bass.

Fine, A. H. (Ed.). (2010). *Handbook on animal-assisted therapy: Theoretical foundations and guidelines for practice* (3rd. ed.). New York: Elsevier.

Gallo-Lopez, L., & Schaefer, C. E. (2005). *Play therapy with adolescents.* New York: Aronson.

Ginsberg, B. G. (1989). Training parents as therapeutic agents with foster/adoptive children using the filial approach. In C. E. Schaefer & J. M. Briesmeister (Eds.), *Handbook of parent training* (pp. 442–478). New York: Wiley.

Ginsberg, B. G. (2004). *Relationship Enhancement family therapy* (2nd ed.). Doylestown, PA: Relationship Enhancement Press.

Guerney, B. G. (1964). Filial therapy: Description and rationale. *Journal of Consulting Psychology, 28*, 303–310.

Guerney, L. F. (1983). Introduction to filial therapy: Training parents as therapists. In P. A. Keller & L. G. Ritt (Eds.), *Innovations in clinical practice: A source book* (Vol. 2, pp. 26–39). Sarasota, FL: Professional Resource Exchange.

Guerney, L. F. (1995). *Parenting: A skills training manual* (5th ed.). North Bethesda, MD: Institute for the Development of Emotional and Life Skills.

Guerney, L. F. (2003). The history, principles, and empirical basis of filial therapy. In R. VanFleet & L. Guerney (Eds.), *Casebook of Filial Therapy* (pp. 1–20). Boiling Springs, PA: Play Therapy Press.

Guerney, L. F., & Ryan. V. (2013). *Group Filial Therapy: The complete guide to teaching parents to play therapeutically with their children.* London: Jessica Kingsley

Hart, J., Shaver, P. R., & Goldenberg, J. L. (2005). Attachment, self-esteem, worldviews, and terror management: Evidence for a tripartite security system. *Journal of Personality and Social Psychology, 88*(6), 999–1013.

Heegaard, M. (1991). *When something terrible happens.* Minneapolis, MN: Woodland Press.

Hughes, D. A. (1997). *Facilitating developmental attachment.* Northvale, NJ: Jason Aronson.

Humber, N., & Moss, E. (2005). The relationship of preschool and early school age attachment to mother–child interaction. *American Journal of Orthopsychiatry, 75*(1), 128–141.

Jackins, H. (1994). *The human side of human beings: The theory of re-evaluation counseling* (3rd ed.). Seattle, WA: Rational Island.

James, B. (1994). *Handbook for treatment of attachment-trauma problems in children.* New York: Free Press.

Jernberg, A. M., & Booth, P. B. (1999). *Theraplay* (2nd ed.). San Francisco: Jossey-Bass.

Johnson, S. (2005). So now we know what love is—It's all about attachment. *Family Psychologist, 21*(2), 13–14.

Kaduson, H. G. (1994). Play therapy for children with attention-deficit hyperactivity disorder. In H. G. Kaduson, D. Cangelosi, & C. Schaefer (Eds.), *The playing cure* (pp. 197–227). New York: Rowan & Littlefield.

Knell, S. M. (1993). *Cognitive-behavioral play therapy.* Northvale, NJ: Jason Aronson.

Ladd, G. W., & Ladd, B. K. (1998). Parenting behaviors and parent–child relationships: Correlates of peer victimization in kindergarten? *Developmental Psychology, 34*(6), 1450–1458.

La Greca, A. M., Silverman, W. K., Vernberg, E. M., & Roberts, M. C. (Eds.). (2002). *Helping children cope with disasters and terrorism.* Washington, DC: American Psychological Association.

Landreth, G. L. (2012). *Play therapy: The art of the relationship* (3rd ed.). New York: Taylor & Francis.

Landreth, G. L., & Bratton, S. C. (2006). *Child Parent Relationship Therapy: A 10-session filial therapy model.* New York: Taylor & Francis.

Leathers, S. J., Spielfogel, J. E., Gleeson, J. P., & Rolock, N. (2012). Behavior problems, foster home integration, and evidence-based behavioral interventions: What predicts adoption of foster children? *Children and Youth Services Review, 34*(5), 891–899.

Levinson, B. M., & Mallon, G. P. (1997). *Pet-oriented child psychotherapy* (2nd ed.). Springfield, IL: Charles C. Thomas.

Malon, S. (2003). The efficacy of Filial Therapy with kinship care. In R. VanFleet & L. Guerney (Eds.), *Casebook of Filial Therapy* (pp. 209–234). Boiling Springs, PA: Play Therapy Press.

Marvel, F. A., Rodriguez, R. A., & Liddle, H. A. (2005). Attachment and family therapy: Theory informing practice. *Family Psychologist, 21*(2), 10–12.

Marvin, R., Cooper, G., Hoffman, K., & Powell, B. (2002). The Circle of Security project: Attachment-based intervention with caregiver–pre-school child dyads. *Attachment and Human Development, 4*(1), 107–124.

Muir, E., Lojkasek, M., & Cohen, N. J. (1999). *Watch, Wait, and Wonder.* Toronto: Hincks-Dellcrest Institute.

Munns, E. (Ed.). (2000). *Theraplay: Innovations in attachment-enhancing play therapy.* Northvale, NJ: Jason Aronson.

Nilsson, R., Rhee, S. H., Corley, R. P., Rhea, S. A., Wadsworth, S. J., & DeFries, J. C. (2011). Conduct problems in adopted and non-adopted adolescents and adoption satisfaction as a protective factor. *Adoption Quarterly, 14*(3), 181–198.

Ryan, V., & Wilson, K. (1995). Non-directive play therapy as a means of recreating optimal infant socialization patterns. *Early Development and Parenting, 4*(1), 29–38.

Schaefer, C. E. (1994). Play therapy for psychic trauma in children. In K. J. O'Connor & C. E. Schaefer (Eds.), *Handbook of play therapy* (Vol. 2, pp. 297–318). New York: Wiley.

Sheppard, C. H. (1998). *Brave Bart: A story for traumatized and grieving children.* Grosse Pointe Woods, MI: Institute for Trauma and Loss in Children.

Sroufe, L. A. (1983). Infant–caregiver attachment and patterns of adaptation in the preschool: The roots of maladaptation and competence. In M. Perlmutter (Ed.), *Minnesota Symposia in Child Psychology* (Vol. 16, pp. 41–83). Hillsdale, NJ: Erlbaum.

Sroufe, L. A. (1988). The role of infant–caregiver attachment in development. In J. Belsky & T. Nezworski (Eds.), *Clinical implications of attachment* (pp. 18–38). Hillsdale, NJ: Erlbaum.

Sroufe, L. A., & Rutter, M. (1984). The domain of developmental psychopathology. *Child Development, 55,* 17–29.

Sweeney, D. S. (2003). Filial Therapy in foster care. In R. VanFleet & L. Guerney (Eds.), *Casebook of Filial Therapy* (pp. 235–258). Boiling Springs, PA: Play Therapy Press.

Terr, L. (1990). *Too scared to cry: How trauma affects children . . . and ultimately us all.* New York: Basic Books.

Topham, G. L., Wampler, K. S., Titus, G., & Rolling, E. (2011). Predicting parent and child outcomes of a Filial Therapy program. *International Journal of Play Therapy, 20*(2), 79–93.

VanFleet, R. (1994). Filial therapy for adoptive children and parents. In K. O'Connor & C. Schaefer (Eds.), *Handbook of play therapy* (Vol. 2, pp. 371–385). New York: Wiley.

VanFleet, R. (1998). A parent's guide to filial therapy. In L. VandeCreek, S. Knapp, & T. Jackson (Eds.), *Innovations in clinical practice: A source book* (Vol. 16, pp. 457–463). Sarasota, FL: Professional Resource Press.

VanFleet, R. (2003). Filial Therapy with adoptive children and parents. In R. Van Fleet & L. Guerney (Eds.), *Casebook of Filial Therapy* (pp. 259–278). Boiling Springs, PA: Play Therapy Press.

VanFleet, R. (2005). *Filial Therapy transition model for foster children* (Working Paper and Report No. 05-7STC-R). Boiling Springs, PA: Author.

VanFleet, R. (2006). *Introduction to Filial Therapy: A video workshop.* Boiling Springs, PA: Play Therapy Press.

VanFleet, R. (2008). *Play therapy with kids & canines: Benefits for children's developmental and psychosocial health.* Sarasota, FL: Professional Resource Press.

VanFleet, R. (2012). *A parent's handbook of Filial Therapy* (2nd ed.). Boiling Springs, PA: Play Therapy Press.

VanFleet, R. (2014). *Filial Therapy: Strengthening parent–child relationships through play* (3rd ed.). Sarasota, FL: Professional Resource Press.

VanFleet, R., & Faa-Thompson, T. (2010). The case for using animal assisted play therapy. *British Journal of Play Therapy, 6,* 4–18.

VanFleet, R., & Guerney, L. (Eds.). (2003). *Casebook of Filial Therapy.* Boiling Springs, PA: Play Therapy Press.

VanFleet, R., Ryan, S. D., & Smith, S. (2005). Filial Therapy: A critical review. In L. Reddy, T. Files-Hall, & C. E. Schaefer (Eds.), *Empirically based play interventions for children* (pp. 241–264). Washington, DC: American Psychological Association.

VanFleet, R., & Sniscak, C. C. (2003a). Filial Therapy for attachment-disrupted and disordered children. In R. Van Fleet & L. Guerney (Eds.), *Casebook of Filial Therapy* (pp. 279–308). Boiling Springs, PA: Play Therapy Press.

VanFleet, R., & Sniscak, C. C. (2003b). Filial Therapy for children exposed to traumatic events. In R. VanFleet & L. Guerney (Eds.), *Casebook of Filial Therapy* (pp. 113–138). Boiling Springs, PA: Play Therapy Press.

VanFleet, R., Sniscak, C., & Faa-Thompson, T. (2013). *Filial Therapy groups for foster and adoptive parents: Building attachment in a 14 to 18 week family program.* Boiling Springs, PA: Play Therapy Press.

VanFleet, R., Sywulak, A. E., & Sniscak, C. C. (2010). *Child-centered play therapy.* New York: Guilford Press.

Wright, C., & Walker, J. (2003). Using Filial Therapy with Head Start families. In R. VanFleet & L. Guerney (Eds.), *Casebook of Filial Therapy* (pp. 309–325). Boiling Springs, PA: Play Therapy Press.

Youngblade, L. M., & Belsky, J. (1992). Parent–child antecedents of 5-year-olds' close friendships: A longitudinal analysis. *Developmental Psychology, 28*(4), 700–713.

Ziegler, D. (2000). *Raising children who refuse to be raised: Parenting skills and therapy interventions for the most difficult children.* Phoenix, AZ: Acacia Press.

Part III

≈

GROUP PLAY THERAPY

Chapter 14

⌘

Directive Group Play Therapy for Children with Attention-Deficit/Hyperactivity Disorder

Norma Leben

Directive group play therapy is the use of fast-paced structured and semistructured games designed for children diagnosed with attention-deficit/hyperactivity disorder (ADHD) and low self-esteem. Through specifically designed games and a regimen of concurrent reinforcement methods, the therapist sustains the attention of fidgety children; teaches values, social skills, emotional, and life skills; and manages misbehaviors. The group process and games empower and motivate the players, help build their self-esteem, promote self-confidence and teamwork, and facilitates improved handling of interpersonal conflicts. The fun atmosphere dissipates past fear and pain in learning. The learned positive experience is transferable to new social settings and situations.

—NORMA LEBEN

During my undergraduate and master's social work training in the 1970s, my favorite class was social group work. I was influenced by group-work classics of that time such as Konopka (1963), Bernstein (1965), Cartwright and Zander (1968), Trecker (1955), and Yalom (1995), to name only a few. I was also fortunate to have expert group-work teachers who engaged students using experiential, structured exercises to help

325

us understand firsthand all the components of group dynamics and stages of group development. We experienced the power of group dynamics, and clearly saw the changing of thoughts and behaviors.

Earlier, as a youth worker in Hong Kong, I led activity, hobby, and friendship groups for many years. After graduation from graduate school, I continued running groups as well as supervising students with their group work. However, these were not therapy-related groups. It was not until I was the treatment supervisor for a 16-bed small residential treatment center in Texas, when I realized that group work was used as a treatment method.

Before beginning each group, I planned the treatment with games appropriate to meet the residents' developmental needs and interests. However, it became clear to me that with the youngest group of children (ages 5–7), more was needed. The younger children had not developed the self-control that adults had, and the beginning of this group was a teaching moment in that typical means could not work.

THE ORIGINS OF DIRECTIVE
GROUP PLAY THERAPY

It was at that time that directive group play therapy (DGPT) was first utilized. Many of the children in residential treatment had the behaviors associated with children diagnosed with attention-deficit/hyperactivity disorder (ADHD): hyperactivity short attention span, and impulsivity. To plan a group for children with ADHD, it was clear to me that their symptomatic behaviors would have to be a primary focus. In fact, many of these behaviors were reasons why they were sent by their parents, teachers, probation officers, and judges for treatment at the treatment center. In addition to the social group-work training that emphasized the building of relationships and personal growth, there was also a need to incorporate treatment for short attention spans, distractibility, restlessness, feet tapping, talking out of turn, idiosyncratic attention-seeking behavior, and aggressiveness toward themselves, peers, and even the therapist.

In order to deal with these problems, it was clear that children could only learn when they were paying attention (Gaskill & Perry, 2014). Research has revealed that brains of children with ADHD are "wired" differently, with a smaller left hemisphere and weak executive functions. Therefore, these children have a harder time with tasks like paying attention, managing time, following multistep directions, and delaying gratification. Therefore, my approach was to engage their attention first. Perhaps then children with ADHD could be motivated to use appropriate manners, polite language, feeling words, social skills, some etiquette, and better judgment. Because children with ADHD are impulsive, they cannot think before acting, and do not seem to have the natural inclination and patience to learn, every social or life skill must be broken down and taught to them in tiny steps. Therefore the goal for therapeutic interaction should be to sustain the child's interest long enough to look, to listen, and to practice using a feeling word like "frustrated," understanding a value like responsibility or empathy, learning a social skill like "taking turns," or understanding a life motto like "All good things in this world are earned." If children with ADHD can understand, practice, and internalize these "fact bites," then they will have the basic intellectual scaffolding to understand themselves and others, apply rules in different settings, find ways to communicate, and discover ways to build meaningful relationships. By learning to habitually break down every task in life to manageable steps, they will create "mini-successes" and avoid frustration, which can unglue them emotionally.

BOOSTING LOW SELF-ESTEEM IN CHILDREN WITH ADHD

There is a high incidence of maltreatment among children with ADHD (Perry, 1999). Some children with ADHD are reported to have a high threshold for physical pain, so quite often adults in their lives cross the line from discipline to abuse. At school, these children's idiosyncratic behaviors make them targets for bullies. The taunting, name calling, and hurtful personal ridicule increases their feelings of helplessness, which turns inward as self-doubt, depression, and self-hatred. Children can perceive repeated rejection by family, teachers, and foster families or treatment facilities' staff as "nobody wants me." As a result, many children with ADHD appear to be loners, lack a sense of belonging, are fearful of new settings, sensitive to personal feedback, defensive, and do not trust adults.

A play therapist can provide opportunities for group members to *safely* express their real personality during their treatment to help rebuild their self-image. This is done in games by encouraging short constructive feedback from their peers and the therapist. At the end of each group session, there is at least 10 minutes for members to practice listening to and giving honest feedback to each other.

In order to achieve the goals in these groups, I found it was important to get their attention, keep them motivated, and provide feedback about their behavior without being overly critical. Positive reinforcement by giving and withholding chips in this group was used to increase the appropriate behaviors and attention.

CAPTURING INTEREST
WITH FAST-PACED, NOVELTY PLAY

Thomas Phelan's (1993) book *All About Attention Deficit Disorder: Symptoms, Diagnosis and Treatment: Children and Adults* was most helpful, especially when creating structured games. He described how children with ADHD were more likely to pay attention under four conditions:

1. *When it is a novelty item or idea.* The games used (Leben, 2009) included recycled materials, easy to find items in the home, and toys found at garage sales. The children can play rough and "accidentally" break toys. If the games or toys are created from disposable materials, they are easily replaced. Also, when group members see a handful of pinto beans and empty egg cartons on the table, they were immediately curious and asked, "What are those for?" The therapist could reply, "These are for one of our new games I will teach you," knowing that at that moment the therapist had their attention. Only a few store-bought games include surprise novelty in their design. For example, the 50-year-old "Booby-Trap Game" (sold by Gem Color Co. #214 or Parker Brothers; *www.samstoybox.com/toys/BoobyTrap.html*) was so much fun that the boys would behave better for 30 minutes just to "earn" 15 minutes to play it. Balancing items like matchsticks on a soda bottle or stacking alphabet blocks to make a tower are also great examples of including novelty that attract children with ADHD.

2. *When it is something the child is interested in.* Playing games is something that most children with ADHD like to do. To match their temperament and treatment objectives, fast-paced, fun games with only a few, easy to remember rules like my "Bigger–Smaller–Same Game" (Leben, 2009) were very helpful. Children with ADHD prefer games that are engaging with win-win results for every player and that allow spontaneous, creative expression. Even though store-bought games facilitate the social skill of taking turns, many of these children dislike them because such games have too many rules, take too long to play, and only one person can win. Furthermore, many store-bought games promote a superficial participation of moving a marker instead of an opportunity for deeper interactions between members and therapist.

3. *When it is a one-on-one situation.* Resembling a blackjack dealer at a casino table, the therapist can be playing with each child one-on-one, and yet the rest of the group is watching and learning from the therapist's interactions with other players.

4. *When the child feels intimidated.* When children are scared or intimidated, they also will show fewer symptoms of ADHD. The therapist

should remain cordial, respectful, and directive when explaining a game, but should always be in charge. The therapist strictly follows the game rules and dispenses poker chip rewards for appropriate behavior or genuine effort. When loudly dropping a poker chip in a child's bowl, the therapist smiles and offers simultaneous short remarks like "That's good sitting; I like it," or "I like the way you're listening to me," or "Thank you for changing your attitude." Such short feedback statements when accompanied with rewards are exactly what children with ADHD need as guidance.

5. *When the child is rewarded frequently.* Rewarding group members frequently with tokens like poker chips, as well as by making positive comments continuously throughout the session, helps the child remain focused and on task. For children with severe symptoms, start by using dry roasted peanuts (after consulting with their parents about food allergies) as primary reinforcement because after eating one, the players tend to want another, creating an internal drive for appropriate behavior. Then gradually introduce a second plastic bowl and use poker chips as a secondary reinforcement. After two more sessions, transition to using only poker chips. This can help train the children to delay gratification because the group members are required to wait until the end of the group session to redeem their chips for healthy food items like corn nuts, sesame sticks, or baby carrots. Furthermore, having a treasure chest with many small toys and trinkets adds to the motivation and positive reinforcement; for example, a child who earns 27 chips can trade in 20 of those for a small toy car and seven sesame sticks.

It had been observed that the parents of these boys, who might have also had ADHD, love token rewards too. Parents are just as curious about the treasure chest items and will excitedly trade their chips for little tubes of toothpaste and fancy little hotel shampoo bottles.

STAGES OF GROUP DEVELOPMENT

The DGPT model includes the model for stages of development in social work groups (Garland, Jones, & Kolodny, 1965): (1) preaffiliation, (2) power and control, (3) intimacy, (4) differentiation, and (5) separation. In each stage, the group members show characteristic behaviors that help the therapist to assess the group's stage. The stages of vital importance in helping members change are the *intimacy* and *differentiation stages*. However, the group does not just reach those stages by having a certain number of sessions. It is up to the therapist to use facilitation skills and the selection of effective games and activities to encourage interactions to resolve the key dynamics of each stage, thus "pushing" the group to develop.

When children first enter the group they act like strangers and need opportunities to safely feel accepted and see other members' abilities. Games in the *preaffiliation stage* should focus on inclusion and feeling good about participation (Garland et al., 1965, pp. 25–32). When members see a firm, competent leader, offering fun games, food, and rewards, they are more likely to return for more positive experiences.

During the *power and control stage*, group members jockey for status positions and challenge each other and test the leader's authority and rules (Garland et al., 1965, pp. 32–34). The therapist's ability to handle the challenges fairly and calmly is the key to winning members' confidence that he or she is a person they can trust and whose guidance they can accept. For example, the therapist consistently should model the use of polite, clean language. If a member starts swearing or cursing, instead of dealing directly with that member, the therapist can simply look in his direction, followed by giving a chip to each of the other members and saying, "Thank you for using clean language," or "Thank you for respecting yourself and our group," or "Thank you for exercising self-control." After that takes place, then the member who was using foul language is asked if he or she can express him- or herself in a different way. One such member actually said, "I wish all of you would jump into the lake and leave me alone!" The therapist immediately gave him a chip for changing to clean language to express his frustration! Another member said in response, "Yeah, you bet we'd be speaking clean language if we jumped in the water." Everyone laughed, which broke up a tense moment. The therapist then gave out chips to everyone with remarks like "very funny," "good belly laugh," and "a lovely smile!"

In the third stage, *intimacy,* after members know one another better, trust is further built through mutual disclosure and dependence on group norms. The group members feel less defensive, act cohesively when making decisions, and can support each other to change old habits of vocabulary, mannerism, and attitudes (Garland et al., 1965, pp. 35–37).

In the fourth stage, *differentiation,* members feel supported and validated enough to use socially acceptable language to express opinions, adopt more prosocial behavior, and further develop their unique personal identity (Garland et al., 1965, pp. 38–40).

In the final stage, *separation,* the therapist brings the group to a close with play therapy games so that members can evaluate and share their own personal growth in social and emotional skills (Garland et al., 1965, pp. 40–44). Other activities help celebrate the friendships built between members and express possible feelings of loss and sadness (Leben, 2009). It is important to work on planning and implementing the final three group sessions, because there may be cases of abused and traumatized children who have had serial abandonment issues that were never addressed. With the separation stage group activities, children master those moments with greater competency. It is important to make sure that children learn to handle parting moments in the DGPT experience.

OTHER COMPONENTS OF A DGPT GROUP

In addition to theoretical frameworks, there are other components that make DGPT more effective.

Structure

Children with ADHD need and function better with structure, that is, in an environment that is organized and predictable. This is the most important DGPT group component.

1. *Meeting time and place.* Same time, same place every week.
2. *Same set-up.* Every player has a plastic bowl (perhaps recycled, small margarine bowls). In the therapist's corner is a rack of poker chips and a container or two of crunchy snacks.
3. *Seating arrangement.* Sit around a table or on the floor in a close circle so as to facilitate eye contact and assurance of safety. The child who needs the most support should sit on the therapist's right-hand side to benefit from close proximity, a helping hand, and verbal encouragement for participation.
4. *Routine program format.* Check-in with each member, followed by a couple of fast-paced, fun games; a story; sharing and feedback time; and chips redemption.
5. *Game choice.* Reviewing each child's treatment objectives will allow for games that fit, and the therapist should be prepared to switch to another game that promotes better interaction.
6. *Supplies.* Provide clean, well-maintained toys, puppets, and play materials, mostly recycled or second-hand from garage sales or thrift stores.

Short, to-the-Point Language

The therapist should remember that children with ADHD have short attention spans. It is helpful to discipline oneself with a "6-second rule" when an instruction, request, or feedback is spoken. This rule helps to keep the therapist aware that there is about 6 seconds of attention from a child with ADHD. Therefore, it is important to use specific, clear, to-the-point "sound bites" or verbal requests to say what is meant and/or wanted without hesitation. For example, "Good sitting. I like it," "Pay attention," or "Eye contact."

The therapist should make a conscious effort to counteract the children's low self-esteem by giving frequent encouragement within 6-seconds. If at all possible, stay away from the two words "good" and "bad" because they are too general. Instead members are encouraged to use more descriptive language in the feedback segment at the end of each session. For example, if Peter says, "John, you told a *good* story," then the therapist can prompt and have the child say, "John you told an *interesting* story. I enjoyed the funny ending." Another example would be when Ben said, "Simon, you were bad in this session." The therapist prompted Ben and he changed it to say, "Simon, you kicked me under the table several times for no reason at all. I don't appreciate it. I want you to stop that."

Group Size

For novice play therapists, two or three members, definitely no more than four, allows the therapist to give adequate attention to members as well as to make better observations.

Group Duration

At the outset it is a good idea to let potential group members know the planned duration of the group, usually eight to 10 sessions. Knowing the beginning and end dates provides an incentive for their commitment to participate. For schools with 12-week semesters, a 10-session group allows the play therapist time for member recruitment and therapeutic separation. Even if a child can benefit from added sessions, it is preferable to have him or her join another group with different members allowing him or her more practice with various social–emotional skills and problem-solving situations.

Reinventing Group Process to Help Children with ADHD

This approach actually worked to keep members' attention and resulted in more prosocial behavior, which then increased the motivation to create more games.

The DGPT session can illustrate how the boys or girls are closely watching the therapist for nonverbal and verbal cues for how to behave. The therapist's every move purposefully shapes better social–emotional interactions.

CASE ILLUSTRATION: THE YOUNG BOYS' GROUP

The boys at the residential treatment center were gathered for the DGPT sessions. The boys sat at a round table, with a recycled plastic margarine container in front of each boy. Next to the therapist was a rack of poker chips, a bottle of dry roasted peanuts, and a bowl of round cereal pieces for rewards. Other supplies included a stack of playing cards omitting the jack, queen, and king; a container of dry, raw pinto beans; and a rubber band.

The game plan for our 60-minute session included (1) check-in time; (2) two structured games, the "Bigger–Smaller–Same Card Game" and the "Pinto Bean Picture Game" (Leben, 2009); (3) feedback time; and (4) redemption of tokens.

All group sessions start with a *check-in time*. In the first meeting, the check-in time is longer because during the preaffiliation stage it is important for group members to have meaningful opportunities to get to know the therapist and for the members to get to know each other. The check-in time for later sessions are much shorter because the therapist asks each member to pick one to two feeling words from my *Feelings Wheel Game* boards mounted on the wall that describe their current feelings (Leben, 2001). Each feeling word they express will earn one chip.

Check-In Time

THERAPIST: (*as soon as the boys come in and sit down*) John, thank you for good sitting. (*I put a peanut in John's bowl.*) Ben, thank you for good eye contact. (*I put a peanut in Ben's bowl.*) Simon, thank you for looking at me. (*I put a peanut in Simon's bowl.*) Peter, thank you for joining our group. (*I put a peanut in Peter's bowl.*) Thank you for attending this meeting.

We met 2 weeks ago and it didn't go well. I'm sorry about that. Today I would like to try again and start properly this time. Thank you for listening. (*I give every member another round of peanuts.*) So, let's begin by introducing ourselves. I'll go first. My name is Norma, your new social worker. You can either call me Norma or Ms. Norma. I plan to have a play therapy group with you boys every Tuesday after school for 10 weeks. We will then take a 2-week break for the holidays. After that we'll start again. As for now, I want everyone to tell me your name and ask a question about me so we can get acquainted.

BEN: (*jumping up and down and pointing*) I want a cookie now!!

THERAPIST: (*ignoring Ben*) Thank you, John, for waiting. (*I put a chip in John's bowl.*) Thank you, Simon, for good sitting. (*I put a chip in Simon's bowl.*) Thank you, Peter, for listening to me. (*I put a chip in*

Peter's bowl.) Ben, thank you for calming down and sitting properly. (*I put a chip in Ben's bowl.*) John, would you like to go first?

JOHN: My name is John. Are you Japanese?

THERAPIST: Hi, John. Nice meeting you. (*I extend a hand for a handshake.*) Here is a peanut for telling me your name and another peanut for asking a good question. (*I put two peanuts in John's bowl.*) I'm Chinese, not Japanese, because I was born in Hong Kong, China. I'm married and living in Austin.

BEN: My name is Ben. I'm 6 years old. Is peanuts all we have to eat today?

THERAPIST: Hi, Ben. Nice meeting you. (*I extend a hand for a handshake.*) Here is a peanut for telling me your name and a cereal for asking a good question. (*I put a peanut and a cereal in Ben's bowl.*) After the games, we will have a granola bar and juice. When we play games, you'll earn more peanuts or cereal for good behavior! You can eat them right away. And I may give you poker chips too for using good manners and nice words. You may save those poker chips and at the *end of the session* redeem them for more peanuts or go to my treasure chest for a small trinket if you have 20 chips.

PETER: My name is Peter. What do you have in your treasure chest?

THERAPIST: Hi, nice meeting you, Peter. (*I extend a hand for a handshake. I try to put a peanut and a cereal in his bowl, but he points to the peanuts, so I acknowledge his choice and give him two peanuts.*) Well, I have all sorts of trinkets in there. It's for me to know and for you to find out. So let's not worry about them until you earn 20 chips.

SIMON: My name is Simon. We live in the same dorm. Where do you live?

THERAPIST: Hi, Simon. Nice meeting you. (*I extend a hand, but Simon only offers me his four fingers, which he quickly pulls back. He also points only to peanuts, so I give him two.*) I live in my own house off campus, about 10 miles away. I live there with my husband and my two cats, Maple and Tippy.

　　You all asked good questions. Before we play games, I want to tell you my rules. Rules are necessary when two or more people are trying to learn, live, or work together. My rule number 1 is safety for everyone. Rule number 2 is to use words and not fists, so I can help you find the right words to use. Rule number 3 is confidentiality, which is a big word meaning what is shared in this room should not be said again outside. Because that is the way you show respect to one another by not telling personal information to others without their permission first. Rule number 4 is that the toys we play with here will stay in this playroom. If anything is broken, please let me know so that I can either fix it for safe use by other children or discard it. Thank you for listening (*I give every player two peanuts.*) Oh, one last thing (*I reach for the rubber band and hold it with two thumbs*). From time to time, it is my job to stretch your patience and attention (*I stretch out the rubber band several times*). Other things I'm going to stretch out are your creativity, imagination, kindness, and different ways to solve problems. I'm also like a mirror that reflects how you behave and the effect it has on others. You definitely will earn *more* chips when you show me you are learning and growing.

Discussion of the Preaffiliation Stage

It is important to note that while speaking to the boys the therapist rewards frequently. The first several rounds of peanuts or cereal are only for engaging their attention. When I feel that I have their attention I switch to rewarding desirable behaviors. It is more positive to teach proactively than waiting until a player misbehaves and then punish him. When misbehavior occurs, like it did with Ben demanding a cookie, I will manage the situation by rewarding other boys who are acting appropriately rather than focusing on Ben's misbehavior. This encourages all players to stay alert for bonus tokens. I repeatedly demonstrate appropriate words and social skills that group members can copy.

I allow players to ask personal questions about me to model a beginning level of disclosure and trust. Players feel empowered and secure in the process when given honest answers by a kind but firm leader. When leading adolescent groups, players occasionally ask me obnoxious questions to test my boundaries. One time I was asked, "Do you have sex with your husband?" While the rest of the group giggled, I squarely faced this boy and showed him my left hand. "See this wedding ring? We're licensed to have sex." Then I gave each of the other boys a bonus chip for exercising self-control and not asking inappropriate questions so soon after we had just met. I briefly looked away from that boy and continued with the session.

The Bigger–Smaller–Same Game

THERAPIST: Now let's play some games. The first card game we're going to play is called the "Bigger–Smaller–Same Game." I'm the dealer. It's a new game for you. So let's learn it together with a trial run. (*I swiftly shuffle the deck of ordinary playing cards and deal every boy a card, face down.*) I'll play with you one at a time. I'll say "1, 2, 3" and you'll flip your card and I'll put down a card too. If you have a 3 and I have a 2, say "Bigger!" If you have a 2 and I have a 3, say "Smaller." If you have a 3 and I have a 3, say "The same!" I'll give you a chip for every correct answer. Is that clear so far?

GROUP: (*They nod their heads.*) Yes.

THERAPIST: Thanks for paying attention. (*I give every player a poker chip.*) John, you're sitting on my left, so I'll play with you first. Are you ready?

JOHN: Yes.

THERAPIST: OK, 1, 2, 3. Flip your card. What's your answer?

JOHN: You have a 4 and I have a 9! So I'm "bigger!"

THERAPIST: That's a correct answer, John. Here's a chip. (*I put a poker chip in his bowl.*)

JOHN: (*smiling*) Thank you!

THERAPIST: Ben, you're next. Are you ready?

BEN: Yes

THERAPIST: OK, 1, 2, 3. Flip your card! What's your answer?

BEN: You have a 7 and I have a 5, so I'm "smaller!" But I don't like to be smaller. I want to be bigger!

THERAPIST: You have a correct answer, so here is a chip for your correct answer. (*I put a poker chip in his bowl.*)

BEN: I guess that's all right.

THERAPIST: Simon, it's your turn. Are you ready?

SIMON: (*softly and slowly*) Y-e-a-h.

THERAPIST: OK, 1, 2, 3. Flip your card. What's your answer?

SIMON: (*He looks at his cards, not saying anything. He has an 8 and I have a 10. The rest of the boys are squirming and making faces. But Simon doesn't say a word.*)

THERAPIST: John, this is a chip for you for quietly supporting Simon. (*I put a chip in John's bowl.*) Ben, this is a chip for you for being patient. (*I put a chip in Ben's bowl.*) Peter, this is a chip for you for patiently waiting for your turn. (*I put a chip in Peter's bowl.*) Now, Simon, let's look at your cards again. I have 10 and you *only* have an 8. So, is your card bigger, smaller, or the same as mine?

SIMON: (*sheepishly but clearly thinking*) Smaller.

THERAPIST: That's a correct answer, so here is your chip. (*I put a chip in his bowl.*) However, I want to give you a *bonus* chip for spending extra time to look at your problem, think about it, and come up with a right answer all by yourself. I like your effort. (*I put another chip in his bowl.*)

THERAPIST: Peter, thank you for waiting for your turn. Are you ready?

PETER: Yes, I was ready 5 minutes ago.

THERAPIST: OK, 1, 2, 3. Flip your card. What's your answer?

PETER: I have a 10 and you have a 2. I'm way bigger than you.

THERAPIST: That's a correct answer, here's your chip. (*I put a poker chip in his bowl. I continue to play three more game rounds, making sure that each boy takes a turn to go first.*)

    (*I explain a variation two of the game.*) All of you did wonderful with one card. Now, I'm going to show you how to play with two cards. For this variation I'll give everyone two cards. Go ahead and turn your cards over. I'm giving you a little bit more time to look at your cards because you will be doing something more difficult called "making a *choice*." Let's say you have a 3 and a 2, it is your job to decide whether your number is 32 or 23. Is that clear? I think it is John's turn again. Are you ready, John? What is your number? (*I turn over two cards from the deck. I drew a 4 and a 5.*) My number is 45.

JOHN: (*He has a 7 and an 8.*) My number is 87. Your number is 45, so I'm bigger than you! Again!

THERAPIST: That is a correct answer. (*I give a chip.*) However, I like the *choice* you have made in maximizing your two numbers, so this is a bonus chip for that.

JOHN: (*grinning*) Thank you.

THERAPIST: (*I turn over two cards from the deck. I drew a 2 and a 7.*) My number is 72. Ben, what is your number?

BEN: My number is 44. It makes no difference which card goes first. I'm still smaller.

THERAPIST: That's a correct answer, Ben. (*I give a chip.*) However, I like your *choice* of leading your number with a 4 of hearts. I think if you live your life leading your decisions with a heart, you can seldom go wrong, so this is a *bonus* chip for you. (*I put a chip in his bowl.*) Simon, are you ready? What is your number? (*I turn over two cards from the deck, a 6 and an 8.*) My number is 68.

SIMON: My number is 25. I think I'm smaller than you.

THERAPIST: That's a correct answer, Simon. (*I give a chip.*) However, I like your *choice* because you can only count confidently up to 30, so 25 is a number you know well at this time. Here is a *bonus* chip for you. (*I put a chip in his bowl.*)

THERAPIST: Peter, are you ready? What's your number? (*I turn over two cards from the deck.*) Um, I have an ace and a 7, so I choose my number to be 71.

PETER: (*He has a 10 and 4.*) Well, I can play 104 or 410, both bigger than 71.

THERAPIST: True, but what is your final *choice*?

PETER: (*laughing*) My final *choice* is 104 because I don't want to hurt your feelings too much!

THERAPIST: You have a correct answer. (*I give one chip.*) I like your *choice* of considering my feelings, so here is a *bonus* chip for you. (*I put a chip in his bowl.*)

Discussion of the Bigger–Smaller–Same Game

The Bigger–Smaller–Same Game is the first structured game designed for DGPT (Leben, 2009) and the first game played with all new groups because it involves making choices, an essential life skill. Adaptations are made for children of different ages as necessary. For example, with kindergarteners, the jack, queen, and king are taken out because they do not show a number. For elementary school children, they are included, saying each face card counts as 10. For middle and high school children, they are challenged to use three or even four cards to make larger numbers so as to make the game more exciting. With this game the therapist can easily observe their level of math competency.

Even though it is a simple, three-rule game, it is amazing how many different situations can arise. Children with ADHD want to be correct, but because they are impulsive, they are quicker to answer even more without using their brains. Some children try to cheat; for example, lifting a card corner to secretly peek. When this happens, the therapist would take away their cards, returning them to the bottom of the deck, and giving out new cards, all without saying a word. Other children may use tears to try to manipulate the therapist for extra assistance. For these children, the therapist asks the group to wait quietly while the player who is upset tries to think. Then, just as quietly the therapist put chips into their bowls to reward them. Some other children will say anything to earn a chip. The child might coyly tilt their heads, look at the therapist, and guess, "Bigger? Smaller? Bigger? Smaller?" hoping to get the correct answer with my facial expression. To help this child trust his own ability, the therapist would patiently wait with a calm face while rewarding the other members' social skills like "sitting quietly" and values like "tolerance."

During play therapy the therapist can use three kinds of reinforcement: positive reinforcement, negative reinforcement, and random reinforcement. When a child is rewarded for a confident right answer, this is *positive* reinforcement for relying on his own ability. Since he actually spent effort on the task, he is getting a genuine boost to his self-esteem. It helps to drop the chips very loudly in their bowls. In that way, the reward is both visual and audible, putting smiles on their faces. Soon the children do not even have to look at their bowls. They trust the sound of the chip and continue their focus on the game.

When a child tries to manipulate the group process but sees the other group members getting chips for good behavior and he does not, it acts as *negative* reinforcement. He certainly does not want other players to earn more chips. Peer pressure also plays a part in spurring him to take the risk of coming up with his own answer. Children will watch others in order to learn why they are getting rewarded so they can get rewards too.

Giving *bonus* chips is *random reinforcement* because all members are rewarded when least expected. After a child gets the correct bigger–smaller–same answer, the therapist can surprise him with a *bonus* chip for coming up with his own answer; not guessing. The technique that can be used is as follows: I pinch the chip between my thumb and index finger, steadily holding it between the child and myself. Then the therapist leans her body slightly forward, says his name, and calmly states the observation about the quality or special deed he has just done. An intense gaze usually gets the child's complete attention. Just this one technique can increases the child's eye contact and attention span three to five times as compared to the first encounter (reference). After the use of *bonus* chips the first time in the group, suddenly all members become more eager to practice new words, behaviors, values, and social skills.

The Pinto Bean Picture Game

THERAPIST: Next, we're going to play the Pinto Bean Picture Game. I'm giving each of you a handful of pinto beans. The idea of this game is to create a picture with the pinto beans. Give your picture a name after you're done and I'll give you a chip. I want each of you to make three pictures, so get started. (*I observe the members quietly while they move their beans around on the table.*)

JOHN: (*In front of him is a small, shapeless pile of beans.*) I finished my first picture.

THERAPIST: John, what name are you giving to your picture?

JOHN: A tree.

THERAPIST: If you say it's a tree, a tree it is! (*I put a chip in his bowl.*) Now make your second picture.

BEN: I have my first picture. It's a circle.

THERAPIST: Ben, what does a circle remind you of?

BEN: A soccer ball. I love playing soccer.

THERAPIST: Thank you for that soccer ball. Here is a chip for you. (*I put a chip in his bowl.*) Now start your second picture.

PETER: Here's my picture. It's a gun.

THERAPIST: (*Very softly, with barely a sound, I put a chip in his bowl.*) I see, Peter. Now do your second picture. And let me see over here what Simon has drawn.

SIMON: This is an ant! See, it has six legs.

THERAPIST: Yes, Simon, I can see those legs. Here is a chip for paying attention to details. (*I put a chip in his bowl.*) Now do your second picture.

JOHN: I made another picture for you. This is a smiley face.

THERAPIST: Yes, John. I can see the eyes and lips. (*I put a chip in his bowl.*) Now work on your last picture.

PETER: I got my second picture. This is a knife with a long blade.

THERAPIST: Peter, I can see it. (*Very softly, I put a chip in his bowl.*) Whenever you're around knives, I want you to be very careful because they are sharp and dangerous.

PETER: My stepdad keeps a knife in his boot. He likes to sharpen it all the time. Once he threw it in my direction, scaring me to death.

THERAPIST: Wow, I see how a flying, sharp knife might scare you. Thanks for sharing. (*I loudly drop a chip in his bowl.*) Now work on your last picture.

BEN: Here is my second picture. This is a rectangle.

THERAPIST: Ben, what does a rectangle remind you of? (*I put a chip in his bowl.*)

BEN: A letter? No, a card like a birthday card!

THERAPIST: Whose birthday is it?

BEN: My birthday, of course! It's next week.

THERAPIST: Oh, thank you for letting us know. I hope you get a birthday card from home. Perhaps our little group can have cupcakes at our next meeting to help you celebrate.

JOHN:, Peter, Ben, and Simon: Y-e-a! Cupcakes, cupcakes, cupcakes!

SIMON: My turn, Miss Norma. This is a picture of my gerbil. His name is Fluffy. I miss him.

THERAPIST: What a lovely Fluffy! I can see why you love and miss him. (*I loudly put a chip in his bowl.*) Now, please work on your last picture.

JOHN: Miss Norma, this is a picture of my mom. She smokes a lot. See the cigarette hanging on her lips. I told her it's bad for her, but she still keeps on smoking.

THERAPIST: I hear you, John. It sounds like you love her and worry about her, but it's her choice to stop smoking. You tried. Thank you for sharing a story. (*I put a chip in his bowl.*)

PETER: (*His beans are all scattered about.*) My last picture is the front door of my house.

THERAPIST: Tell me more.

PETER: One time, some guys drove by and shot at us from the street, leaving all these holes in the door.

THERAPIST: My goodness. That must be very scary for you and your folks with the loud noise and wood chips all over the place. (*I point at his scattered beans and put a chip in his bowl.*)

PETER: (*He nods his head.*) But the landlord wouldn't give us another door, so my mom put a blanket over it to stop the cold wind blowing into our house.

THERAPIST: So you were scared and cold because of that! No wonder you remember this incident so well. Thank you for sharing your story. Now you can all help me put your beans back into this tub.

BEN: This is a picture of a bike. I want a bike for my birthday.

THERAPIST: That is a good birthday wish. Here is a chip for sharing your wish. (*I put a chip in his bowl.*) However I know for a fact that this agency does not give out bikes for birthdays. Can you ask your family?

BEN: My mom promised me for 2 years! But I still didn't get one.

THERAPIST: I can hear that you're pretty disappointed about that. However, I know the campus has bikes in the shed for high-token children to ride. If you finish your homework early, you could ask your houseparent to check out one for you.

BEN: All right! (*He proceeds to put his beans away without my asking.*)

SIMON: Look, this is a picture of a cinch bug! In fact I have a few in my pocket. (Big grin) You want to see?

THERAPIST: Not really, but here is a chip for your cinch bug picture. (*I put a chip in his bowl.*) Now help me put all your beans back into this tub, please.

Discussion of Pinto Bean Picture Game

As the game transcript illustrates, in the context of making things with their hands, children more freely share what is on their minds, more so than in a direct conversation with adults. In my groups, I use many nontraditional materials like pinto beans in picture making so children can use their creativity to express past concerns and feelings. In my experience, many children with ADHD do not like to use paper and pencil unless they are required to do so, as in the case of homework. Pinto beans are organic media, very comforting to the touch, and definitely not expensive. Using pinto beans to form pictures and shapes is probably a novel concept to most children. The Pinto Bean Picture Game takes just a few minutes for a player to create images that serve as a focus for sharing memories, thus encouraging self-disclosure in the group. I ask each child to make three pictures so I can look for themes. For example, Peter made a gun, a knife, and the door of his house hit by bullets. Young children especially do not have the ability to tell a complete story from beginning to end. However, they are able to remember particular scenes in their past or express worries about the future. In the case transcript, I validated the feelings associated with the child's own picture descriptions. If nothing else, it is empowering to arrange the pinto beans any way he likes, decide on a picture title, and be rewarded with a chip for his creativity. Even if it is an imperfect pinto bean picture, a child can make it disappear with a brush of his hand, erasing any evidence that can be judged by anyone.

One of my favorite experiences playing the Pinto Bean Picture Game was the time a kid with ADHD, who just loved to eat anything, asked me if he could eat the pinto beans. He grabbed a few beans and opened his mouth ready to eat some. I said, "You could, but we might have to end our group soon!" "Why?" he asked. I looked at him and said, "Because if you eat uncooked, raw beans, you'll start passing gas in no time! I don't want to be around to sniff it!" He threw the beans in his hand back to his pile and said, "No-o-o, I want to stay and play longer." I gave him a chip for a wise decision and a bonus chip to him and all the other group members for "exercising their self-control!"

Group Feedback Time

THERAPIST: It is almost closing time! For the last 10 minutes of every session, we will share honest feedback to each other about how we have done in *just this past hour*. Only helpful friends are courageous enough to give feedback. You cannot make people change, but if you give concrete feedback out of respect and kindness, the receiver can decide what to do with it—to change or not to change.

This is how we're going to do it. I am putting a tall stack of chips in the middle of the table. As helpful friends, you'll take turns and give feedback to each other by awarding these chips. You cannot give more than three or less than one chip. Stay away from using the words "good" and "bad" because usually they are not clear enough to help.

I'll give you my feedback at the end of the session. So who would like to start first?

JOHN: Me, me, me. Ben, I'll give you three chips because you're my best friend.

THERAPIST: John, let's stay focused on what we've done today, just in the last hour. Try again.

JOHN: I'll give you *three* chips, Ben, because you know your numbers for the first game, and thanks to you, we may have cupcakes for next meeting. Simon, I'll give you *three* chips also because you used manners and took your turn. Peter, you know your numbers well too, but I can only give you *two* chips because you were wiggling a lot in the first game making my eyes tired just looking at you.

PETER: (*sounding defensive*) But, Simon was holding up traffic!

THERAPIST: Peter, as a receiver of feedback, please remain humble. When you sound defensive, friends can choose not to give you feedback, so you're actually getting less goodies in life. If you want to get three chips from John next time, maybe sitting still more often will get you three chips. Even though this moment may not sit well in your heart, say "Thank you" anyways to show that you're gracious in listening to honest opinion from friends.

PETER: (*mumbling*) Thanks.

BEN: John, you play good.

THERAPIST: Ben, remember to stay away from the words *good* and *bad*. Try to say something you saw.

BEN: John, I like you because you're smart and almost always the first one to say the correct answer or finish your picture. I'll give you three chips. Simon, you are the youngest in the dorm, but you listened to Ms. Norma and could keep up with us. I'll give you three chips too. Peter, you must show more patience. But I think you are honest in telling things about your stepdad and door of your house, so I'll give you three chips too.

PETER: John, we both like numbers and you're as fast as me. Your mom smokes and so does my stepdad. That is a *nasty* habit. I'll give you three chips for sharing. Ben, you are in a good mood because you have a birthday next week. I like riding bikes too. Let's finish homework early every day and we can ride together on campus. You get three chips from me today. Simon. You're OK. You stayed in this room the whole time today without running off like last time. I'll give you three chips.

THERAPIST: Now it is my turn to give you guys my feedback. John, you're quite a leader. You listened and focused on getting your task done.

Keep up with the good work. Here are three chips for you. (*pause*) Ben, you have a big heart. You care for others' feelings and give honest feedback. I definitely want to give these three chips to you. (*pause*) Peter, I guess that you feel restless whenever you do not feel safe or maybe when you don't know what is expected of you. I believe you have good intentions and willingness to share your life stories. I just love it when you could take my redirection about receiving feedback and thanked John afterward. You're improving in front of my eyes, and here are three chips for you.

Chip Redemption Time

THERAPIST: Well, boys, the session is officially over. Please count your chips in rows of five so that you'll quickly know how many chips you have earned. Tell me the numbers of chips before going to the treasure chest. Then come back to me for more peanuts, a granola bar, and a juice box. Let's be on task because your staff is waiting.

   (*with raised voice over scurrying of busy feet*) Remember to think of a name for our group next time. See you next week, same time, and same place. Bye.

Discussion of Feedback Time and Chip Redemption Time

Group members need help in giving feedback. With modeling and coaching, they can learn new vocabulary to share their opinions. In my experience of *Feedback Time*, group members take very seriously the task of awarding chips and expressing their reasons. They are empowered with the time and attention received from the group. They will speak honestly as peers knowing that in the group the therapist can help smooth out their words to be more diplomatic for the listener.

Encouraging members to decide on a group name, in general, is a catalyst to pushing towards Stage 3, group intimacy. A group name reflects the members' identity and sense of belonging. In their second session, this young boys group decided that they were the Tuesday-after-school "Amigos Club."

If the therapist can quickly complete most of the tasks needed for the Preaffiliation Stage, and even the Power and Control Stage, it will make more time for therapeutic work in the Intimacy and Differentiation Stages. In the first session, only two games might be played. However, in a 10-week group, from the second session onward, I use *The Feelings Wheel Game* (Leben, 2001) on the wall as a guide for check-in time. In later sessions, the therapist can add story time and additional structured games for different target behaviors. It is also allowed to let members propose games spontaneously if they address their target behaviors.

CASE ILLUSTRATION: PRETEEN GROUP

One summer, I had the consent of four parents to put together a middle school prep group for four boys diagnosed with ADHD. I had previously worked separately with each family. I convinced the parents that a weekly, eight-session, 2-hour Thursday morning group would be beneficial for all the boys in terms of preparing them for their big transition from elementary school to middle school. Middle school demands include heavy book bags, combination locks that need nimble fingers to open, more academic subjects, more loose papers to organize, voice and hormonal changes, pretty girls, and newfound freedoms. Both the parents and boys were anxious about middle school being less structured with less supervision from adults. Plus, these boys were physically much shorter than their peers. All these boys needed more general readiness skills: sitting still, raising their hands rather than blurting out questions or answers, walking with more confidence, being respectful to teachers, and being assertive to peers without aggressiveness.

It was the boys' third group session. After we finished playing the "Snow Picture Game" (Leben, 2009) and everyone was helping to return the super lightweight foam packing peanuts, which they endearingly called "Ghost Poop" back to the bag, Juan shouted, "I have an idea for a new game!" He asked every member to put a foam peanut on their heads and whoever could keep it the longest without dropping would get a bonus chip. All the boys liked his idea. I responded by saying, "How about if I make the deal sweeter? What if for each round the first one who drops his peanut still gets one chip? But because you are sitting still longer, the second one will get two chips, the third one will get three chips, and the one who keeps it the longest will get four chips." At that point, everyone was really motivated to put a foam peanut on their heads.

Next, we played the "Feelings Wheel Game" (Leben, 2001). Suddenly all four were little gentlemen sitting up straight and still around me, at least for a few seconds. Many foam peanuts fell and chips were earned while we played. However, the boys' motivation remained high, the foam peanuts remained on their heads longer and longer. They each earned the four-chip reward many times. I was impressed by how this spontaneously invented game reinforced sitting still with positive peer pressure and group culture.

During feedback time they were thrilled with the heaping bowls of chips they earned and congratulated each other for sitting still longer than before. As feedback to them I said, "You're all growing up in front of my eyes. Juan, you spontaneously suggested a fun game, which others can recognize and play. Romeo, Chris, and Tom, you were supportive and encouraged each other to do better. In your case, sitting very still is good preparation for middle school. I'm so proud of you and everyone gets three chips from me for extra effort and attentively listening to my feedback." Then they all zoomed off to my treasure chest to redeem their chips for little toys.

After all these years, I am still deeply touched by this moment because it exemplifies positive peer pressure, group cohesiveness, and accepting a member-initiated, original game interactively coming together to fulfill several treatment objectives.

TROUBLESHOOTING INAPPROPRIATE BEHAVIORS IN THE GROUP

The boys' behaviors I describe above are simple ones to manage. However, in my over 30 years of working with groups of boys with ADHD, there were much harder, difficult boys who were difficult to manage. Since my intention is to keep the group experience positive, I do not take away chips, reprimand, or send them away. However, there are a few considerations and favorite measures that work for me, as described below:

1. To be sure, not all children with ADHD will benefit from DGPT right away. If a specific child needs lots of attention, it may be best to first work with him one-on-one for several sessions to develop a trusting relationship. This assures the child a familiar adult is present for support, perhaps preventing possible acting-out behavior.

2. If a member is screaming or talking too loudly, use peer pressure by rewarding chips to all other members with "Thank you for using your inside voice." Or if a member says, "It's boring! I don't want to play anymore," put chips in the bowls of other members with remarks like "Thank you for still wanting to play with me." "Thank you for showing tolerance to your peers," or "Thank you for showing patience."

3. Especially when working with children the therapist doesn't know yet from residential treatment centers or group homes or with aggressive members having severe ADHD symptoms, it is a good idea to consider using a helper or cotherapist for the first few sessions. Sometimes school events, news from home, or health issues cause members extra emotional distress. As a safety issue, I would request their houseparent, campus secretary, or even an intern to sit by the door with a timer. Most of the time, this adult can just observe. When a group member acts out, he would be asked to go sit on the floor (literally "grounded") next to the adult for 1 minute

while the game continues. After the timer bell rings, the player may return. If he acts out a second time, he must sit next to the adult on the floor for 2 minutes. Once again, after the timer rings, he can return. But if it happens a third time, the child would be required to sit quietly with this adult for the rest of the session. For every minute of "good sitting" the helper can award one chip. Sometimes, just having time to himself is exactly what this member needed in the first place. My philosophy is to offer opportunities to earn chips for "calming down."

ADDITIONAL THOUGHTS ON SUCCESSFUL DGPT

Modifications can be made to use this method in settings other than residential treatment centers. Although the group-work methods remain the same, adaptation for group size and various combinations of members can be carried out. Some suggestions are as follows:

1. *Partnering with parents is a must.* I prefer to meet parents alone first before starting play therapy with their child. My goal is to strengthen their parenting skills, which might include choice of words, gestures, and a structured daily routine to bring about positive changes in their child in two sessions. Divorced parents are requested to attend the parent education together or at least to take turns bringing the child and participating in the sessions.

For parent education, I provide each parent with a folder filled with psychoeducational material, as follows:

- Current criteria for ADHD diagnosis.
- The importance of healthy food choices to nourish the brain.
- Strengthening parent–child relationship with feeling words.
- Literature on how the brain works.
- Left brain executive functions, defined as mental processes that deal with self-regulation, paying attention, organization, time management, productivity, and task completion.
- The five conditions parents can use to get their child's attention.
- The 6-second rule of communication.
- A list of age- and grade-appropriate social skills.
- Why children misbehave and how to design creative logical consequences to help them change bad habits.
- Characteristics to look for in teachers who work well with children who have ADHD

Also included are instructions on how parents should start up a token economy system like my *Smiley System for Compliance and Responsibility*

Training for Children (Leben, 2013) to provide a 24/7 visual structure with ways for children to earn Smileys by means of regular chores, and daily routines for getting ready for school, meals, homework, and bedtime. My goal is that parents will learn to be consistent with discipline issues.

2. *Be creative in recruiting group members.* In a private practice setting, it may be harder to find three or four children to start an ADHD group. So, I have tried to be creative in recruiting members. For a family, I include one or both parents with the child and another sibling or a big teddy bear on another chair to form a group. I have also formed groups with two different single moms and their children. No matter what group size or mix of adults and children, the individuals still learn from the group peer pressure and interactive experience.

Duration for family groups can be more flexible, with eight to 14 sessions. The focus is on the child's target behavior and family members' relationships. After the first phase, I'll give the family a therapy vacation for 6 months. However, the parents can call either to have a refresher course to strengthen old skills, resolve new issues, or learn new skills for the next school grade.

3. *Treatment duration for children with ADHD.* Based on my experience as a residential treatment center supervisor and a foster mom of 40 children in my therapeutic foster group home for a total of 15 years, I believe the optimum duration for minimum treatment for a child with ADHD is two academic years and a structured summer program in between with DGPT groups running every 8 to 10 weeks. This provides four seasons and several anniversaries of past traumas that require the child to adjust. Many parents can be coached to provide a structured home program and to set up a strict daily routine for their children with ADHD.

Children diagnosed with ADHD need constant structure, especially during summer vacation; otherwise, they regress. I recommend that diligent parents start planning their home summer program in February. Then in the last week of school, parents will be ready with an organized summer program with every day planned. My supervised activities were comprised of a daily school hour, independent living skills training, lunch preparations, quiet reading time, weekly library visits, hobby groups, swimming at the community pool, outdoor exercise activities, and special car trips. The eight-session weekly DGPT should be also part of the structured summer program. Throughout the day, children earn chips with the token economy system for good behavior and performance. Earned tokens are redeemed weekly for allowance and the total number of tokens accumulated during the summer can earn out-of-town trips to beaches, amusement parks, the zoo, or even a special destination like Disneyland as reward for persistence and accomplishments.

4. *Consistency.* The final element in successful DGPT is consistency from all the adults involved in the children's lives at home, school, and in the community to reinforce treatment goals.

Case Illustration

A mom called requesting play therapy for Anna, her 9-year-old daughter diagnosed with severe ADHD symptoms. During the intake interview, the mom said that her daughter had already been seen for 3 years by another therapist, and that the mom was not allowed to participate in the sessions. She also reported that she was never told about Anna's progress. Now her patience had run out, and she just wanted Anna to see a different therapist. While assuring her that she certainly could change, I requested she have the other therapist sign a consent form so we could consult together about her daughter. I explained to her that with my DGPT method, she or her husband *were expected* to take part in the play therapy sessions.

In my first meeting with the mom and Anna, I introduced my play therapy method. I asked them if they had any questions to ask me. Mom shook her head, but Anna looked at me with earnest eyes and said, "I saw my last therapist for 3 years. I remember seeing two other therapists for months too. Can you tell me if I am really, really, really sick? Why else would I need to go see doctors for so many years?" It was hard for me to believe Anna asked such a candid question, not knowing why she had to be dragged to therapy for so many years. It bothered me that the lack of communication among adults gave Anna the wrong impression that she was very sick. I dropped a plastic chip in her bowl and said, "That's for asking an excellent question because you have every right to know about the progress of your treatment. I'm happy to tell you that usually the first phase of my work with you may last no more than 3 months. In fact, if your mom, teacher, and I see that you are paying better attention, earning better grades, following instruction after one request, taking your meds on time, and going to bed without prompting, we might even end sooner. After this first phase, I'll give you a therapy vacation until your mom calls me to schedule for more sessions, usually no more than six. After that, I will leave it to your mom to call me whenever she thinks we need to work on any more personal or school issues, that sort of thing." Anna was listening carefully and nodding her head. I put another plastic chip in her bowl and said, "That's for paying excellent attention. I like that!" Needless to say, I learned that even a 9-year old child wanted to know how many treatment sessions would be necessary and when they would end.

TREATMENT EFFECTIVENESS

Throughout my career, I have made various attempts to measure the effectiveness of DGPT methods. The findings were as follows:

While I worked in residential treatment programs, I kept a record of how many tokens were earned each session by each group member. Usually from the first to the last session, there was a steady climb in the number of earned chips, meaning that members were using more and more prosocial behaviors. If a member had a sudden drop in chips for a session, it was a clear indication of a major discrepancy in behaviors.

In a suburban school-based program near Austin, Texas, I asked the school district for permission to work with four elementary-school boys with the most ADHD symptoms. I was referred a second grader, two third graders, and one fourth grader. At the beginning I had the intake meeting with each child's teacher and parent to learn about what target behaviors they wanted the boys to improve. After an 8-week DGPT group, all teachers reported increases in the students' grades and decreases in disruptive behaviors. The parents reported increases in the boys' response to their first requests for chores and completion of homework with fewer hassles.

In a trial study at an Austin, Texas, charter school, I conducted weekly 30-minute DGPT group sessions for four very hyperactive kindergarteners from two classes. At the time of referral, I asked teachers to write a description of each child's classroom problem behaviors. Toward the end of the 8 sessions, I observed that the group members could sit still longer and were more willing to talk and share what was on their minds. Their teachers' final evaluations reported that the children showed more self-control during recess, talked more among themselves, and played less aggressively with other peers. However, I felt the 30-minute period allowed by the school was insufficient for major impact.

In an inner-city elementary school in Austin, I conducted a 10-week, 45-minute DGPT group for four second-graders diagnosed with ADHD symptoms (two boys and two girls from two different classes.) The school social worker helped me design a self-evaluation form that included a 5-point scale with drawings of facial expressions for unhappy, mildly unhappy, neutral, mildly happy, and happy. When the students walked in they marked their initial feeling in the check-in column, then at the group's end, before they went back to their classroom, they marked their feelings again in the check-out column. After 10 sessions, the overall improvement in mood every week as reported by the students was up an average of two levels. In addition, the group members' two teachers were asked to rate the children on 65 social skills using a 7-point scale from "nonexistent" to "consistently observed." They gave an initial assessment and again after the 10 DGPT sessions were done. All four children improved an average of 1, 2, or even 4 points on 63 of the 65 social skills rated.

School psychologists and counselors who use this method in the Unites States and Hong Kong have shared with me that DGPT process and games are very helpful when they lead school groups for hyperactive students. Furthermore, by seeing students in groups, they can now include three times as many children exhibiting ADHD symptoms than working with similar students individually. The skills learned from DGPT are clearly observed to be transferred to the home and school settings. This kind of efficiency is exciting to school administrators who are faced with increasing demands from parents of students needing social and emotional services.

USING DGPT WITH OTHER POPULATIONS

In the past 30 years, I have also worked with many children with such comorbid diagnoses as autism spectrum disorder (ASD). Treatment of children with my DGPT method has usually yielded positive results. While doctors and scientists are still searching for the neurobiological causes for ASD, therapists are treating ASD symptoms. However, I am encouraged by parents' feedback that weekly DGPT sessions help their children to become more aware of social skills and making friends in weeks.

In my Hong Kong teacher and counselor workshops, I am often asked about the issue of increasing numbers of students who exhibit social and/ or emotional challenges, yet are not formally diagnosed. In Hong Kong, after 2007, these students were labeled as having Special Education Needs. Every school has one school social worker whose responsibility is to supposedly work with Special Education Needs students one-on-one, but they are overwhelmed by the range of behavioral problems. Since applying my DGPT methods in school programs, many school social workers shared their success in promoting more prosocial behaviors. It is apparent to me that DGPT methods have been applicable to children in both the American and Chinese cultures.

In 2011, I was invited to work with one agency's social workers providing residential care and convalescence to elderly clients with various degrees of dementia and Alzheimer's. Because the regular recreational activities program did not sustain residents' interest, they asked me to teach them DGPT structured games that they could try with residents in weekly groups. After two or three sessions, the members in these small groups seemed to have regained some prosocial qualities including looking people in the eyes, leaving their dorm rooms more often, engaging in peer conversation more readily, and showing a happier general disposition. The social workers admitted they started as nonbelievers, but were amazed how a handful of colorful poker chips and adapted DGPT games could motivate their elderly residents. Like children with ADHD, it seems reasonable to me that withdrawn elderly residents also suffer from diminished executive functions. Every year when I return to Hong Kong I teach these social workers new games and am excited to hear their success stories with the elderly.

SUMMARY AND CONCLUSIONS

The DGPT method evolved from working with children in residential treatment centers. While it is clinically observed to be quite successful, I am hopeful that others will someday conduct evidence-based studies to document its effectiveness because after practicing and sharing this method for over 30 years in the United States and internationally, I believe that it has its place in short-term treatment methods for children with ADHD.

REFERENCES

Bernstein, S. (1965). *Explorations in group work: Essays in theory and practice.* Boston: Boston University School of Social Work.

Cartwright, D., & Zander, A. (1968). *Group dynamics: Research and theory* (3rd ed.). London: Tavistock.

Garland, J. A., Jones, H., & Kolodny, R. (1965). A model for stages of development in social work practice. In S. Bernstein (Ed.), *Explorations in group work: Essays in theory and practice* (pp. 19–51). Boston: Boston University.

Gaskill, R., & Perry, B. (2014). The neurobiological power of play: Using the neurosequential model of therapeutics to guide play in the healing process. In C. Malchiodi & D. A. Crenshaw (Eds.), *Creative arts and play therapy for attachment problems* (pp. 178–194). New York: Guilford Press.

Konopka, G. (1963). *Social group work: A helping process.* Englewood Cliffs, NJ: Prentice Hall.

Leben, N. (2001). *The feelings wheel game.* Pflugerville, TX: Morning Glory Treatment Center for Children.

Leben, N. (2009). *Directive group play therapy: 60 structured games for the treatment of ADHD, low self-esteem, and traumatized children.* Pflugerville, TX: Morning Glory Treatment Center for Children.

Leben, N. (2013). *Smiley system for compliance and responsibility training for children.* Pflugerville, TX: Morning Glory Treatment Center for Children.

Perry, B. D. (1999). Bonding and attachment in maltreated children: Consequences of emotional neglect in childhood. *CTA Parent and Caregiver Education Series, 1*(3).

Phelan, T. (1993). *All about attention deficit disorder: Symptoms, diagnosis and treatment: Children and adults.* Glen Ellyn, IL: Parentmagic.

Trecker, H. B. (1955). *Social group work.* New York: Whiteside.

Yalom, I. D. (1995). *The theory and practice of group psychotherapy.* New York: Basic Books.

Chapter 15

❧

Integrated Play Groups®
for Children on the
Autism Spectrum

Pamela Wolfberg

*W*ith the incidence of autism spectrum disorder (ASD) rising at an unprecedented rate worldwide (Centers for Disease Control and Prevention, 2014), we face a growing need for effective, intensive, and culturally responsive therapeutic intervention. ASD is a complex neurodevelopmental disorder that presents in early childhood and persists over the lifespan. Diagnostic criteria include discrepancies in social interaction and social communication and restrictive, repetitive patterns of behavior, interests, and activities (American Psychiatric Association, 2013). The notion of a spectrum derives from the understanding that there are diverse manifestations of autism that correspond to varying degrees of support that are needed for an individual to function at his or her full potential. Among the characteristics shared by children across the spectrum are pervasive problems with social and imaginary play.

This chapter introduces the Integrated Play Groups® (IPG) model as a form of short-term play therapy for children on the autism spectrum (for overviews, see Wolfberg, 2009; Wolfberg, Bottema-Beutel, & DeWitt, 2012). The IPG model is an empirically validated approach designed to address the complex problems children with autism experience in play while building relationships with typical peers in natural settings. Specifically, an IPG brings together children with autism in mutually engaging play experiences with more capable peer play partners while guided by a qualified adult facilitator. The therapeutic approach is multidimensional, encompassing methods for program and environmental design, assessment, and intervention that build on children's play interests and emerging capacities for social and imaginary play.

The IPG model has evolved over the years to keep pace with rapid changes in the field. It has come to be recognized among evidence-based practices for children on the autism spectrum (American Speech–Language–Hearing Association, 2006; Disalvo & Oswald, 2002; Iovannone, Dunlap, Huber, & Kincaid, 2003; National Autism Center, 2009; Wong, Odom, Hume, Cox, Fettig, et al., 2014). A growing body of research demonstrates the efficacy of the IPG model for children across the autism spectrum representing diverse ages, abilities, socioeconomic groups, languages, and cultures (for a synopsis of this research, see Wolfberg, 2015). Outcomes of a recent large-scale study suggest that children with autism are capable of making significant progress in a 12-week IPG intervention, which represents a relatively short period of time for program delivery (Wolfberg, Dewitt, Young, & Nguyen, 2014). The aim of this chapter is to describe the IPG model and its therapeutic benefits for children on the autism spectrum. The chapter begins with an overview of the IPG model's conceptual foundation focused on addressing the challenge of play for children with autism. The next section describes the methods used to implement the IPG model in diverse settings. The chapter concludes with a case vignette of an IPG in practice and closing remarks.

ADDRESSING THE CHALLENGE
OF PLAY FOR CHILDREN WITH AUTISM

The IPG model was designed with consideration of the unique and complex challenges children with autism encounter in play (for an in-depth review, see Wolfberg, 2009). Hallmarks of autism include disparities in the development of spontaneous play that manifest in both symbolic and social forms. Childhood characteristics include a lack of varied, socially imitative, and imaginative play and difficulties socializing and forming relationships with peers appropriate to developmental level. The challenge of play for children with autism is inextricably linked to what Wing and Gould (1979) describe as a "triad of impairments" in socialization, communication, and imagination.

While prevailing developmental issues are largely influenced by factors related to genetics and the brain, with specialized intervention children with autism can make considerable progress relative to the level of severity they present (Minschew & Williams, 2014). However, without appropriate intervention children with autism are exposed to other risk factors that may compound difficulties in these areas while affecting their quality of life. Thus, how children with autism develop and experience play may be influenced by multiple factors.

Developmental Differences in Play

The spontaneous play of children with autism differs in form, function, and degree of complexity as compared to the play of typically developing children (Boucher & Wolfberg, 2003; Libby, Powell, Messer, & Jordan, 1998). In typical development, play emerges along a continuum and becomes increasingly diverse, creative, and socially coordinated with age. In contrast, children with autism exhibit a restricted play repertoire that includes pursuing repetitive and stereotyped activities apart from others (Hobson, Hobson, Malik, Kyratso, & Calo, 2013). They often become intensely absorbed in one or a few preferred activities that may last hours, and continue over months and even years. Some children gravitate to conventional toys and play themes while others display unique interests focused on unusual objects or arcane topics.

Within the symbolic domain, children with autism show delays and qualitative differences in their play development (Hobson, Lee, & Hobson, 2009). Research suggests that children with autism display a specific impairment in symbolic pretend play (i.e., representation of objects, events, self, and others) that likely extends to functional play (i.e., conventional use and association of objects) (Baron-Cohen, 1987; Jarrold & Cohn, 2011). Overall, they engage in higher rates of object manipulation as opposed to either functional or symbolic pretend play. They are less likely to spontaneously produce pretend play that includes (1) object substitutions, (2) attributing absent or false properties to objects, and (3) representing imaginary objects, events, or themes as if they are present and real (Baron-Cohen, 1987; Leslie, 1987). Children with milder forms of autism further experience difficulties comprehending and producing more sophisticated forms of play that involve role playing or improvisation using complex narrative (Jarrold & Cohn, 2011).

Within the social domain, children with autism present distinct problems engaging in play with peers (Carter, Davis, Klin, & Volkmar, 2005; Jordan, 2003). While with growing exposure to peers, social play typically increases in frequency, duration, and complexity, the social play of children with autism is impacted by difficulties in social communication. Research suggests that children with autism initiate play with peers less often and with less consistency than developmentally matched peers (Corbett, Schupp, Simon, Ryan, & Mendoza, 2010). When they make attempts to interact with their peers, their social approach may be subtle, obscure, or poorly timed (Wolfberg, Zercher, Lieber, Capell, Matias, et al., 1999). Children with autism present social play styles that may differ across settings and over time. A child whose style is *aloof* may appear to withdraw or maintain a distance from peers. A child with a *passive* style may watch, follow, or willingly be led by peers, but rarely initiates play on his or her own. A child whose style is *active and odd* will make obvious attempts to engage peers that are idiosyncratic or one-sided—such as by talking excessively about one topic (Wing & Gould, 1979).

Sociocultural Influences on Play

In addition to developmental factors, sociocultural factors may also significantly influence the play experiences of children with autism. Difficulties often arise from the common misconception that children with autism lack an inherent desire and are incapable of learning how to play and socialize with peers. In fact, research suggests that children with autism do show evidence of an innate drive to play and socialize with peers (Chamberlain, Kasari, & Rotheram-Fuller, 2007; Kasari, Rotheram-Fuller, Locke, & Gulsrud, 2012). Moreover, with appropriate support, they show many of the same capacities for play as typical children (Boucher, 1999). However, what does make children with autism different from typical peers are the idiosyncratic ways in which they display their play interests and abilities.

Peer perceptions impact the extent to which children with autism may be included in or excluded from the play experiences that dominate their age group (Corbett, Schupp, Simon, Ryan, & Mendoza, 2010; Kasari et al., 2012; Wolfberg et al., 1999). Without explicit guidance, they are more likely to be excluded by peers who lack a framework for interpreting their unconventional behavior as productive and meaningful attempts to initiate play. In social situations, peers often neglect children with autism by ignoring them. Children with autism are also often rejected, and many become targets of bullying by peers (Heinrichs, 2003). As an outgrowth of repeated scenarios like this, children with autism make fewer attempts to engage in play with peers and many give up trying altogether. This, in turn, leads to an increase in solitary engagement in stereotyped activities, which further separates them from the peer group.

Connecting Theory with Practice

The IPG model connects theory with practice to support children with autism in their development and experience of play with typical peers. The IPG model is grounded in sociocultural theory drawing on the work of Russian psychologist Lev Vygotsky (1966, 1978). Vygotsky ascribed profound importance to the role of play as both mirroring and leading development. In particular, he viewed imaginary play as a significant social activity through which children acquire capacities to symbolize, socialize, and ultimately construct cultural meaning.

Vygotsky further stressed that it is through social interaction with others that learning takes place within a child's "zone of proximal development" (ZPD). He defines the ZPD as "the distance between the actual developmental level as determined by independent problem solving, and the level of potential development as determined through problem solving under guidance or in collaboration with more capable peers" (Vygotsky, 1978, p. 86).

Consistent with Vygotsky's theory, Rogoff (1990) proposed the notion of guided participation as a natural process through which children learn and develop while engaging in meaningful activity with the assistance and challenge of social partners whose skill and status vary. Thus there are gains to be made by both novices and experts who learn from one another in a reciprocal fashion.

In practice, the overarching aims of the IPG model are to facilitate mutually enjoyed and reciprocal play among novice players (children with autism) and expert players (typical peers/siblings) while expanding and diversifying novice players' social and symbolic play repertoires. Another aim is for the children to mediate their own play experiences with minimal adult support. Finally, the IPG model aims to demystify autism for typical peers by fostering understanding and acceptance of children's unique ways of relating, communicating, playing, and thinking. Thus, the adult's purpose is to act as a guide who is observant, responsive, and respectful to each player and the group as a whole. Table 15.1 provides a summary of the key features of the IPG model, which are discussed in the following section.

IMPLEMENTING THE IPG MODEL

Initiating the IPG Program

An IPG is tailored for each novice player while incorporated as a component of an existing educational/therapy plan. Upon request, information is shared so that the parents/primary caregivers along with other members of the interdisciplinary team can assess whether an IPG intervention is right for the child. The following are prerequisites and guidelines for making an informed decision.

Child Prerequisites

- At least 3 up to 11 years of age (preschool through elementary age).
- Diagnostic profile consistent with autism spectrum.

TABLE 15.1. Key Components of the IPG Model

IPG model component	Description
Overarching aims	Foster spontaneous, mutually enjoyed, and reciprocal play. Expand/diversify social and symbolic play repertoires. Children mediate their own play experiences with minimal adult support. Demystify autism by fostering understanding and acceptance of children's unique ways of relating, communicating, playing, and thinking.
Conceptual foundation	Developmentally based approach grounded in sociocultural theory.
Program and environmental design	
Service delivery	Preschool–elementary ages (3–11 years). Customized as part of education/therapy program. Facilitated by qualified adult provider trained in IPG model.
Schedule	12-week IPG program cycle. Two sessions per week for 30–60 minutes.
Group composition	Three to five players. Higher ratio of expert to novice players: • Novice players—children on autism spectrum. • Expert players—typical peers/siblings.
Play setting	Natural integrated site in school, home, or community. Specially designed play space—wide range of high-interest, age-, and developmentally appropriate materials conducive to social and imaginative play.
IPG assessment Observation framework	Naturalistic observation of children at play: • Social play styles • Symbolic dimension of play • Social dimension of play • Communicative functions and means • Play preferences—diversity of play.
Assessment tools	Play Questionnaire Play Preference Inventory IPG Observation Profile of Individual Play Development Record of Monthly Progress in IPG (with sample goals) IPG Summative Report.
IPG Intervention Session structure	Consistent, predictable schedule, routines ,and rituals. Systematic use of visual supports (picture–word symbols, written words, photographs, drawings) used as labels, transitional devices, depict schedule, provide guidelines, and tips.
Guided participation practices	Nurturing play initiations. Scaffolding play. Social–communication guidance. Play guidance in the ZPD.

- Individualized education/therapy program (individualized education plan/individualized family service plan) in place with appropriate support services.
- Positive behavior support plan for children with significant behavior issues.

Parent–Professional Team Agreement

- Child presents developmental differences that impact capacity to spontaneously play and socialize with peers.
- Child will potentially benefit from an intensive inclusive peer play intervention to address the above areas of need.

Once there is agreement, the next step is to identify a qualified IPG provider if one is not yet readily available at the program site. An IPG provider is designated as qualified after having completed a mandatory advanced training and supervision program (Wolfberg, 2003, 2014).

Setting Up the IPG Program

Thoughtful and careful planning is needed to set up an effective IPG program in a selected site. Programs are carried out over a minimum period of 12 weeks, during which time the children meet twice weekly for 30- to 60-minute sessions. An IPG is composed of three to five players with a higher number of expert to novice players. Keeping in mind the prerequisites, novice players include children of all abilities across the autism spectrum. Expert players include typical peers and siblings who demonstrate competent social, communication, and play abilities and who express an interest and willingness to participate.

Expert players are recruited on a voluntary basis with parent consent. The recruitment of expert players will vary from program to program, depending upon whether or not typically developing children are already present on the site. It is preferable to recruit players who are already familiar with and show an interest in one another. If this is not possible, then the goal should be to recruit players who have the potential of becoming a part of the child's natural peer network.

A number of factors may also be considered in the formation of the group. With respect to age, there are differing benefits in bringing children together who are close in age and who are of different ages. There are no particular benefits to groups being of a single or mixed gender, but gender may be a consideration based on children's preferences. While it goes without saying that there is no need to match children in terms of their developmental level, it may be beneficial when they have shared interests. If an adult is not familiar with a child's primary language and culture, it might be helpful to include a peer in the group who has a similar background. While it is not always possible to know the social play styles of all the children in advance, it may be worth noting that a mix of certain styles may be preferable for certain children. Some of the styles that have been observed include:

- Quiet, passive, reserved
- Loud, active, outgoing
- Take charge, leaders
- Doting, nurturers
- Clowns, teasers

An important part of setting up and delivering the IPG program is to offer *autism demystification* activities (Wolfberg, McCracken, & Tuchel, 2014). Originated by Heather McCracken of the Friend 2 Friend Social Learning Society, these activities are designed to foster understanding, acceptance, and empathy for the unique ways in which individuals with autism play, relate, communicate, think, and learn. Friend 2 Friend (F2F) programs are delivered in an age-appropriate and sensitive manner. When conducting sessions, the children with autism participate right alongside their typical peers. Never is a particular child identified as having autism; however, a child with autism may choose to self-disclose this information. F2F programs for younger children include puppet presentations (live or on video) while a simulation game is offered to older populations. Additional demystification activities (e.g., sharing books, holding discussions) are also facilitated as a part of the IPG session over the course of the program.

Setting Up the IPG Environment

The IPG environment is designed to be safe, familiar, and predictable while accommodating children's diverse interests, abilities, and needs. It is best to have a consistent play space that is designated for regular and extended use. The play space may be located in any number of locations—for example, in a classroom, therapy room, or corner of a living room in the home. As opposed to a large and open area, the play space is intentionally restricted in size and has boundaries that are clearly defined.

High-interest play materials that are especially conducive to social interaction and imaginative play are purposely selected. These may include a variety of sociodramatic, constructive, and sensory toys and props. Play materials also need to be both age- and developmentally appropriate. For example, if a 5-year-old child with autism tends to shake things for play, fill cereal boxes with beans so that he or she may participate with the other children in the pretend theme of grocery shopping.

Conducting IPG Assessments

The IPG model includes a comprehensive set of assessment tools and techniques that are introduced in the field manual (Wolfberg, 2003). A digital binder that includes a schedule of assessments is also provided to IPG master guides. The assessment process requires astute observation and interpretation of various aspects of the children's play development and experience. Each observer must be sensitive to the unique qualities rather than the purported deficiencies reflected in the children's play. The assessment process is key for setting appropriate goals for children, designing effective intervention strategies, and monitoring the children's progress over time.

Several key areas are covered in the assessment process. Within the symbolic dimension of play are the developmentally based *manipulation, functional,* and *symbolic/pretend* domains. These play domains represent acts that are directed toward objects or signify specific events. The observed acts range from simple forms of sensory–motor and exploratory play to more complex and imaginative forms of play.

Within the social dimension of play are the developmentally based domains of *isolate (solitary), onlooker (orientation), parallel (proximity), common focus (reciprocal),* and *common goal (cooperative).* These play domains are representative of the child's distance from and involvement with one or more peers, ranging from brief and fleeting encounters to coordinated and sustained interactions in play with peers.

Social communication is also assessed with a focus on the child's *communicative functions* (e.g., requests for objects, peer interaction and affection, protests, declarations, and comments) and *communicative means* as expressed verbally and nonverbally (e.g., facial expressions; eye gaze; proximity; manipulating a peer's hand, face or body; showing or giving objects; gaze shift; gestures; intonation; vocalization; nonfocused or focused echolalia; and one-word or complex speech/sign) (adapted from Schuler & Fletcher, 2002).

The play preferences of novice players are also assessed in order to identify play interests that create opportunities for mutual enjoyment with the other players. Play preferences include a child's attraction to and engagement with objects, play activities and play themes, and preferred playmates (prefers no one in particular, prefers one or more peers). Determining the number and range of play preferences provides an additional measure for diversity of play. Figure 15.1 shows the *Profile of Individual Play Development* (revised version), which is an example of an IPG assessment used to compile observational data and document children's progress over time (Wolfberg, 2003).

Profile of Individual Play Development

Child's Name:	Evaluator:
IPG Setting:	Start Date:
Play Guide:	End Date:

Play Domains	Week						Key Observations
	4	8	12	16	20	24	
Social Play Style							
Active–Odd							
Passive							
Aloof							
Other (describe)							
Symbolic Dimension of play							
Symbolic–Pretend							
Functional							
Manipulation–Sensory							
Not Engaged							
Social Dimension of Play							
Common Goal							
Common Focus							
Parallel–Proximity							
Orientation–Onlooker							
Isolate							
Communication—Functions/Means							
Rate of Social Initiation—Responsiveness							
High							
Moderate							
Low							
Quality of Social Initiation—Responsiveness							
Clear intent							
Unclear intent							
Play Preferences—Diversity of Play							
Range of Play Interests							
Highly Diverse							
Moderately Diverse							
Limited–Restricted							
Number of Play Interests							

Comments:

Key: X, Prevailing characteristic   **E,** Emerging characteristic

FIGURE 15.1. Example of an IPG assessment tool.

Structuring the Play Session

Predictable support structures that capitalize on the way children with autism think and learn are integral to the IPG intervention. The play session is structured around predictable routines and rituals. Opening rituals (e.g., greeting, song, brief discussion of plans) and closing rituals (e.g., brief discussion of events and future plans, goodbyes) are tailored to the ages and abilities of the players. Sharing snacks or small meals are often incorporated in longer sessions. These rituals are meant to be relatively brief so that the bulk of the session is devoted to play.

The systematic use of visual supports comprising picture–word symbols and/or written words are often used to label the play space and materials, support transitions, depict the schedule, display guidelines for expected behavior, offer tips for playing together, and provide social communication cues. Photographs and drawings are also used to foster a group identity through recurring activities. For example, the children come up with a name and logo for their group. Children then receive an identification badge that includes their photograph, group name, and logo. They also create a poster depicting their group that is displayed during each play session.

Applying Guided Participation Practices

As previously articulated, guided participation is what defines the IPG intervention. The focus is on fostering opportunities for novice and expert players to coordinate play activities while also challenging novice players to practice new and increasingly complex forms of play. The metaphor of a lotus flower has been used to describe the process of guided participation. Each petal represents a practice that layers one upon the other while supporting the flower as a whole.

Nurturing play initiations is a practice that involves recognizing the sometimes subtle or obscure ways children initiate play. All initiations are interpreted as purposeful and adaptive, as the child's meaningful attempt to play with and beside peers. A play initiation may be expressed in conventional or unconventional ways. Acts that are directed to oneself, peers, and materials are indicators of an initiation. A child's unusual fascinations or idiosyncratic patterns of communication are also interpreted as initiations. To nurture an initiation requires modeling a response and translating for the peers the child's intention so that they may respond to the child in affirmative and productive ways. These responses may then serve to stimulate reciprocation on the part of the child as well as to shape further play interactions. Ultimately, this provides a point of departure for the novice and expert players to establish a joint focus and coordinate play activities.

Scaffolding play (a concept inspired by Rogoff, 1990) is a key practice.

This involves the adult moving in, out, and around the players to regulate the amount and type of support provided in relation to their needs. If any child is unengaged or isolated from the other players for a noticeable period, the adult steps in to provide intensive support. This high level of support may involve directing and modeling the play for the children—for example, by arranging props, assigning roles, scripting parts, and stimulating play using rhythm, ritual, and affect cues. As the children begin to engage in the play beside or with one another, this is a sign for the adult to move to the periphery while redirecting the children to focus on each other and not the adult. This type of support may include posing leading questions, commenting on activities, offering suggestions, and giving subtle reminders to the children using verbal and/or visual cues. Once the children are clearly absorbed in the play, the adult retreats even further and remains on the sidelines. At this point the adult's role is to stand by as a "secure base" with whom the players can check in as needed. Scaffolding requires the adult to be especially observant of the key moments for stepping in without intruding and moving out to allow the play to unfold in natural ways.

Social communication guidance prepares the children to elicit one another's attention and sustain reciprocal interactions using verbal and nonverbal means. The objective for expert players is to interpret and respond to unique forms of communication in meaningful ways so that novices may be included. The objectives for the novice players are twofold: to interpret and respond to the complex ways in which expert players communicate and to learn how to communicate in more conventional ways themselves. There are a variety of strategies to guide social communication that include making use of visual supports. Similar to nurturing initiations, one strategy is to identify those moments when a child attempts to communicate but fails to receive a response from another child. In this moment the adult models an appropriate response while explaining to the peers what the child was attempting to communicate. Visual supports may also be used to support communication. Graphic symbols or written words may be used to depict a single step (e.g., "look," "show," "take turns") or a series of steps (e.g., "Say your friend's name, show your friend the doll, say 'let's pretend we have babies' ").

Play guidance in the ZPD focuses on immersing the children in play experiences that slightly challenge them within their ZPD. Identifying a child's present and emerging capacities across symbolic and social domains of play offers a starting point for each child. A variety of strategies are used to support each child along the developmental continuum including orienting, mutual imitation, joint focus, joint action, role enactment, and role playing. These strategies afford the children opportunities to participate in increasingly complex and sophisticated play activities, themes, and roles. They can take a part in the play even if they do not fully comprehend it.

For example, a child who is inclined to repeatedly line up objects can take the role of store clerk who lines up the toys on the shelf for the others to purchase. Ultimately, repeated exposure to these types of group play experiences stimulates the child to explore and diversify existing play routines.

CASE ILLUSTRATION

The following vignette features Nikko, an 8-year-old boy who originally received a diagnosis of Asperger's syndrome (now referred to as ASD Level 1). Nikko attends a public elementary school where he is fully included in the fourth-grade class. Based on an evaluation by his interdisciplinary team, it was determined that Nikko would potentially benefit from participation in an inclusive peer play intervention to address his peer socialization and play needs. An IPG was formed for Nikko as a part of the afterschool program on his school campus. A school district therapist, who had completed training to become a qualified IPG master guide, facilitates the IPG with three of Nikko's typically developing classmates. The IPG meets twice weekly for 60 minutes over a 12-week period. The sessions take place in a playroom that is used for individual play therapy during the school day and the IPG after school.

IPG assessments indicate that Nikko has an active–odd social play style. He expresses a genuine desire for peer companionship, but has had little success in developing a mutual friendship. His peers frequently ignore his attempts to engage them for social interaction and play. Nikko has a tendency to initiate in a one-sided and idiosyncratic fashion without consideration of his peers' perspectives. He typically approaches peers by asking them if they have seen a particular movie, and then proceeds to recite lines from the movie no matter what the response.

Nikko's play interests are consistent with themes generated from his most beloved movies. His current favorite is the Harry Potter movie series based on the books by J. K. Rowling. He enjoys collecting figurines and other paraphernalia represented in these movies. He spends much of his time organizing these toys and generating lists that depict the characters and key events.

The goals and objectives identified for Nikko focus on the following areas:

1. To maximize development in social play with peers, Nikko will demonstrate a common focus and common goals in play by (a) engaging in reciprocal social exchanges, (b) jointly planning and carrying out a common agenda, (c) and negotiating and comprising around divergent interests.

2. To maximize representational abilities (i.e., flexible imagination

and creative expression), Nikko will demonstrate symbolic pretend play at an advanced level by role-playing scripts (real or invented) with age-appropriate props, self, peers, and/or imaginary characters.

3. To maximize social–communicative competence, Nikko will expand his language expression in play with peers by (a) carrying on conversations and (b) narrating sociodramatic pretend play scripts.

4. To expand and diversify his repertoire of spontaneous play preferences/interests, Nikko will demonstrate (a) an increased number and (b) variety of self-selected play interests.

The IPG session opens with a ritual greeting and a recap of the last session. The therapist asks the children to come up with ideas and a plan of what they would like to play together. She prepares to write the different ideas on the board. Nikko immediately tells Lakesha, Annaluna, and Joachim (expert players) that the plan for the day is to make a Harry Potter movie. The therapist reminds the group (for Nikko's sake), "One of the goals of play groups is to 'cooperate'—that means each member may make a suggestion, which may be different from one's own suggestion."

The therapist guides the group by suggesting, "So Nikko, you mentioned you want to make a Harry Potter movie. Why don't you ask the others what they'd like to play?" While facing the therapist, Nikko begins to speak. The therapist quietly redirects him by pointing to a visual cue that depicts two people facing each other with talking bubbles above their heads. The caption reads "Look at your friends when talking to them." Nikko faces Lakesha and asks, "What do you want to play?" Lakesha suggests putting on a puppet show. Annaluna says she'd like to do the same. Joachim begins to speak, but Nikko interrupts. The therapist quietly points to another visual cue with the caption "Take turns when speaking." Nikko pauses as Joachim continues and suggests drawing a space station.

The therapist writes the different ideas on the board and asks the children if they can think of a way to combine their different ideas. Joachim suggests drawing Hogwarts School instead of a space station. Lakesha and Annaluna suggest making popsicle stick puppets of Harry Potter characters. Nikko adds that he will be Harry Potter and assigns the other children roles. "Joachim, you be Ron Weasley, Lakesha, you be Hermione, and Annaluna, you be Professor McGonagall." Annaluna protests, "I want to be Hermione, not professor whatchamacallit." Lakesha suggests, "Why don't we be twin Hermiones?" Nikko protests loudly, "No! There can only be one Hermione, don't you know the movie?" Lakesha shrugs and asks Nikko if there is another girl role that she can have. Without missing a beat, Nikko excitedly suggests, "Okay, you can be Helena Ravenclaw, she is the Grey Lady, you know, her mother is Rowena Ravenclaw. She stole her diadem and tried to hide it and then she got killed by the Bloody Baron and she's the ghost now." Lakesha responds, "Wow, you really know a lot. That sounds so cool—I wanna be the ghost."

The therapist next asks the children what materials they will need and how they will make their creations. Upon request, the therapist brings an assortment of art materials. As the children make their creations, the therapist occasionally interjects to guide the conversation with leading questions and comments.

The therapist stands back as the children next begin acting out a simple script directed by Nikko. Nikko begins to cite lines from the scene while holding the Harry Potter puppet. He then tells Lakesha and Annaluna exactly the lines each of their characters should say. They deviate from the script and begin hitting each other's stick puppet while screaming excitedly. Nikko protests, "Hey, that is not what Hermione and Rowena Ravenclaw are supposed to do." Nikko begins to walk away with his puppet in hand, reciting lines to himself.

The therapist gently reminds all of the children (for Nikko's sake) that another goal of the playgroup is to be creative and use your imagination – that means it is OK to change the story so that it is different from the original. Nikko turns around but remains at a distance from the other players, watching them. Now Joachim joins the girls and initiates another battle with the puppets. Joachim then lifts the drawing he and Nikko made into the air and states, "Hogwarts is flying to outer space." Meanwhile, Lakesha fixes her puppet's hair while Annaluna begins picking up random toys.

The therapist mentions that Nikko is a great director since he has vast knowledge and memory of all the Harry Potter movies. She hands Annaluna a clapboard and tells her she can clap it when Nikko says "Action." This draws Nikko back and he yells "Action." Joachim pretends his puppet is going to Hogwarts on a space station. Nikko appears a bit uneasy, but then responds, "OK, all of you guys go to outer space, but Harry Potter has to wear his invisibility cloak."

During the closing ritual, the therapist holds a discussion with the group. Annaluna suggests that the next time they meet they should write their own movie script so Harry Potter can have new adventures. Nikko says, "OK, then let's see if Hogwarts can be in the ocean this time." The other players enthusiastically make suggestions for how they can accomplish this in the next session. Joachim suggests that they make surfboards, to which Nikko responds, "Yes, and they can all wear wetsuits, too!"

SUMMARY AND CONCLUSIONS

This chapter introduced Integrated Play Groups, an inclusive therapeutic model designed to address the unique peer socialization and play needs of children on the autism spectrum. The IPG model offers opportunities for children with autism to learn and develop while participating in mutually engaging activities with peers. While originally developed for younger children (preschool to elementary school age), there have been innovative extensions of the IPG model for various age groups, including adolescents and adults. For example, drama, visual arts, filmmaking, physical movement, and other high-interest, culturally valued activities are being used (see, e.g., Bottema-Beutel, 2011; Fuge & Berry, 2004; Julius, Wolfberg, Jahnke, & Neufeld, 2012; Schaefer & Attwood, 2003; Wolfberg et al., 2012).

Owing to the collective efforts of many professionals and families, there is an increasing interest in applying the principles and practices of the IPG model to support children, adolescents, and adults with autism in diverse settings. Training, research, and global outreach efforts offered by the Autism Institute on Peer Socialization and Play (*www.autisminstitute. com*) have resulted in widespread adoption of its practices by government and nongovernment organizations in the public and private sector around the world. Many university programs are utilizing books and related publications focused on the IPG model in courses aimed at preparing professionals to work with children with autism in educational and therapeutic settings. By adding to the wealth of short-term play therapy options that are covered in this volume, I hope that this chapter will be beneficial to those seeking to help children on the autism spectrum.

REFERENCES

American Psychiatric Association. (2013). *Diagnostic and statistical manual of mental disorders* (5th ed.). Arlington, VA: Author.

American Speech–Language–Hearing Association. (2006). Guidelines for speech–language pathologists in diagnosis, assessment, and treatment of autism spectrum disorders across the life span. Available at *www.asha.org/policy/GL2006–00049.htm.*

Baron-Cohen, S. (1987). Autism and symbolic play. *British Journal of Developmental Psychology, 5*(2), 139–148.

Bottema-Beutel, K. (2011). The negotiation of footing and participation structure in a social group of teens with and without autism spectrum disorder. *Journal of Interactional Research in Communication Disorders, 2,* 61–83.

Boucher, J. (1999) Interventions with children with autism-methods based on play [Editorial]. *Child Language Teaching and Therapy Journal, 15*(1), 1–5.

Boucher, J., & Wolfberg, P. J. (Eds.). (2003). Special issue on play. *Autism: The International Journal of Research and Practice, 7*(4), 339–341.

Carter, A., Davis, N. O., Klin, A., & Volkmar, F. (2005). Social development in autism. In F. Volkmar, R. Paul, A. Klin, & D. Cohen (Eds.), *Handbook of autism and pervasive developmental disorders* (3rd ed., pp. 312–334). Hoboken, NJ: Wiley.

Centers for Disease Control and Prevention. (2014). Autism spectrum disorders (ASD). Retrieved May 30, 2014, from *www.cdc.gov/ncbddd/autism/index.html.*

Chamberlain, B., Kasari, C., & Rotheram-Fuller, E. (2007). Involvement or isolation?:

The social networks of children with autism in regular classrooms. *Journal of Autism and Developmental Disorders, 37,* 230–242.

Corbett, B. A., Schupp, C. W., Simon, D., Ryan, N., & Mendoza, S. (2010). Elevated cortisol during play is associated with age and social engagement in children with autism. *Molecular Autism, 1*(13), 1–12.

DiSalvo, C., & Oswald, D. (2002). Peer-mediated interventions to increase the social interaction of children with autism: consideration of peer expectancies. *Focus on Autism and Other Developmental Disabilities, 17,* 198–207.

Fuge, G., & Berry, R. (2004). *Pathways to play! Combining sensory integration and integrated play groups.* Shawnee Mission, KS: Autism Asperger.

Heinrichs, R. (2003). *Perfect targets: Asperger syndrome and bullying—Practical solutions for surviving the social world.* Shawnee Mission, KS: Autism Asperger.

Hobson, J. A., Hobson, P., Malik, S., Kyratso, B., & Calo, S. (2013). The relation between social engagement and pretend play in autism. *British Journal of Developmental Psychology, 31,* 114–127.

Hobson, R. P., Lee, A., & Hobson, J. A. (2009). Qualities of symbolic play among children with autism: A social–developmental perspective. *Journal of Autism and Developmental Disorders, 39*(1), 12–22.

Iovannone, R., Dunlap, G., Huber, H., & Kincaid, D. (2003). Effective educational practices for students with autism spectrum disorders. *Focus on Autism and Other Developmental Disabilities 18,* 150–165.

Jarrold, C., & Conn, C. (2011). The development of pretend play in autism. In *Oxford handbook of the development of play* (pp. 308–321).

Jordan, R. (2003). Social play and autistic spectrum disorders. *Autism: The International Journal of Research and Practice, 7*(4), 347–360.

Julius, H., Wolfberg, P. J., Jahnke, I., & Neufeld, D. (2012). Integrated play and drama groups for children and adolescents with autism [Final report]. Alexander von Humboldt TransCoop Research Project, University of Rostock, Germany, with San Francisco State University.

Kasari, C., Roheram-Fuller, E., Locke, J., & Gulsrud, A. (2012). Making the connection: randomized controlled trial of social skills at school for children with autism spectrum disorders. *Journal of Child Psychology and Psychiatry, 53*(4), 431–439.

Leslie, A. M. (1987). Pretence and representation: The origins of "theory of mind." *Psychological Review, 94,* 412–426.

Libby, S., Powell, S., Messer, D., & Jordan, R. (1998). Spontaneous play in children with autism: A reappraisal. *Journal of Autism and Developmental Disorders, 28,* 487–497.

Minschew, N. J., & Williams, D. L. (2014). Brain-behavior connections in autism. In K. Buron & P. J. Wolfberg (Eds.), *Learners on the autism spectrum: Preparing highly qualified educators and related practitioners* (2nd ed.). Shawnee Mission, KS: Autism Asperger.

National Autism Center. (2009). *Addressing the Need for Evidence-based Practice Guidelines for Autism Spectrum Disorders* (National Autism Center's National Standards Project: Findings and conclusions).

Rogoff, B. (1990). *Apprenticeship in thinking.* New York: Oxford University Press.

Schaefer, S., & Atwood, A. (2003). *The effects of sensory integration therapy paired with integrated play groups on the social and play behaviors of children with autistic spectrum disorder.* Unpublished master's thesis, San Jose State University, San Jose, CA.

Schuler, A., & Fletcher, C. (2002). Making communication meaningful: Cracking the language interaction code. In R. Gabriels & D. Hill (Eds.), *Autism: From research to individualized practice* (pp. 41–52). London: Jessica Kingsley.

Vygotsky, L. S. (1966). Play and its role in the mental development of the child. *Soviet Psychology, 12*, 6–18. (Original work published 1933)

Vygotsky, L. S. (1978). *Mind in society: The development of higher psychological processes.* Cambridge, MA: Harvard University Press.

Wing, L., & Gould, J. (1979). Severe impairments of social interaction aud associated abnormalities in children Epidemiology and classification. *Journal of Autism and Childhood Schizophrenia, 9*, 11–29.

Wolfberg, P. J. (2003). *Peer play and the autism spectrum: The art of guiding children's socialization and imagination* (Integrated Play Groups Field Manual). Shawnee, KS: Autism Asperger.

Wolfberg, P. J. (2009). *Play and imagination in children with autism* (2nd ed.). New York: Teacher's College Press.

Wolfberg, P. J. (2014). *Integrated play groups apprenticeship program: Advanced training and supervision for preparing qualified IPG providers.* Autism Institute on Peer Socialization and Play. Retrieved May 13, 2014, from from *www.autisminstitute.com.*

Wolfberg, P. J. (2015). Integrated play groups: Supporting children with autism in essential play experiences with typical peers. In L. Reddy, C. Schaefer, & L. File-Hall (Eds.), *Empirically-based play interventions for children* (2nd ed.). Washington, DC: American Psychological Association

Wolfberg, P. J., Bottema-Beutel, K., & DeWitt, M. (2012). Integrated play groups: Including children with autism in social and imaginary play with typical peers, *American Journal of Play, 5*(1), 55–80.

Wolfberg, P. J., DeWitt, M., Young, G., Nguyen, T., & Bottema-Beutel, K. (submitted for publication). *Integrated play groups: Promoting symbolic play and social engagement in children with autism with typical peers across settings* (working title).

Wolfberg, P. J., McCracken, H., & Tuchel, T. (2014). Fostering peer play and friendships: Creating a culture of inclusion. In K. Buron & P. J. Wolfberg (Eds.), *Learners on the autism spectrum: Preparing highly qualified educators and related practitioners* (2nd ed.). Shawnee Mission, KS: Autism Asperger.

Wolfberg, P. J., Zercher, C., Lieber, J., Capell, K., Matias, S. G., Hanson, M., et al. (1999). "Can I play with you?": Peer culture in inclusive preschool programs. *Journal for the Association of Persons with Severe Handicaps, 24*(2), 69–84.

Index

Note. Italics in page numbers indicates figures or tables.